Pearson's *Nursing Notes*
FUNDAMENTALS

Calculating Medication Dosages

Formula 1

$$\frac{\text{dose ordered (desired)}}{\text{dose on hand (have)}} \times \text{amount available (quantity)} = \text{amount to give}$$

Formula 2 (ratio and proportion)

$$\frac{\text{dose ordered}}{\text{dose on hand}} = \frac{x}{\text{quantity available}}$$

Formula 3 (dimensional analysis)

Rule 1: Multiplying one side of an equation by a conversion factor will not change the value of the equation.

Rule 2: Set up the problem so that all labels cancel from the numerator and denominator except the label desired in the answer.

Calculating IV Drip Rates

$$\frac{\text{volume (of fluid)}}{\text{time (in minutes)}} \times \text{drop factor} = \text{flow rate}$$

Critical Points in Measuring Vital Signs

Temperature	To convert Fahrenheit to centigrade: (degrees in F – 32) X $^5/_9$.
	To convert centigrade to Fahrenheit: (degrees in C X $^9/_5$) + 32.
	Ensure no eating or drinking within last 20 minutes for oral temp. to avoid errors.
	Follow manufacturer directions if electronic measuring devices used.
	Wear gloves and use lubricating gel if taking a rectal temperature.
Heart rate	Measure apical rate for 1 full minute at apex (5th intercostal space [ICS], mid-clavicular line [MCL]).
	Measure radial rate for 30 seconds and multiply by 2 if heart rate regular; if irregular, measure for 1 full minute and take an apical rate as well.
Respiratory rate	Measure respiratory rate for 1 minute; note pattern also; try to be unobtrusive because rate can change if client is nervous or self-conscious; also take note of any oxygen therapy the client is receiving.
Blood pressure	Measure in both arms initially to determine differences between sides.
	Measure orthostatic blood pressures in lying, sitting, and standing positions.
	Have arm resting at heart level and use a proper size cuff (cuff width = $^2/_3$ length of client's upper arm).
	Ensure no smoking in last 15–20 minutes to avoid false high readings.
	Wait at least 1–2 minutes or more between repeat readings to avoid false highs.
	Compare readings obtained from electronic measuring device with that obtained using a sphygmomanometer each shift or per agency policy.
Oxygen saturation	Keep pulse oximeter unit plugged into electrical outlet when not in use.
	Put probe on digit/earlobe with adequate circulation to avoid false low readings. Consider measuring O_2 sat whenever client has a lung disorder or otherwise compromised respiratory status.

Areas to Auscultate Heart Sounds

RSB, 2nd ICS
LSB, 2nd ICS
LSB, 3rd ICS
LSB, 4th ICS
MCL, 5th ICS

Sequence for Auscultating Lungs

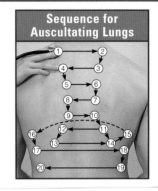

Adult Reference Ranges for Common Laboratory Tests

Coagulation Studies	*Prothrombin time (PT):* 10–13 seconds; 1.5–2.0 times the control in seconds for anticoagulant therapy
	Activated partial thromboplastin time (APTT): 20–35 seconds (1.5–2.5 times the control in anticoagulant therapy)
	Partial thromboplastin time (PTT): 60–70 seconds; 1.5–2.5 times the control in anticoagulant therapy
	International normalized ratio (INR): 2.0–3.0 for most anticoagulation needs
Electrolytes	*Sodium (Na$^+$):* 135–145 mEq/L; *Potassium (K$^+$):* 3.5–5.1 mEq/L
	Chloride (Cl$^–$): 95–105 mEq/L
	CO_2 combining power: 22–30 mEq/L; 22–30 mmol/L
	Calcium, total (Ca^{++}): 9–11 mg/dL, 4.5–5.5 mEq/L, 2.3–2.8 mmol/L
	Calcium (ionized): 4.25–5.25 mg/dL, 2.2–2.5 mEq/L, 1.1–1.24 mmol/L
	Magnesium (Mg^{++}): 1.8–3.0 mg/dL, 1.5–2.5 mEq/L
Glucose	*Fasting (FBS):* 70–110 mg/dL (serum, plasma); 60–100 mg/dL (whole blood); 70–120 mg/dL (elderly); panic values: < 40 or > 700 mg/dL
	Fingerstick glucose (self-monitoring device): 60–100 mg/dL
Hematology	*White blood cells (WBC):* 5,000–10,000 mm^3 or 4,500–11,500/mm^3
	Neutrophils: 1,935–7,942 (absolute count) or 45–75%
	Red blood cells (RBC): 4.5–5.3 million or (10^6)/mm^3 (men), 4.1–5.1 million or (10^6)/mm^3 (women)
	Hemoglobin (Hgb): 13–18 grams/100mL (men), 12–16 grams/100mL (women)
	Hematocrit (Hct): 37–49 % (men), 36–46 % (women)
	Platelet count: 150,000–400,000/mm^3
Renal Function Studies	*Blood urea nitrogen (BUN):* 5–25 mg/dL
	Serum creatinine: 0.5–1.5 mg/dL
Therapeutic Drug Levels	*Digoxin (Lanoxin):* 0.5–2.0 ng/mL; *Phenytoin (Dilantin):* 10–20 mcg/mL
	Theophylline derivatives: 10–20 mcg/mL

Therapeutic Communication Techniques

Listening	Maintain eye contact and have open, receptive body posture
Broad opening	"What would you like to talk about today?" "What brought you to the hospital?"
Restating	"You say the doctor told you that you will need surgery?" "What I hear you saying is…"
Clarification	"I'm not sure what you mean. Could you tell me again?"
Reflection	"You're feeling anxious and upset, and it's related to the conversation you just had with the cardiologist?"
Focusing	"Let's focus more on your relationship with your mother."
Sharing perceptions	"You look upset, but you are saying you don't mind that your discharge from the hospital has been delayed."
Identifying themes	"I've noticed that in all the relationships you describe, you've been hurt by your partner. Do you think this is an underlying issue?"
Silence	Sitting with a client or group of clients and nonverbally communicating interest and presence

PEARSON

Pearson Reviews & Rationales: Nursing Fundamentals 3rd Edition. Copyright 2014 by Pearson Education, Inc.

Center for Disease Control (CDC) Precautions

Tier 1: Standard Precautions (use for all clients)

Handwashing	Wash hands before contact with each client, during care as needed (even if wearing gloves) to prevent cross-contamination of body sites, and after touching blood, body fluids, secretions, excretions, and contaminated items (with or without gloves).
	Use a plain (nonantimicrobial) soap for routine handwashing; use an antimicrobial agent or a waterless antiseptic agent as per agency policy.
Gloves	Wear gloves (clean, nonsterile adequate) whenever contact is expected with blood, body fluids, secretions, excretions, mucous membranes and nonintact skin, and contaminated items.
	Always change gloves between clients and between tasks and procedures on the same client after contact with material that may contain a high concentration of microorganisms.
	Remove gloves promptly after use, before touching noncontaminated items and environmental surfaces, and before going to another client; wash hands.
Face protection (mask, goggles, face shield)	Wear a face shield, or wear goggles and a mask that covers both the nose and the mouth during procedures and client care activities that are likely to generate splashes or sprays of blood, body fluids, secretions, or excretions to provide protection of the mucous membranes of the eyes, nose, and mouth.
Gowns and other protective apparel	Wear a gown to prevent contamination of clothing and skin from blood and body fluid exposures.
	Gowns specially treated to make them impermeable to liquids and leg/shoe covers provide greater skin protection when splashes or large quantities of infective material are present or anticipated.
	Remove soiled gown as soon as possible, and wash hands to avoid transfer of microorganisms.
Others	Clean and reprocess reusable equipment before using it on another client.
	Follow agency procedure for routine cleaning and disinfection of surfaces and for handling spills of blood and body fluids.
	Avoid contamination of self with soiled linen by folding contaminated areas to the inside, holding linen away from the body, and placing it directly into the laundry receptacle.
	Avoid recapping needles; use scoop technique if recapping is necessary; discard used syringes and needles immediately into a puncture-proof container while holding the needle pointed away from self; do not bend or break needles.

Tier 2: Transmission Based Precautions (use when indicated)

Airborne Precautions:	Use Standard Precautions.
Use when small (<5 µm) pathogen-infected droplet nuclei may remain suspended in air over time and travel distances greater than 3 feet	Place client in private room or with a client with the same infection but no other infection (cohorting).
	If possible, use room equipped with negative pressure ventilation, outside venting, and 6–12 air exchanges per hour.
	Keep the door to the room closed.
Examples: varicella, measles, tuberculosis	Wear a special approved particulate filter mask (N95) whenever entering room of all clients with tuberculosis or when staff or visitors not exposed to rubeola or varicella must enter room.
	Limit visitors and caretakers to those already immune if chicken pox (varicella) or measles are involved.
	Keep client in room; place surgical mask on client if transport is necessary.
	Follow additional agency guidelines for preventing transmission of tuberculosis.
Droplet Precautions:	Use Standard Precautions.
Use with large (>5 µm) pathogen-infected droplets that travel 3 feet or less via coughing, sneezing, etc. or during procedures (suctioning)	Place client in private room or with a client with the same infection but no other infection (cohorting).
	When private room or cohorting is unavailable, keep a distance of 3 feet or more between the infected client and other clients or visitors.
	Special ventilation is not necessary and the door may remain open.
Examples: Haemophilus influenzae, Neisseria meningitides, others	Wear a mask when working within 3 feet of the client or entering the room according to agency policy.
	Limit the transport of the client from the room and then mask the client, if possible.
	Additional recommendations for specific pathogens may also apply.
Contact Precautions:	Use Standard Precautions.
Use with known or suspected microorganisms transmitted by direct hand-to-skin client contact or indirect contact with surfaces or care items in the environment	Place client in private room or use cohorting; consult agency infectious disease department as needed.
	Wear gloves when entering the room; change gloves after contact with infective material; remove gloves before leaving room and wash hands immediately with antimicrobial agent or waterless antiseptic agent; then ensure that hands do not touch potentially contaminated room surfaces or items.
Examples: Clostridium difficile, diphtheria (cutaneous), herpes simplex (mucocutaneous or neonatal), impetigo, pediculosis, scabies, zoster (disseminated, immunocompromised host), viral/hemorrhagic infections (Ebola, Lassa, Marburg), others	Wear a clean, nonsterile gown when entering room if clothing may have substantial contact with client, environmental surfaces or items, or if client is incontinent, or has diarrhea, ileostomy, colostomy, or wound drainage not contained by a dressing; remove gown before leaving the room; then ensure that clothing does not contact potentially contaminated environmental surfaces.
	Limit to essential purposes client transport from room; if transport needed, maintain precautions to minimize the risk of pathogen transmission to other clients and environmental surfaces or equipment.
	When possible, dedicate the use of noncritical client-care equipment to a single client or cohort colonized with the same pathogen; if use of common equipment or items is unavoidable, adequately clean and disinfect them before use on another client.
	Additional recommendations for specific pathogens may also apply.

Source: Courtesy of Centers for Disease Control and Prevention.

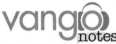

Hear it. Get It.

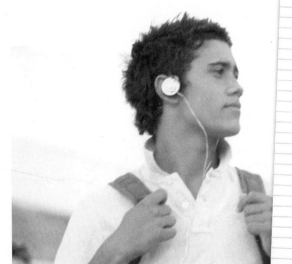

Study on the go with VangoNotes.

Just download chapter reviews from your text and listen to them on any mp3 player. Now wherever you are-- whatever you're doing--you can study by listening to the following for each chapter of your textbook:

Big Ideas: Your "need to know" for each chapter

Practice Test: A gut check for the Big Ideas-- tells you if you need to keep studying

Key Terms: Audio "flashcards" to help you review key concepts and terms

Rapid Review: A quick drill session -- use it right before your test

VangoNotes.com

Pearson Nursing Reviews & Rationales

Nursing Fundamentals

Third Edition

SERIES EDITOR

MaryAnn Hogan, MSN, RN

Clinical Assistant Professor
School of Nursing
University of Massachusetts–Amherst
Amherst, Massachusetts

CONSULTING EDITORS

Sara Bolten, MSN, RN

Nursing Instructor
McKendree College
Louisville, Kentucky

Geralyn Frandsen, EdD, RN

Professor of Nursing
Maryville University
St. Louis, Missouri

Bonita Longo, MS, RN

Nursing Education Consultant
Springfield, Ohio

PEARSON

Boston   Columbus   Indianapolis   New York   San Francisco   Upper Saddle River
Amsterdam   Cape Town   Dubai   London   Madrid   Milan   Munich   Paris   Montréal   Toronto
Delhi   Mexico City   São Paulo   Sydney   Hong Kong   Seoul   Singapore   Taipei   Tokyo

Director of Readypoint™: Maura Connor
Executive Editor: Jennifer Farthing
Developmental Editor: Victoria Gaudette
Editorial Assistant: Deirdre MacKnight
Director, Digital Product Development: Alex Marciante
Media Product Manager: Travis Moses-Westphal
Vice President, Director Sales & Marketing: David Gesell
Senior Marketing Manager: Phoenix Harvey
Marketing Coordinator: Michael Sirinides
Director of Media Production: Allyson Graesser
Media Project Manager: Rachel Collett

Managing Editor, Production: Patrick Walsh
Production Liaison: Maria Reyes
Production Editor: GEX Publishing Services
Manufacturing Manager: Lisa McDowell
Art Director/Cover Designer: Christopher Weigand
Cover Designer: Candace Rowley
Cover Image: Rob Marmion/Shutterstock.com
Composition: GEX Publishing Services
Printer/Binder: Edwards Brothers Malloy
Cover Printer: Lehigh/Phoenix Color Hagerstown

Notice: Care has been taken to confirm the accuracy of the information presented in this book. The authors, editors, and the publisher, however, cannot accept any responsibility for errors or omissions or for the consequences for application of the information in this book and make no warranty, express or implied, with respect to its contents.

The authors and the publisher have exerted every effort to ensure that drug selections and dosages set forth in this text are in accord with current recommendations and practice at time of publication. However, in view of ongoing research, changes in government regulations, and the constant flow of information relating to drug therapy and drug reactions, the reader is urged to check the package inserts of all drugs for any change in indications of dosage and for added warnings and precautions. This is particularly important when the recommended agent is a new and/or infrequently employed drug.

The authors and publisher disclaim all responsibility for any liability, loss, injury, or damage incurred as a consequence, directly or indirectly, of the use and application of any of the contents of this volume.

Library of Congress Cataloging-in-Publication Data

Nursing fundamentals / [edited by] MaryAnn Hogan ; consulting editors,
Sara Bolten, Geralyn Frandsen, Bonita Longo. -- 3rd ed.
    p. ; cm. -- (Pearson nursing reviews & rationales)
  Includes bibliographical references and index.
  ISBN 978-0-13-308359-0 (pbk. : alk. paper) -- ISBN 0-13-308359-4
(pbk. : alk. paper)
  I. Hogan, Mary Ann, MSN. II. Series: Pearson nursing reviews & rationales
series.
  [DNLM: 1. Nursing Process--Examination Questions. 2. Nursing
Process--Outlines. 3. Nursing Care--Examination Questions. 4. Nursing
Care--Outlines. WY 18.2]

  610.73076--dc23
                    2012026112

10 9 8 7 6 5 4 3 2 1

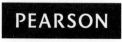

ISBN 10: 0-13-308359-4
ISBN 13: 978-0-13-308359-0

Contents

Welcome to the Pearson Nursing Reviews & Rationales Series!

This series has been specifically designed to provide a clear and concentrated review of important nursing knowledge in the following content areas:

- Anatomy & Physiology
- Nursing Fundamentals
- Nutrition & Diet Therapy
- Fluids, Electrolytes, & Acid–Base Balance
- Medical-Surgical Nursing
- Pathophysiology
- Pharmacology
- Maternal-Newborn Nursing
- Child Health Nursing
- Mental Health Nursing
- Health & Physical Assessment
- Leadership & Management

The books in this series are designed for use either by current nursing students as a study aid for nursing course work, for NCLEX-RN® exam preparation, or by practicing nurses seeking a comprehensive yet concise review of a nursing specialty or subject area.

This series is truly unique. One of its most special features is that it has been developed and reviewed by a large team of nurse educators from across the United States and Canada to ensure that each chapter is edited by a nurse expert in the content area under study. The series editor, MaryAnn Hogan, designed the overall series in collaboration with a core Pearson team to take full advantage of Pearson's cutting edge technology. The consulting editors for each book, also experts in that specialty area, then reviewed all chapters and test questions submitted for comprehensiveness and accuracy. Finally, MaryAnn Hogan reviewed the chapters in each book for consistency, accuracy, and applicability to the NCLEX-RN® Test Plan.

All books in the series are identical in their overall design for your convenience. As an added value, each book comes with a comprehensive support package, including access to additional questions online, complete eText, and a tear-out *NursingNotes* card for clinical reference and quick review.

What's New in this Edition

- Completely updated review material reflecting the 2013 NCLEX-RN® Test Plan.
- Online access to NursingReviewsandRationales. com where students can complete quizzes on the computer to practice for the NCLEX® experience.
- Includes a fully searchable eText version of the book as well as valuable note-taking and highlighting tools.
- 550 updated or brand-new NCLEX®-style practice test questions.
- Features new alternate-item format questions.
- Includes the latest test prep advice from MaryAnn Hogan, trusted expert in what nursing students need to know.

Study Tips

Use of this book should help simplify your review. To make the most of your valuable study time, also follow these simple but important suggestions:

1. Use a weekly calendar to schedule study sessions.
   - Outline the timeframes for all of your activities (home, school, appointments, etc.) on a weekly calendar.
   - Find the "holes" in your calendar, which are the times when you can plan to study. Add study sessions to the calendar at times when you can expect to be mentally alert and follow your plan!
2. Create the optimal study environment.
   - Eliminate external sources of distraction, such as television, telephone, etc.
   - Eliminate internal sources of distraction, such as hunger, thirst, or dwelling on items or problems that cannot be worked on at the moment.
   - Take a break for 10 minutes or so after each hour of concentrated study both as a reward and an incentive to keep studying.

3. Use pre-reading strategies to increase comprehension of chapter material.
   - Skim read the headings in the chapter (because they identify chapter content).
   - Read the definitions of key terms, which will help you learn new words to comprehend chapter information.
   - Review all graphic aids (figures, tables, boxes) because they are often used to explain important points in the chapter.
4. Read the chapter thoroughly but at a reasonable speed.
   - Comprehension and retention are actually enhanced by not reading too slowly.
   - Do take the time to reread any section that is unclear to you.
5. Summarize what you have learned.
   - Use the accompanying online resource, NursingReviewsandRationales.com, to test yourself with hundreds of NCLEX-RN®-style practice questions.
   - Review again any sections that correspond to questions you answered incorrectly or incompletely.

Test-Taking Strategies

Test-taking strategies accompany the rationales for every question in the series. These strategies will assist you to select the correct answer by breaking down the question, even if you don't know the correct response. Use the following strategies to increase your success on nursing tests or examinations:

- Get sufficient sleep and have something to eat before taking a test. Avoid concentrated sweets before a test, however, to avoid rapid upward and then downward surges in your blood glucose. Avoid also high-fat foods that will make you sleepy.
- Take deep breaths during the test as needed. Remember, the brain requires oxygen and glucose as fuel.
- Read the question carefully, identifying the stem, all the options, and any critical words or phrases in either the stem or options.
  - Critical words in the stem such as "most important" indicate the need to set priorities, since more than one option is likely to contain a statement that is technically correct.
  - Remember that the presence of red flag words such as "never" or "only" in an answer option is more likely to make that option incorrect.

- Determine who is the client in the question; often this is the person with the health problem, but it may also be a significant other, relative, friend, or another nurse.
- Decide whether the stem is a true response stem or a false response stem. With a true response stem, the correct answer will be a true statement, and vice-versa.
- Determine what the question is really asking, sometimes referred to as the core issue of the question. Evaluate all answer options in relation to this issue, and not strictly to the "correctness" of the statement in each individual option.
- Eliminate options that are obviously incorrect, then go back and reread the stem. Evaluate those remaining options against the stem once more to make a final selection.
- If two answers seem similar and correct, try to decide whether one of them is more global or comprehensive. If one option includes the alternative option within it, it is likely that the more global option is the correct answer.

The NCLEX-RN® Licensing Examination

Upon graduation from a nursing program, successful completion of the NCLEX-RN® licensing examination is required to begin professional nursing practice. The NCLEX-RN® exam is a Computer Adaptive Test (CAT) that ranges in length from 75 to 265 individual (stand-alone) test items, depending on your performance during the examination. The blueprint for the exam is reviewed and revised every three years by the National Council of State Boards of Nursing using the results of a job analysis study of new graduate nurses practicing within the first six months after graduation. Each question on the exam is coded to a *Client Need Category* and an *Integrated Process*.

Client Need Categories. There are four categories of client needs, and each exam will contain a minimum and maximum percent of questions from each category. Each major category has subcategories within it. The *Client Need* categories according to the NCLEX-RN® Test Plan effective April 2013 are as follows:

- Safe, Effective Care Environment
  - Management of Care (17–23%)
  - Safety and Infection Control (9–15%)
- Health Promotion and Maintenance (6–12%)
- Psychosocial Integrity (6–12%)
- Physiological Integrity
  - Basic Care and Comfort (6–12%)

- Pharmacological and Parenteral Therapies (12–18%)
- Reduction of Risk Potential (9–15%)
- Physiological Adaptation (11–17%)

Integrated Processes. The integrated processes identified on the NCLEX-RN® Test Plan effective April 2013, with condensed definitions, are as follows:

- Nursing Process: a scientific problem-solving approach used in nursing practice; consisting of assessment, analysis, planning, implementation, and evaluation.
- Caring: client–nurse interaction(s) characterized by mutual respect and trust and

that are directed toward achieving desired client outcomes.

- Communication and Documentation: verbal and/or nonverbal interactions between nurse and others (client, family, health care team); a written or electronic recording of activities or events that occur during client care.
- Teaching/Learning: facilitating client's acquisition of knowledge, skills, and attitudes that lead to behavior change.

More detailed information about this examination may be obtained by visiting the National Council of State Boards of Nursing website at www.ncsbn.org and viewing the *2013 NCLEX-RN® Test Plan.*[1]

---

[1]Reference: National Council of State Boards of Nursing, Inc. 2013 *NCLEX-RN© Test Plan.* Effective April, 2013. Retrieved from https://www.ncsbn.org/2013_NCLEX_RN_Test_Plan.pdf.

HOW TO GET THE MOST OUT OF THIS BOOK

Each chapter has the following elements to guide you during review and study:

Chapter Objectives describe what you will be able to know or do after learning the material covered in the chapter.

Objectives

➤ Explain the process utilized in obtaining a health history.
➤ Identify the preparation required for physical assessment.
➤ Describe the process used to complete a physical assessment.
➤ Document health assessment findings using correct medical terminology.
➤ Identify common alterations in assessment findings characteristic of selected pathophysiologic processes.

 NCLEX-RN® Test Prep

Use the accompanying online resource, NursingReviewsandRationales, to test yourself with hundreds of NCLEX®-style practice questions.

Review at a Glance Contains a glossary of critical terms used in the chapter, with definitions provided up-front and available at your fingertips, to help you stay focused and make the best use of your study time.

Review at a Glance

auscultation utilizes sense of hearing and a stethoscope to detect normal and abnormal sounds produced by body, including gastrointestinal tract, arteries, heart, and lungs

health history a process used by health care professionals to obtain complete relevant information about a client's physical, psychosocial, and spiritual health

inspection utilizes sense of sight to visually observe all areas of body to assess pathology, color, level of comfort, anxiety, and any visual signs that provide clues to client's health status; determining odor is also included under inspection

palpation utilizes sense of touch to examine client's body, using pressure of hands and fingers to assess masses,

elevations, temperature, organ position, and any abnormal findings; palpation can be deep or light depending on area being examined; ulnar surfaces of hands and fingers are most commonly used for palpation

percussion utilizes pressure from hands and fingers to generate sounds that will elicit clues about density of underlying tissues or organs

Pretest provides a 10-question quiz as a sample overview of the material covered in the chapter and helps you decide in what areas you need the most—or the least—review.

PRETEST

1 When taking a health history, the nurse should focus on which of the following?

1. Completing the process in a timely manner
2. Using therapeutic communication skills to identify the client's health care status
3. Documenting objective data using the client's own words
4. Attempting to have no interruptions from family members who are present

Practice to Pass questions are open-ended, stimulate critical thinking, and reinforce mastery of the chapter information.

▶ Practice to Pass

The nurse needs to interview a client. What approaches should the nurse take to obtain information most effectively?

!

NCLEX® Alert identifies concepts that are likely to be tested on the NCLEX-RN® examination. Be sure to learn the information highlighted wherever you see this icon.

Case Study, found at the end of the chapter, provides an opportunity for you to use your critical thinking and clinical reasoning skills to "put it all together." It describes a true-to-life client case situation and asks you open-ended questions about how you would provide care for that client and/or family.

Case Study

A client who is a married 56-year-old female secretary has decided to retire after working for 30 years in an office located in an old warehouse in the city. She has 5 children who have moved out of the house. The youngest is preparing to leave for college in another state. The client is 5' 8" tall and weighs 184 pounds. She has smoked one pack of cigarettes per day since she was 15 years old. Her husband is a bus driver in the inner city.

She has come to the clinic to see her primary health care provider. She has had some difficulty sleeping at night and has had to use 2 pillows to breathe comfortably. She has noticed some respiratory congestion and has treated it with cough syrup. She has been afebrile but cannot seem to comfortably catch her breath. She has also noticed that her rings and shoes are a bit tight, but she attributes this to her recent weight gain. The client states, "I have not been eating much, but I seem to be gaining some weight. I no longer have the energy that I once had. Maybe I am getting old."

1. What would the nurse do first to gain the client's confidence?

2. How would the nurse approach the health history?

3. The client's symptoms "cross over" several body systems. Describe how the nurse can link the symptoms and develop appropriate nursing diagnoses.

4. The client's husband has entered the room, and he wants to take the client home. He seems angry and agitated. She begins to get dressed even though the health assessment and history are not yet completed. Describe how his agitation can impact the client's symptoms.

5. The client begins to breathe heavily and appears to be in respiratory distress. She states that she feels "one of her spells coming on." What are the next steps that the nurse should take?

For suggested responses, see pages 305–306.

Posttest provides an additional 10-question quiz at the end of the chapter. It provides you with feedback about mastery of the chapter material following review and study. All pretest and posttest questions contain comprehensive rationales for the correct and incorrect answers, and are coded according to cognitive level of difficulty and NCLEX-RN® Test Plan categories of client need and integrated process.

POSTTEST

1 Prior to taking the health history, the nurse should first do which of the following?

1. Establish a rapport with the client.
2. Offer the client a beverage of choice.
3. Establish that insurance coverage exists.
4. Ask the client to disrobe and put on a gown.

NCLEX-RN® Test Prep: NursingReviewsandRationales.com

For those who want to prepare for the NCLEX-RN®, practicing online will help you become more familiar with the computer-based testing experience, especially for the new alternate item formats such as audio, media-enhanced, hot spot, and exhibit questions. With this new edition, use the code printed inside the front cover of the book to access Nursing Reviews & Rationales, which offers 550 practice questions using all NCLEX®-style formats. This includes the practice questions found in all chapters of the book as well as 30 additional questions per chapter. Nursing Reviews & Rationales allows you to choose two ways to prepare for the NCLEX-RN®. Both approaches personalize your practice experience according to what stage you are at in your NCLEX® preparation:

Nursing Reviews & Rationales includes the eText version of *Pearson Nursing Fundamentals* Third Edition. This eText is fully searchable and includes features like note-taking, highlighting, and more. The eText allows you to take your review with you anywhere you have an internet connection to NursingReviewsandRationales.com.

Pearson NursingNotes Card

This tear-out card provides a reference for frequently used facts and information related to the subject matter of the book. This is designed to be useful in the clinical setting, when quick and easy access to information is so important!

About the Nursing Fundamentals Book

Chapters in this book cover "need-to-know" information about foundational concepts in nursing. The first three chapters of the book provide a review of core processes and skills, including nursing process, physical assessment, and communication. Next, a chapter on professional standards explores the roles of the nurse, ethical and legal considerations in practice, and principles of managing client care. Concepts related to health promotion throughout the lifespan are the focus of the next chapter. The remaining chapters in the book provide a review of key aspects of nursing practice, including the skills needed for safe practice, meeting basic human needs, managing pain, caring for clients with special needs or undergoing surgery, and an overview of medication and IV therapy. Mastery of the information in this book and effective use of the test-taking strategies described will help you be confident and successful in testing situations, including the NCLEX-RN®, and in actual clinical practice.

Acknowledgements

This book is a monumental effort of collaboration. Without the contributions of many individuals, this edition of *Nursing Fundamentals: Reviews and Rationales* would not have been possible. Thank you to all the contributors and reviewers who devoted their time and talents to the third edition. The contributors for this edition are Sara Bolten, MSN, RN; Geralyn Frandsen, EdD, RN; and Bonita Longo, MS, RN. The reviewers for this edition are JoAnn Marshall, MSN, RN, Associate Professor, Macon State College, Macon, Georgia; and Marisue Rayno, RN, EdD, Faculty, Luzern Community College, Nanticoke, Pennsylvania.

Thanks also to the contributors and reviewers who assisted with the previous editions of this book: Mary Jean Ricci, MSN, RN, Assistant Professor, Holy Family University, Bensalem, Pennsylvania; Donna Taliaferro, PhD, Associate Professor, University of Missouri–St. Louis, St. Louis, Missouri; Judy E. White, RNC, MA, MSN, Southern Union Community College, Opelika, Alabama; Donna Bowles, EdD, MSN, RN, Indiana University, New Albany, Indiana; Ellise D. Adams, CNM, MSN, ICCE, CD (DONA), Calhoun Community College, Decatur, Alabama; Gina M. Ankner, MSN, RN, CS-ANP, University of Massachusetts-Dartmouth, North Dartmouth, Massachusetts; Mary T. Boylston, RN, MSN, CCRN, Eastern College, St. Davids, Pennsylvania; Ellen G. Christian, MS, RN, University of Massachusetts-Dartmouth, North Dartmouth, Massachusetts; Arlene M. Coughlin, RN, MSN, Holy Name Hospital School of Nursing, Teaneck, New Jersey; Lourdes A. D. de la Cruz, MSCHN, MHSc, RN, Sheridan College Brampton, Ontario, Canada; Jean Vanderbeek, MS, APRN, BC, Miami University Department of Nursing, Oxford, Ohio; Heidi S. Walker, RN, BSN, Ashtabula, Ohio;

Marilyn L. Weitzel, MSN, RN, University of South Alabama, Mobile, Alabama; Clara W. Boyle, PhD, Salem State College, Salem, Massachusetts; Carol Feingold, MS, RN, University of Arizona, Tucson, Arizona; Peggy L. Hawkins, RN, PhD, College of Saint Mary, Omaha, Nebraska; Beverly K. Hogan, MSN, RN, CS, University of Alabama, Birmingham, Alabama; Patricia Koller, MSN, RN, Milwaukee Area Technical College, Milwaukee, Wisconsin; Kenyann Lucas, RN, MS, Texarkana College, Texarkana, Texas; Terran R. Mathers, MSN, RN, Spring Hill College, Mobile, Alabama; Patricia Marrow, RN, BSN, Daytona Beach Community College, Daytona Beach, Florida. Their work will surely assist both students and practicing nurses alike to extend their knowledge in the area of nursing fundamentals.

I owe a special debt of gratitude to the wonderful team at Pearson Nursing for their enthusiasm for this project, as well as their good humor, expertise, and encouragement as the series developed. Maura Connor, Director of ReadyPoint™, was unending in her creativity, support, encouragement, and belief in the need for this series. Jennifer Farthing, Executive Editor, Readypoint™ coordinated this revision with insight, talent, and zeal, and fostered a culture of true collaboration and team work. Victoria Gaudette, Developmental Editor, devoted many long hours to coordinating different facets of this project. Her high standards and attention to detail contributed greatly to the final "look" of this book. Editorial Assistant, Deirdre MacKnight, helped to keep the project moving forward on a day-to-day basis, and I am grateful for her efforts as well. A very special thank you goes to the designers of the book and the production team, led by Patrick Walsh, Managing Editor and Maria Reyes, Project Manager, who brought the ideas and manuscript into final form.

Thank you to the team at GEX Publishing Services, led by Project Coordinator Michelle Durgerian, for the detail-oriented work of creating this book. I greatly appreciate their hard work, attention to detail, and spirit of collaboration.

Finally, I would like to acknowledge and gratefully thank my children Michael Jr., Kathryn, Kristen, and William, who sacrificed precious hours of family time so this book could be revised. I would also like to thank my students, past and present, for continuing to inspire me with their quest for knowledge and passion for nursing. You are the future!

–MaryAnn Hogan

The Nursing Process

1

Chapter Outline

Overview of the Nursing
   Process
Critical Thinking and Problem
   Solving

Assessment
Nursing Diagnosis
Planning
Implementation

Nursing Responsibilities While
   Implementing Care
Evaluation

Objectives

➤ Outline the 5 steps of the nursing process.
➤ Identify characteristics of the nursing process.
➤ Identify 3 methods of problem solving.
➤ Discuss methods utilized to collect assessment data.
➤ Identify the steps used in the diagnostic process.
➤ Define the different categories of nursing diagnoses and
   collaborative problems.
➤ Describe the development of measurable client outcomes.
➤ Select nursing interventions that assist the client to achieve
   health outcomes.
➤ Identify 10 responsibilities in implementing nursing care.
➤ List the steps necessary for the evaluation process.

NCLEX-RN® Test Prep

Use the accompanying online resource,
NursingReviewsandRationales, to test
yourself with hundreds of NCLEX®-style
practice questions.

Review at a Glance

assessment the process of
collecting, organizing, validating, and
documenting information about a client's
health status
collaborative problem
physiological complication that the
nurse monitors to detect onset
of changes in client status but for which
the nurse cannot independently initiate
definitive treatment
cue any piece of data or information
that influences a decision
delegating transferring to
a competent individual the responsibility
and authority for performing a selected
nursing task in a selected situation; nurse
retains accountability for delegation and
supervises the care provider
diagnosis involves critical analysis
and interpretation of assessment data,

as it is used in nursing; may also be
called analysis
evaluation planned, ongoing,
purposeful activity in which client and
nurse determine client's progress toward
achievement of outcome goals
goals expected client outcomes
of care that can be measured within
a specific time frame
implementation phase of nursing
process in which the nursing care plan is
put into action
inference nurse's judgment or
interpretation of cues, such as
judging a blood pressure to be lower
than normal
nursing diagnosis nurse's clinical
judgment about a client's responses to
actual or potential health problems or
state of wellness

nursing process a systematic,
rational method of planning and providing
nursing care
objective data include measurable
and observable data that can be detected
by someone other than the client
planning a deliberate, systematic
process that involves critical thinking,
problem solving, and decision making
carried out in collaboration with the
client and family
subjective data data that originate
from client, are not measurable, and
include client's thoughts, beliefs, feelings,
perceptions, and sensations
supervising provision by the
nurse of guidance or direction,
evaluation, and follow-up of assistive
personnel for accomplishment of a
delegated nursing task

PRETEST

1 A client comes to the walk-in clinic with reports of abdominal pain and diarrhea. While taking the client's vital signs, the nurse is implementing which phase of the nursing process?

1. Assessment
2. Diagnosis
3. Planning
4. Implementation

2 The nurse is measuring the client's urine output and straining the urine to assess for stones. Which of the following should the nurse record as objective data?

1. The client reports abdominal pain.
2. The client's urine output was 450 mL.
3. The client states, "I didn't see any stones in my urine."
4. The client states, "I feel like I have passed a stone."

3 When evaluating an older adult client's blood pressure (BP) of 146/78 mmHg, the nurse takes which action before determining whether the BP is normal or represents hypertension?

1. Compare this reading against defined standards.
2. Compare the reading with one taken on another client of the same age.
3. Determine if there are gaps in the vital signs data in the client's record.
4. Compare the current measurement with previous ones.

4 Which of the following behaviors by the nurse demonstrates that the nurse is participating in critical thinking? Select all that apply.

1. Admitting not knowing how to do a procedure and requesting help
2. Using clever and persuasive remarks to support an opinion or position
3. Delaying the formation of a nursing diagnosis for a client when there is a conflict between subjective and objective data in the assessment
4. Finding a quick and logical answer, even to complex questions
5. Gathering 3 assistants to help transfer the client to a stretcher after noting the client weighs 300 pounds.

5 The nurse has documented the following outcome goal in the care plan: "The client will transfer from bed to chair with 2-person assist." The charge nurse tells the nurse to add which missing element to complete the goal?

1. Client behavior
2. Conditions or modifiers
3. Performance criteria
4. Target time

6 The nurse who documents on the client's care plan an outcome goal that states "Client will report that his anxiety is relieved within 20 to 40 minutes following administration of lorazepam (Ativan)" is engaged in which step of the nursing process?

1. Assessment
2. Planning
3. Implementation
4. Evaluation

7 When the client resists taking a liquid medication that is essential to treatment, stating "It just feels so slimy in my mouth. I can't stand to take it," the nurse demonstrates critical thinking by taking which action first?

1. Omitting this dose of medication and waiting until the client is more cooperative
2. Suggesting to the client that the medication can be diluted in a beverage to decrease the unpleasant sensation.
3. Informing the client that the medication must be taken regardless of how it feels in the mouth
4. Notifying the provider that the client has refused the medication

8 A female night charge nurse in the ICU has cared for critically ill clients for over 20 years. She is widely recognized within the facility for her intuition and clinical judgment skills and her ability to analyze complex client problems and to assist other nurses in planning care. According to Benner's Model of Skill Acquisition, this nurse is practicing at which level?

1. Novice
2. Competent
3. Expert
4. Proficient

9 The nurse assigned to care for a postoperative client has asked an unlicensed assistive person (UAP) to help the client ambulate in the hall. Before delegating this task, the nurse must do which of the following? Select all that apply.

1. Assess the client to be sure ambulation with assistance is an appropriate care measure.
2. Ask the client if he or she is ready to ambulate.
3. Ask whether the UAP has time to assist the client.
4. Ask the charge nurse whether UAP have ambulated the client during this shift.
5. Ask the UAP to report back on how the client tolerated ambulation.

10 The nurse makes the following entry on the client's care plan: "Goal not met. Client refuses to ambulate, stating, 'I am too afraid I will fall.'" The nurse should take which of the following actions?

1. Notify the health care provider.
2. Reassign the client to another nurse.
3. Reexamine the nursing orders.
4. Write a new nursing diagnosis.

➤ *See pages 22–24 for Answers and Rationales.*

I. OVERVIEW OF THE NURSING PROCESS

A. Definition of the *nursing process*

1. A systematic, rational method of planning and providing nursing care for individuals, families, groups, and communities
2. Requires critical thinking
3. Enables nurse to identify a client's actual and potential health care needs, define **goals** (aims or ends; expected outcomes) with the client, establish a plan of care to meet those goals, implement the plan, and evaluate its effectiveness in improving client's health
4. Provides a framework for a nurse's responsibility and accountability

5. Consists of 5 sequential and interrelated steps or phases: **A**ssessment, **D**iagnosis, **P**lanning, **I**mplementation, **E**valuation (ADPIE) (see Table 1-1 for an overview of the steps of the nursing process)

Table 1-1 Overview of the Nursing Process

Component and Description	Purpose	Activities
Assessing		
Collecting, organizing, validating, and documenting client data	To establish a database about the client's response to health concerns or illness and the ability to manage healthcare needs	Establish a database: • Obtain a nursing health history • Conduct a physical assessment • Review client records • Review nursing literature • Consult support persons • Consult health professionals Update data as needed Organize data Validate data Communicate and document data
Diagnosing		
Analyzing and synthesizing data	To identify client strengths and health problems that can be prevented or resolved by collaborative and independent nursing interventions To develop a list of nursing and collaborative problems	Interpret and analyze data Compare data against standards: • Cluster or group data (generate tentative hypotheses) • Identify gaps and inconsistencies Determine client's strengths, risks, and problems Formulate nursing diagnoses and collaborative problem statements Document nursing diagnoses on the care plan
Planning		
Determining how to prevent, reduce, or resolve identified client problems; support client strengths; and implement nursing interventions in an organized, individualized, and goal-directed manner	To develop an individualized care plan that specifies client goals or desired outcomes and related nursing interventions	Set priorities and goals/outcomes in collaboration with client Write goals or desired outcomes Select nursing strategies or interventions Consult with other health professionals Write nursing orders and nursing care plan Communicate care plan to relevant health care providers
Implementing		
Carrying out the planned nursing interventions	To assist the client to meet desired goals or outcomes; promote wellness; prevent illness and disease; restore health; and facilitate coping with altered functioning	Reassess the client to update the database Determine need for nursing assistance Perform or delegate planned nursing interventions Communicate what nursing actions were implemented: • Document care and client responses to care • Give verbal reports as necessary
Evaluating		
Measuring the degree to which goals or outcomes have been achieved and identifying factors that positively or negatively influence goal achievement	To determine whether to continue, modify, or terminate the plan of care	Collaborate with client and collect data related to desired outcomes Judge whether goals or outcomes have been achieved Relate nursing actions to client outcomes Make decisions about problem status Review and modify the care plan as indicated or terminate nursing care Document achievement of outcomes and modification of the care plan

B. Steps of the nursing process
1. **Assessment** (overview of components)
   a. A process of systematically collecting, organizing, validating and documenting data (information) about the health status of an individual, family, group, or community
   b. All phases of the nursing process rely on accurate and complete data
   c. A thorough assessment is an ongoing process that uses multiple sources and continues throughout the nurse–client relationship
2. **Diagnosis** (overview of components)
   a. May also be called "analysis"
   b. Involves critical analysis and interpretation of assessment data
   c. Identifies actual or potential health problems, risks, and strengths
   d. Is the process that results in formulating a **nursing diagnosis** (a statement representing a clinical judgment about client responses to actual or potential health problems or state of wellness) and creation or design of a care plan
   e. Provides the basis for selecting nursing interventions to achieve outcomes
3. **Planning** (overview of components)
   a. A deliberate, systematic process that involves decision making and problem solving
   b. Steps
      1) Prioritize problems and diagnoses
      2) Set outcome goals with client in a specific time frame
      3) Identify interventions that will address client's health problem and achieve outcome goal(s)
      4) Document the plan of care including nursing interventions.
   c. Involves formulating client goals and designing the nursing strategies (interventions) required to prevent, reduce, or eliminate the client's health problems
   d. Planning for discharge begins at the time of admission
   e. The nurse establishes a written care plan to use in client care
   f. Planning is an ongoing process
4. **Implementation** (overview of components)
   a. The phase of the nursing process in which the nursing care plan is put into action
   b. May also be called "intervention"
   c. Consists of carrying out interventions or **delegating** nursing interventions, which involves assigning aspects of care for a client to another individual while retaining accountability for that care
   d. Nursing interventions are specific strategies designed to assist the client in achieving outcome goals
   e. Interventions are designed to prevent, reduce, or eliminate the client's health problems
   f. Includes documenting or recording nursing activities and the resulting client responses
5. **Evaluation** (overview of components)
   a. Is a planned, ongoing, purposeful activity in which client and nurse determine client's progress toward achievement of outcome goals
   b. Compares client response to outcome goals to determine whether, or to what degree, goals have been met
   c. Based on evaluation, the care plan is either continued, modified, or terminated
   d. Evaluation may be:
      1) Ongoing: done while or immediately after carrying out a nursing intervention
      2) Intermittent: performed at specified intervals, such as twice a week
      3) Terminal: performed to indicate client's condition at time of discharge

C. Figure 1-1 illustrates the sequence and interrelationships among the steps of the nursing process

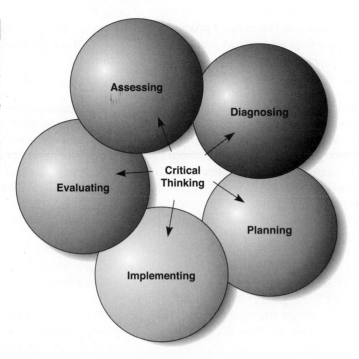

Figure 1-1

The nursing process in action

Berman, Audrey J.; Snyder, Shirlee, *Kozier & Erb's Fundamentals of Nursing*, 9th Ed. © 2012. Reprinted and Electronically reproduced by permission of Pearson Education, Inc., Upper Saddle River, New Jersey.

D. Characteristics of the nursing process
   1. Person-centered
      a. Process is open and flexible to meet the unique needs of client, family, group, and community
      b. Emphasizes client problems rather than nursing problems
      c. Assessment identifies unique characteristics of the client used to individualize the approach to care
   2. Emphasizes feedback
      a. Theoretically based in systems theory and uses feedback to:
         1) Reassess a problem or an outcome
         2) Identify the need to revise the care plan
      b. A cyclical and dynamic process rather than a static one
   3. Facilitates creativity
      a. Merges conscious, intuitive, and spontaneous thinking to solve nursing problems
      b. Encourages nurse to bring together seemingly unrelated information, find connections, and formulate an effective plan of care
      c. Develops solutions to problems in the rapidly changing health care environment
   4. Foundation of nursing practice
      a. Framework in which nurses use their knowledge and skill to assist clients to manage potential and/or actual health problems or maintain wellness
      b. Professionally recognized as a series of planned actions taken by nurses when planning and providing client care

II. CRITICAL THINKING AND PROBLEM SOLVING

A. Benner's model of skill acquisition applied to critical thinking (Source: Benner, Patricia, *From Novice to Expert: Excellence and Power in Clinical Nursing Practice*, Commemorative Edition, 1st Edition, Prentice Hall 2000.)

1. Novice: uses rules to perform correctly in client care situations
2. Advanced beginner: recognizes common patterns and benefits from assistance in setting priorities; begins to develop professional habits
3. Competent: recognizes own thinking and analyzes problems (often after 2 to 3 years of experience)
4. Proficient: uses increasingly intuitive thinking; perceives a clinical situation "as a whole," rather than its individual aspects, with speed and accuracy (generally takes 3 to 5 years of experience)
5. Expert: does not need analytical principles to understand a situation; intuition becomes prominent in thinking (usually takes 5 or more years of experience; this stage may or may not be achieved by all nurses)

B. Concept mapping

1. Uses graphic figures to illustrate both linear and nonlinear relationships and represent critical thinking
2. Is used to help bridge the gap between theory and nursing practice and to improve understanding of complex phenomena
3. Helps nurses organize and make sense of large amounts of information from multiple sources to improve clinical decision making

C. Trial-and-error problem solving

1. Problem solving in which a number of approaches are tried until a successful one is found
2. Lacks precision and may be time consuming if failures occur
3. Approaches are tried without carefully evaluating the situation, available options, and potential consequences of each option
4. Client may suffer harm if an approach is inappropriate

D. Scientific method as used in nursing for problem solving

1. Logical, organized, and systematic approach used to discover relationships between what is observed and its explanation
2. Follows a logical sequence of steps
   a. Identify the problem
   b. Define it carefully
   c. Review the literature
   d. Determine data-gathering methodology
   e. Collect data
   f. Generate solution(s)
   g. Execute solution(s)
   h. Evaluate results
3. Is most effective in controlled situations
4. The profession's unique use of the scientific method
   a. Involves interaction between client and nurse as they work together
   b. Used to identify potential or actual health care needs, set goals, and devise a plan to meet client needs, and evaluate its effectiveness
5. Process is not always linear or sequential and the steps overlap
6. Critical thinking and decision making are important activities in the modified scientific method used in nursing (see Table 1-2)
   a. Nurse applies nursing knowledge and knowledge from other disciplines to resolve client problems
   b. Deals with stressful environments
   c. Creatively resolves nursing care dilemmas with a course of action
7. Evaluation and feedback are essential steps
8. A nurse who effectively uses nursing process must be proficient and comfortable with all the steps

Table 1-2	Examples of Critical Thinking in the Nursing Process
Nursing Process Phase	**Critical-Thinking Activities**
Assessing	Making reliable observations Distinguishing relevant from irrelevant data Distinguishing important from unimportant data Validating data Organizing data Categorizing data according to a framework Recognizing assumptions Identifying gaps in data
Diagnosing	Finding patterns and relationships among cues Making inferences Suspending judgment when lacking data Stating the problem Examining assumptions Comparing patterns with norms Identifying factors contributing to problem
Planning	Forming valid generalizations Transferring knowledge from one situation to another Developing criteria for evaluation Hypothesizing Making interdisciplinary connections Prioritizing client problems Generalizing principles from other sciences
Implementing	Applying knowledge to perform interventions Testing hypotheses
Evaluating	Deciding whether hypotheses are correct Making criterion-based evaluations

Source: Berman, Audrey J.; Snyder, Shirlee, *Kozier & Erb's Fundamentals of Nursing*, 9th Ed. © 2012. Reprinted and Electronically reproduced by permission of Pearson Education, Inc., Upper Saddle River, New Jersey.

III. ASSESSMENT *(SEE FIGURE 1-2)*

A. Collection of data: objective and subjective

1. Review of clinical record
   a. Client records contain information collected by many health care team members, such as demographics, past medical history, diagnostic test results, and consultations
   b. Reviewing the client's record before beginning an assessment prevents the nurse from repeating questions that have already been asked and identifies information that needs clarification
2. Interview
   a. Purpose of an interview is to gather and provide information, identify problems or concerns, and provide teaching and support
   b. Goals of an interview are to develop a rapport with client and to collect data
   c. An interview has 3 major stages
      1) Opening: purpose is to establish rapport by creating goodwill and trust; this is often achieved through self-introduction, nonverbal gestures (a handshake), and small talk about the weather, local sports team, or recent current events; the interview's purpose is also explained to client at this time

Figure 1-2

Assessment components

Berman, Audrey J.; Snyder, Shirlee, *Kozier & Erb's Fundamentals of Nursing, 9th Ed.* © 2012. Reprinted and Electronically reproduced by permission of Pearson Education, Inc., Upper Saddle River, New Jersey.

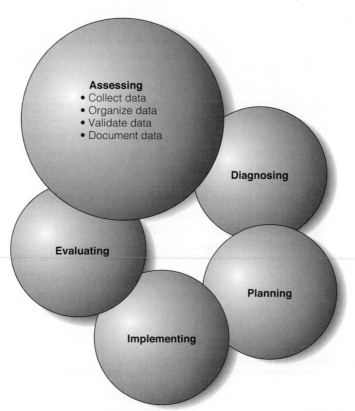

Practice to Pass

The client says, "I have a pain in my chest." Write a closed-ended and an open-ended question the nurse could ask to find out more about this reported symptom.

2) Body: during this phase, the client responds to open- and closed-ended questions asked by nurse

3) Closing: either client or nurse may terminate the interview; it is important for the nurse to try to maintain rapport and trust that was developed thus far during the interview process

d. Types of questions

1) Closed-ended questions used in directive interview

a) Require short factual answers (e.g., "Do you have pain?")

b) Often can be answered with a "yes" or "no"

c) Answers usually reveal limited amounts of information

d) Useful with clients who are highly stressed and/or have difficulty communicating

2) Open-ended questions used in nondirective interview

a) Encourage clients to express and clarify their thoughts and feelings (e.g., "How have you been sleeping lately?")

b) Specify the broad area to be discussed and invite longer answers

c) Useful at the start of an interview to encourage therapeutic communication or to encourage a descriptive or detailed answer

3) Leading questions

a) Direct the client's answer (e.g., "You don't have any questions about your medications, do you?")

b) Suggest what answer is expected

c) Can result in client giving inaccurate data to please the nurse

d) Can limit client choice of topic for discussion

3. Nursing history

    a. Collection of information about the effects of client's illness on daily functioning and ability to cope with this stressor (the human response)

    b. Subjective data

        1) Not measurable or observable

        2) Obtained from client (primary source), significant others, or health professionals (secondary sources)

        3) Include client's thoughts, beliefs, feelings, perceptions, and sensations; for example, the client states, "I have a headache"

        4) Refer to Table 1-3 for additional examples of subjective data

    c. Objective data

        1) Can be detected by someone other than client

        2) Include measurable and observable client behavior or information; for example, a blood pressure reading of 190/110 mmHg

        3) Refer again to Table 1-3 for additional examples of objective data

4. Physical assessment

    a. Systematic collection of information about body systems through use of observation, inspection, auscultation, palpation, and percussion

    b. A body system format for physical assessment is found in Box 1-1

Table 1-3 **Examples of Subjective and Objective Data**

Subjective	Objective
"I feel weak all over when I exert myself."	Blood pressure 90/50 Apical pulse 104 Skin pale and diaphoretic
Client states he has a cramping pain in his abdomen; states, "I feel sick to my stomach."	Vomited 100 mL green-tinged fluid Abdomen firm and slightly distended Active bowel sounds auscultated in all 4 quadrants
"I'm short of breath."	Lung sounds clear bilaterally; diminished in right lower lobe
"He doesn't seem so sad today," wife states.	Cried during interview
"I would like to see the chaplain before surgery."	Holding open Bible Has small silver cross on bedside table

Source: Berman, Audrey J.; Snyder, Shirlee, *Kozier & Erb's Fundamentals of Nursing*, 9th Ed. © 2012. Reprinted and Electronically reproduced by permission of Pearson Education, Inc., Upper Saddle River, New Jersey.

Box 1-1

Suggested Format for Physical Assessment

- General head-to-toe assessment
- Integumentary system
- Head, ears, eyes, nose, throat
- Breast and axillae
- Thorax and lungs
- Cardiovascular system
- Nervous system
- Abdomen and gastrointestinal system
- Anus and rectum
- Genitourinary system
- Reproductive system
- Musculoskeletal system

Box 1-2	• Health perception–health management

Gordon's Functional Health Problems

- Health perception–health management
- Nutritional–metabolic
- Elimination
- Activity–exercise
- Sleep–rest
- Cognitive–perceptual
- Self-perception–self-concept
- Role–relationship
- Sexuality–reproductive
- Coping–stress tolerance
- Value–belief

5. Psychosocial assessment
   a. Gordon's Functional Health Patterns Model is helpful for gathering and organizing both physical and psychosocial data (see Box 1-2)
   b. The developmental theories of Erikson, Freud, Havighurst, Kohlberg, and Piaget also may be helpful for guiding data collection
6. Consultation
   a. The nurse collects data from multiple sources: primary (client) and secondary (family members, support persons, health care professionals, and records)
   b. Consultation with individuals who can contribute to client's database is helpful in obtaining the most complete and accurate information about a client
   c. Supplemental information from secondary sources (any source other than client) can help verify information, provide information for a client who cannot do so, and convey information about client's status prior to admission
7. Review of literature
   a. A professional nurse engages in continued education to maintain knowledge of current information related to health care and nursing practice
   b. Reviewing professional journals and textbooks can help provide additional data to support or help analyze the client database

B. Patterns approach to assessment
1. Gordon's functional health patterns
   a. The 11 functional health patterns (FHPs) guide the collection of data about common patterns of behavior that contribute to health, quality of life, and achievement of human potential
   b. The 11 FHPs are applicable to all clients; see Box 1-3
2. Human response patterns
   a. Human responses are the biological, psychological, social, and spiritual reactions to an event or stressor
   b. The 9 human response patterns reflect the whole person in interaction with the environment (see Box 1-3)

IV. NURSING DIAGNOSIS

A. The nursing diagnosis step of the nursing process involves data analysis and identification of problems, risks, and strengths, and it leads to development of nursing diagnoses (see Figure 1-3)
B. Analysis and interpretation
1. The most common diagnostic system used is that of the North American Nursing Diagnosis Association International (NANDA-I)
2. Involves 3 activities that are sequential and continuous
   a. Compare data against standards, identifying significant **cues** (data that influence a decision)

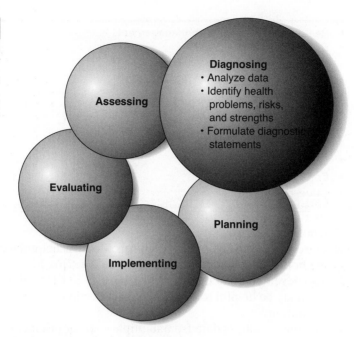

Figure 1-3

Diagnosing components

Berman, Audrey J.; Snyder, Shirlee, *Kozier & Erb's Fundamentals of Nursing*, 9th Ed. © 2012. Reprinted and Electronically reproduced by permission of Pearson Education, Inc., Upper Saddle River, New Jersey.

Box 1-3

Human Response Patterns

- **Exchanging:** mutual giving and receiving
- **Communicating:** sending messages
- **Relating:** establishing bonds
- **Valuing:** assigning relative worth
- **Choosing:** selection of alternatives
- **Moving:** activity
- **Perceiving:** reception of information
- **Knowing:** meaning associated with information
- **Feeling:** subjective awareness of information

Source: Berman, Audrey J.; Snyder, Shirlee, *Kozier & Erb's Fundamentals of Nursing*, 9th Ed. © 2012. Reprinted and Electronically reproduced by permission of Pearson Education, Inc., Upper Saddle River, New Jersey.

    b. Cluster the cues and generate tentative hypotheses
    c. Identify gaps and inconsistencies
C. Making and validating inferences (nurse's judgment or interpretation of cues)
    1. Skillful assessment minimizes gaps and inconsistencies in data
    2. Double-check to ensure data is complete and correct
    3. Clarify all inconsistencies before making inferences
D. Comparing cues and clusters of cues with defining characteristics
    1. Nurses compare client data to standards and norms to identify significant and relevant cues
    2. Significant cues vary from norms of the client population; they indicate a change in client status or indicate a developmental delay
    3. Data clustering involves making inferences about data; it is a process of determining relatedness of facts and whether patterns are present
    4. Data may be clustered inductively by combining all data collected to form a pattern; or deductively by using a framework (e.g., FHPs) and clustering data into defined categories
E. Identifying related factors
    1. A nursing diagnosis may consist of two parts joined by "related to" clause (see Table 1-4), especially if it is a risk diagnosis and not an actual diagnosis

Table 1-4 Design of a 2-Part Nursing Diagnostic Statement

Human Response (Label)	Related to	Related Factor(s) or Risk Factor(s)
What needs to change		*What is contributing to problem*
Risk for impaired tissue integrity	related to	Imposed immobility (bed rest)
Suggests outcomes		*Suggests interventions*
Client will remain free of pressure ulcers throughout hospitalization.		Reposition client every 2 hours.

   a. Part I—human response: naming or labeling the problem (actual or potential)
   b. Part II—related factors: factors contributing to or probable causes of the human response (problem)
2. Human responses are the biological, psychological, social, and spiritual reactions to an event or a stressor such as disease or injury
3. The related factors are the etiology component of a nursing diagnosis; they are the condition(s) or circumstance(s) that influence, precede, or contribute to the development of a diagnosis or increase a person's vulnerability to a diagnosis
4. An example could be "Risk for Infection related to low white blood cell count"
5. Related factors identify one or more probable causes of the health problem and provide direction for required nursing interventions
6. The PES (problem, etiology, signs and symptoms) format may be used for actual (not risk) nursing diagnostic statements
   a. These nursing diagnostic statements may be written as 3-part statements
   b. The 3 parts include the human response, the related factors, and the actual defining characteristics experienced by the client (which are listed after the clause "as evidenced by")

F. **Choosing the nursing diagnosis**
1. Review the parts of a nursing diagnosis
   a. *Label*: the name for the diagnosis
   b. *Definition*: clear description of the diagnosis
   c. *Related factors or risk factors*: conditions or circumstances that contribute to development of a diagnosis or factors that increase one's vulnerability to a diagnosis
   d. *Defining characteristics*: critical behaviors and signs and symptoms that are manifestations of the diagnosis (one or more of these needs to be present to choose the diagnosis)
2. A nursing diagnosis should be concise, related to only one problem, and written clearly
3. Document the nursing diagnosis on the client's care plan using agency-approved format
4. Follow agency policy and guidelines for initiating, updating, and resolving nursing diagnoses on the client's care plan

G. **Types of Nursing Diagnoses**
1. Actual
   a. Client demonstrates defining characteristics of a problem
   b. Nurse intervenes to resolve or help client cope with the problem
   c. Contains 3 parts: the label, related to or risk factors, and defining characteristics (as evidenced by)
   d. Example: Activity Intolerance related to prolonged immobility as evidenced by verbal report of fatigue and increased heart rate when ambulating in hall

!

Practice to Pass

Write a diagnostic statement for each of the following clients.

• A client with type 2 diabetes who states that she has not been taking her medication because it does not make her feel any better and she has difficulty remembering when to take it.

• A 90-year-old client with left-sided hemiparesis who has a red, broken area on the skin over his coccyx and cannot turn himself in bed.

Table 1-5	Collaborative Problems		
Disease or Situation	**Complication**	**Related to**	**Etiology**
Potential complication of childbirth	Hemorrhage	Related to	1. Uterine atony 2. Retained placental fragments 3. Bladder distention
Potential complication of diuretic therapy	Dysrhythmia	Related to	Low serum potassium

Source: Berman, Audrey J.; Snyder, Shirlee, *Kozier & Erb's Fundamentals of Nursing,* 9th Ed. © 2012. Reprinted and Electronically reproduced by permission of Pearson Education, Inc., Upper Saddle River, New Jersey.

    2. High-risk
        a. A problem is likely to develop based on assessment of risk factors
        b. Nurse intervenes to reduce risk factors or increase protective factors
        c. Contains 2 parts: the label and related to or risk factors
        d. Example: Risk for Infection related to hospitalization and central line placement
    3. Wellness or health promotion
        a. Client is presently healthy but wishes to achieve a higher level of function
        b. Nurse intervenes to promote growth or maintenance of the healthy response
        c. Has only one part: the label
        d. Example: Readiness for Enhanced Nutrition
H. Collaborative problems
    1. Definition: a potential problem the nurse manages using both independent and interdependent interventions
    2. Example: potential complication of head injury: loss of consciousness, epidural or subdural hematoma, seizures
    3. Usually occurs when a disease is present or a treatment is prescribed
    4. Clients with similar disease or treatments will have the same potential for complications, which must be managed collaboratively; however, their responses to the condition will vary, so a broad range of nursing diagnoses will apply
        a. Example: a client with asthma will always be at risk for lowered oxygen saturation; however the client's response to this condition will be unique based on his or her developmental level, past experiences, and family configuration
        b. Refer to Table 1-5 for several examples of a **collaborative problems**

V. PLANNING

    A. Consists of developing the plan of care that will assist client in the identified area of concern (nursing diagnosis)
    B. Involves client and family: client participation in the care planning process will help ensure that selected outcomes are reasonable and that client will work toward goal achievement
    C. Has 3 components (see Figure 1-4)
        1. The identified problems or nursing diagnoses must be prioritized according to level of importance; frequently Maslow's hierarchy, physiological condition, and client preference are taken into account when setting priorities; psychological condition of client may also be considered when setting priorities
        2. Goals or desired outcomes must be formulated within a specific time frame; these are necessary to determine whether the plan of care is effective, once implemented
            a. Outcomes are derived from the nursing diagnosis
            b. Outcomes should identify desirable human responses
            c. Outcomes define specific behaviors that demonstrate that the problem has been reduced, prevented, or eliminated and/or the client has adapted to changes in his or her health status

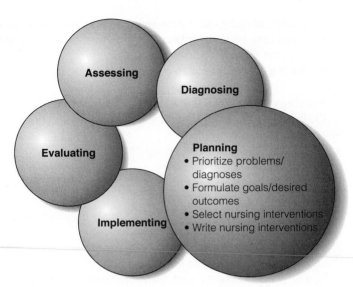

Figure 1-4

Planning components

Berman, Audrey J.; Snyder, Shirlee, *Kozier & Erb's Fundamentals of Nursing*, 9th Ed. © 2012. Reprinted and Electronically reproduced by permission of Pearson Education, Inc., Upper Saddle River, New Jersey.

Practice to Pass

Write expected outcomes for the following nursing diagnosis: Risk for Fluid Volume Deficit related to decreased oral intake and increased insensible losses secondary to tachypnea and fever.

 d. Outcome goals must include client behavior, target time, conditions or modifiers, and performance criteria

 e. Outcomes should be *SMART* (specific, measurable, appropriate, realistic, timely) (Table 1-6)

 f. Example: client will ambulate independently in hall with a walker by 4/10/13

3. Nursing interventions or nursing orders (a nursing intervention that has all the specificity of a provider prescription) must be written to guide the actions of health care providers when implementing care

VI. IMPLEMENTATION

 A. Types of nursing interventions

  1. Independent

   a. Interventions that nurses are licensed to implement for a client by virtue of their education and experience; they may be broad statements that indicate actions to be taken; some interventions are called *nursing orders* when they are very specific (see Section B that follows)

   b. May be performed by a nurse without a health care provider prescription

   c. Example: assess for decreased skin integrity or pressure ulcers

  2. Interdependent

   a. Also called *collaborative* interventions

   b. Are carried out by a nurse in cooperation with other health care team members

Table 1-6	**Outcomes Should Be SMART**	
S	Specific	Indicate how nurse will know that client's response has changed.
M	Measurable	Address what client will do, when this will be accomplished, and to what extent.
A	Appropriate	Include client in formulating outcomes.
R	Realistic	Consider client's present and potential capabilities.
T	Timely	Include a time estimate for outcome attainment.

Practice to Pass

The nurse is working with a nursing assistant to care for an elderly man who has had a stroke but is now stable. He is very thin and immobile. In shift report, the nurse heard that he has a reddened area on his coccyx. If the nurse decides to delegate the bed, bath, and hygiene measures to the nursing assistant, what instructions should the nurse provide?

    c. Example: carrying out a provider's prescription to assist client with ambulating in hall; this may be accomplished in collaboration with physical therapists on the health care team

B. Components of a correctly written nursing order

    1. Date

        a. Nursing orders are dated when they are written

        b. Orders are reviewed periodically depending on client needs

    2. Specific action verb

        a. An action verb starts the nursing order

        b. The verb should be precise

    3. Prescribed activity: content of the order is the "where" and "what" of the prescribed action

    4. Time units or frequencies: the time element indicates when, how long, or how often the intervention should be implemented

    5. Signature of nurse: accountability is accepted when the nurse signs name and title to the nursing order he or she has written

    6. Example: 3/22/13 Assist client with repositioning every 1–2 hours N. Nurse, RN

VII. NURSING RESPONSIBILITIES WHILE IMPLEMENTING CARE (FIGURE 1-5)

    A. Review planned interventions for appropriateness

        1. Focus strategies on eliminating or modifying the cause of the nursing diagnosis

        2. Characteristics of interventions

            a. Realistic, safe, and consider the client's age, health status, and condition

            b. Achievable with available resources

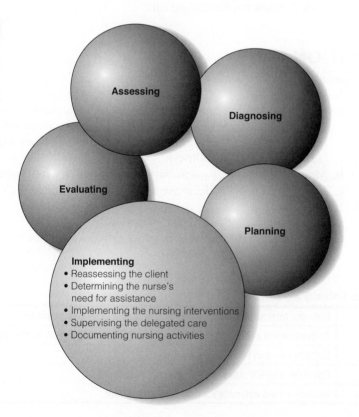

Figure 1-5

Implementation components

Berman, Audrey J.; Snyder, Shirlee, *Kozier & Erb's Fundamentals of Nursing*, 9th Ed. © 2012. Reprinted and Electronically reproduced by permission of Pearson Education, Inc., Upper Saddle River, New Jersey.

Assessing

Diagnosing

Evaluating

Planning

Implementing
- Reassessing the client
- Determining the nurse's need for assistance
- Implementing the nursing interventions
- Supervising the delegated care
- Documenting nursing activities

   c. Congruent with client's values, beliefs, and culture, and acceptable to the client
   d. Based on nursing science and knowledge or rationale from other sciences
   e. Lies within established standards of care, the state Nurse Practice Act, professional organizations, and policies of institution

B. Setting Priorities
   1. Time management and organizational skills facilitate effective nursing care
      a. Plan to get organized before caregiving begins
      b. Put time management down in written form when beginning to coordinate care (e.g., list tasks due at specific times)
      c. Plan the day around the most complex client
      d. Identify the busiest times on the unit; do not plan treatments or interventions at those times
   2. Assess the capabilities of the staff and make assignments that fit corresponding strengths
   3. Use assertive communication techniques (direct and honest but without impeding the rights of others)
   4. Plan time for documentation as care is given; delayed documentation is less likely to be accurate and complete, and could cause confusion in the plan of care if care that has been given is interpreted as omitted because it was not documented

C. Engaging in collaboration
   1. Complexity of care planning necessitates working with others to provide quality client care and improve outcomes
   2. Table 1-7 outlines the dimensions of nurses' collaboration with clients, peers, other health care professionals, professional nursing organizations, and legislators
   3. Is increasingly important as boundaries of health care professions change
   4. Key elements
      a. Establish trusting relationships
      b. Use effective communication

Table 1-7	The Nurse as a Collaborator
With Clients	Acknowledges, supports, and encourages clients' active involvement in health care decisions Encourages a sense of client autonomy and an equal position with other members of the health care team Helps clients set mutually agreed-upon goals and objectives for health care Provides client consultation in a collaborative fashion
With Peers	Shares personal expertise with other nurses and elicits the expertise of others to ensure quality client care Develops a sense of trust and mutual respect with peers that recognizes their unique contributions
With Other Health care Professionals	Recognizes the contribution that each member of the interdisciplinary team can make by virtue of his or her expertise and view of the situation Listens to each individual's views Shares health care responsibilities in exploring options, setting goals, and making decisions with clients and families Participates in collaborative interdisciplinary research to increase knowledge of a clinical problem or situation
With Professional Nursing Organizations	Seeks out opportunities to collaborate with and within professional organizations Serves on committees in state (or provincial) and national nursing organizations or specialty groups Supports professional organizations in political action to create solutions for professional and health care concerns
With Legislators	Offers expert opinions on legislative initiatives related to health care Collaborates with other health care providers and consumers on health care legislation to best serve the needs of the public

      c. Develop mutual respect

      d. Demonstrate good decision-making skills

      e. Manage conflict

   5. To fulfill a collaborative role, nurses must assume accountability and authority in their practice areas

D. Supervising delegated care

   1. Delegating and **supervising** (providing guidance or direction, evaluation, and follow-up after delegation) are integrated processes

      a. Once the nurse delegates, he or she must supervise

      b. Need to know the delegation rules and regulations of the Nurse Practice Act in the state in which employed

      c. Review the delegation policies of the institution and the job descriptions of nursing team members

      d. Assess the client to be sure delegation is appropriate for his or her care

   2. Check that the person to whom the task is delegated has the knowledge and skill to carry it out safely and effectively

      a. The registered nurse is legally responsible for seeing that delegated tasks are performed properly

      b. Appropriate delegation involves assigning people duties within the scope of their practice

      c. Set expectations clearly and verify that the person understands the instructions

      d. Offer and receive feedback effectively

      e. Adequate supervision of licensed practical/vocational nurses (LPN/LVN) and unlicensed personnel (UAP) is a responsibility of the registered nurse

E. Providing direct care

   1. Nurses use 3 major types of interventions in providing direct care to the client

      a. Interpersonal: verbal and nonverbal activities involved in communication

      b. Technical/psychomotor: "hands-on" skills or procedures

      c. Cognitive: involves critical thinking and problem solving to provide safe care

   2. The nurse is responsible to act in a reasonable and prudent manner using the nursing process

F. Providing counseling

   1. Help clients recognize and cope with stressful psychological or social problems

   2. Develop and improve interpersonal relationships and promote personal growth

   3. Provide emotional, intellectual, and psychological support

   4. The nurse primarily counsels healthy clients with adjustment difficulties

G. Involving the client

   1. Nurses do not plan *for* the client but partner *with* the client and family to formulate a plan of care

      a. Consider client's health and mental status

      b. Protect client's right to autonomy in decision making supported in *Patient's Bill of Rights* (Source: The U.S. Department of Health and Human Services.)

      c. Assess client's readiness to learn and participate in care

   2. Clients are more motivated and successful in meeting goals they consider important

H. Teaching client and family

   1. Client education is an essential aspect of nursing practice and an independent nursing function

   2. *Patient's Bill of Rights* mandates client education as a right of all clients

   3. Develop and carry out a teaching plan to promote, protect, and maintain health after assessing each client's individual learning needs

I. Making referrals
1. Help clients use resources to meet their health care needs
2. Requires knowledge of community resources and the ability to solve problems
3. Referrals should present a clear picture of the client and his or her health care needs

J. Documenting care
1. Nurses must accurately document all care, including each step of the nursing process, in the client's record
   a. Documentation must be legible, in ink, and include time, date, and appropriate signature
   b. Assessments, medications, and treatments should be documented immediately to safeguard the client against duplication and provide accurate, up-to-date information available to all health care professionals
   c. The nurse is accountable for using the health care agency's designated documentation system appropriately
2. Documentation is a legal nursing responsibility
   a. Client's record is a legal document and admissible in court
   b. Confidentiality is important; the American Nurses Association (ANA) Code of Ethics describes the nurse's responsibility to maintain client's right to privacy by judiciously protecting information of a confidential nature

VIII. EVALUATION

A. **Is the final step of the nursing process**
B. **May or may not be an end point; if problem is not resolved, then reassessment needs to occur**
C. **Has various components (see Figure 1-6)**
D. **Refer back to client's planned outcomes**
E. **Evaluate client's condition, comparing to outcomes**
   1. Compare client's current health status with the outcomes defined on the care plan

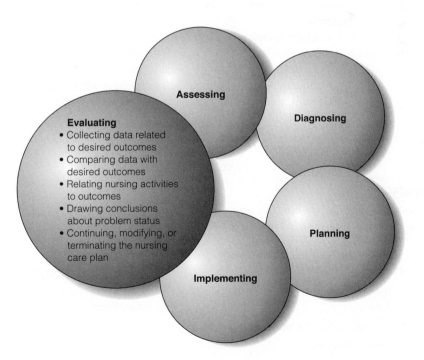

Figure 1-6

Evaluation components

Berman, Audrey J.; Snyder, Shirlee, *Kozier & Erb's Fundamentals of Nursing*, 9th Ed. © 2012. Reprinted and Electronically reproduced by permission of Pearson Education, Inc., Upper Saddle River, New Jersey.

Evaluating
- Collecting data related to desired outcomes
- Comparing data with desired outcomes
- Relating nursing activities to outcomes
- Drawing conclusions about problem status
- Continuing, modifying, or terminating the nursing care plan

Assessing

Diagnosing

Planning

Implementing

2. Determine if the outcome was or was not achieved
   a. If client's current human response is consistent with the desired outcome, the goal was met
   b. If client's current human response is not consistent with the desired outcome, the goal was not met
3. Evaluation is systematic and ongoing, helping to revise the diagnosis, interventions, and/or outcome goals

F. Summarize results
1. Write an evaluation statement that provides a conclusion (goal was or was not met) and supporting data (human responses to support conclusion)
2. Example: "3/8/13 Goal met. Client ambulated 80 ft in hall with walker."

G. Identify reasons outcomes not achieved
1. Outcome goal was not appropriate
2. Collection of new assessment data may reveal that outcome was not specific, measurable, appropriate, realistic, or timely
3. Client may need more time to achieve desired outcome
4. It may be more appropriate to set outcomes at increasing levels of difficulty; example: client states pain is $\leq 6/10$ on day 1, $\leq 4/10$ on day 2, $\leq 2/10$ on day 3

H. Corrective action to modify plan
1. Reassess client for additional or incomplete data
2. Make a judgment about the problem status and use new data to analyze whether the diagnosis is appropriate for the client
3. Outcome goals may need to be revised to be more realistic and attainable
4. Nursing interventions should be examined to ensure the best interventions were selected to assist client toward a more optimal level of functioning
5. A revised diagnosis will require new interventions
6. The manner in which the nursing interventions were implemented may have interfered with achieving the outcome
7. The diagnosis, outcome(s), and/or interventions may need to be changed or additional diagnoses, outcomes, and/or interventions may need to be added

I. Document
1. Client's responses to interventions and any changes made to the care plan should be documented according to agency policy
2. To discontinue a diagnosis once it has been resolved, follow agency documentation procedures, which can include: highlight it with yellow highlighter or marker, then write initials and date; some forms may require the nurse to put date and initials in "Date Resolved" column

---

Practice to Pass

The nurse has formulated the nursing diagnosis, "Disturbed sleep pattern related to cough, pain, and fever as evidenced by temp 101.8°F, constant bronchospastic cough and verbal complaint of "I cannot get to sleep; my chest hurts when I cough." The identified outcome is, "Client will sleep for at least 5 uninterrupted hours and report feeling rested in the morning." What criteria will the nurse use for outcome evaluation? Be specific.

Case Study

A client has just arrived on the nursing unit from the postanesthesia care unit (PACU) following a hysterectomy this morning. She is reporting pain and nausea. You are the nurse assigned to care for her.

1. What critical assessment data do you need to identify and collect?
2. Formulate a nursing diagnosis based on your assessment data.
3. Write 2 outcome goals for the nursing diagnosis.
4. Describe 3 nursing interventions to assist the client in achieving the outcome goal.
5. What criteria would you use to evaluate the effectiveness of the nursing interventions?

For suggested responses, see page 299.

POSTTEST

1. In developing a plan of care for a client with chronic hypertension, which nursing activity would be most important?

   1. Set incremental goals for blood pressure reduction.
   2. Instruct the client to make dietary changes by reducing sodium intake.
   3. Include the client and family when setting goals and formulating the plan of care.
   4. Assess past adherence to medication regimens.

2. Which nurse is demonstrating the assessment phase of the nursing process?

   1. The nurse who observes that the client's pain was relieved with pain medication.
   2. The nurse who turns the client to a more comfortable position.
   3. The nurse who asks the client how much lunch he or she ate.
   4. The nurse who works with the client to set desired outcome goals.

3. The client states, "My chest hurts and my left arm feels numb." The nurse interprets that this data is of which type and source?

   1. Subjective data from a primary source
   2. Subjective data from a secondary source
   3. Objective data from a primary source
   4. Objective data from a secondary source

4. The nurse feels a client is at risk for skin breakdown because he has only had clear liquid intake for the last 10 days (and essentially no protein intake). The nurse would formulate which diagnostic statement that would best reflect this problem?

   1. Imbalanced Nutrition: Less than Body Requirements related to clear liquid diet
   2. Impaired Skin Integrity related to no protein intake
   3. Risk for Impaired Skin Integrity related to malnutrition
   4. Imbalanced Nutrition: Less than Body Requirements related to current illness

5. The nurse would place which correctly written nursing diagnostic statement into the client's care plan?

   1. Cancer related to cigarette smoking
   2. Impaired Gas Exchange related to aspiration of foreign matter as evidenced by oxygen saturation of 91%.
   3. Imbalanced Nutrition: More than Body Requirements related to overweight status
   4. Impaired Physical Mobility related to generalized weakness and pain

6. Which of the following outcome goals has the nurse designed correctly for the postoperative client's plan of care? Select all that apply.

   1. Client will state pain is less than or equal to a 5 on a 0 to 10 pain scale.
   2. Client will have no pain.
   3. Client will state pain is less than or equal to a 4 on a 0 to 10 pain scale within 24 hours.
   4. Client will state pain is less than or equal to a 3 on a 0 to 10 pain scale by time of discharge.
   5. Client will be medicated every 4 hours by the nurse.

7 The nurse questions if the dosage of a medication is unsafe for the client because of the client's weight and age. The nurse should take which of the following actions at this time? Select all that apply.

1. Administer the medication as prescribed by the provider.
2. Call the provider to discuss the prescription and the nurse's concern.
3. Administer the medication, but chart the nurse's concern about the dosage.
4. Give the client half of the dosage and document accordingly.
5. Withhold the dose at this time.

8 Which activity would be appropriate for the nurse to delegate to unlicensed assistive personnel (UAP)?

1. Taking vital signs of clients on the nursing unit
2. Assisting the health care provider with an invasive procedure
3. Adjusting the rate on an infusion pump
4. Evaluating achievement of client outcome goals

9 In giving a change-of-shift report, which type of client information communicated by the nurse is most appropriate?

1. Vital signs are stable.
2. Client is pleasant, alert, and oriented to time, place, and person.
3. The chest x-ray results were negative.
4. Client voided 250 mL of urine 2 hours after urinary catheter removal.

10 Twenty minutes after administering pain medication to the client, the nurse returns to ask if the client's level of pain has decreased. The nurse documents the client's response as part of which phase of the nursing process?

1. Diagnosis
2. Planning
3. Implementation
4. Evaluation

➤ *See pages 24–25 for Answers and Rationales.*

ANSWERS & RATIONALES

Pretest

1 **Answer: 1** **Rationale:** The first step in the nursing process is assessment, the process of collecting data. All subsequent phases of the nursing process (diagnosis, planning, implementing, and evaluating) rely on accurate and complete data gathered in the assessment. **Cognitive Level:** Applying **Client Need:** Basic Care and Comfort **Integrated Process:** Nursing Process: Assessment **Content Area:** Fundamentals **Strategy:** The critical words are *vital signs*. Recall that vital signs give information or assessment data about the client to choose correctly, or recall that a basic nursing assessment of any ill client will include measurement of vital signs. **Reference:** Berman, A., & Snyder, S. J. (2012). *Kozier & Erb's fundamentals of nursing: Concepts, process, and practice* (9th ed.). Upper Saddle River, NJ: Pearson Education, p. 181.

2 **Answer: 2** **Rationale:** Objective data is measurable data that can be seen, heard, or felt and verified by the nurse. In this case, the objective data is the measurement of the urine output. Any client statements or reported symptoms are subjective data. **Cognitive Level:** Applying **Client Need:** Basic Care and Comfort **Integrated Process:** Communication and Documentation **Content Area:** Fundamentals **Strategy:** The critical words are *objective data*. Recall that objective data must be measurable and verified by the nurse. **Reference:** Berman, A., & Snyder, S. J. (2012). *Kozier & Erb's fundamentals of nursing: Concepts, process, and practice* (9th ed.). Upper Saddle River, NJ: Pearson Education, p. 183.

3 **Answer: 1** **Rationale:** Analysis of the client's blood pressure (BP) requires knowledge of the normal BP range for an older adult. The nurse compares the client's data against identified standards to determine whether this reading is normal or abnormal. Comparing this client to another client of similar age will not aid in determining whether this client's blood pressure (BP) is within expected ranges. Gaps in the record will not aid in interpreting the current measurement. Comparing the reading to previous ones will give additional client data, but the comparison alone will not determine whether the blood pressure (BP) is normal. **Cognitive Level:** Applying **Client Need:** Basic Care and Comfort **Integrated Process:** Nursing Process: Diagnosis **Content Area:** Fundamentals **Strategy:** Knowledge of the diagnosis phase of the nursing process would direct you to compare data collected in the assessment process against established standards or norms before drawing a conclusion about the significance of this data. **Reference:** Berman, A., & Snyder, S. J. (2012). *Kozier & Erb's fundamentals of nursing: Concepts, process, and practice* (9th ed.). Upper Saddle River, NJ: Pearson Education, p. 203.

4 **Answers: 1, 3, 5** **Rationale:** Critical thinking is the process of purposeful, self-regulatory judgment. It requires that the nurse suspend judgment when data is incomplete or inconclusive. Critical thinking in nursing is self-directed, supporting what nurses know and making clear what they do not know. It is important for nurses to recognize when they lack the knowledge they need to provide safe care for a client. It is a cognitive process that involves problem solving and decision making, not the persuasion of others. Critical thinking requires the nurse to thoughtfully apply knowledge from multiple disciplines to organize complex data and make a sound clinical decision. This may not always be done quickly. Gathering assistants to help with the transfer would demonstrate good critical thinking by the nurse in evaluating the data (client's weight) and planning care based on the data available. **Cognitive Level:** Applying **Client Need:** Safety and Infection Control **Integrated Process:** Nursing Process: Diagnosis **Content Area:** Fundamentals **Strategy:** Critical words in the question are *critical thinking.* Recall that critical thinking is a process involving evaluation of data to enhance problem solving. **Reference:** Berman, A., & Snyder, S. J. (2012). *Kozier & Erb's fundamentals of nursing: Concepts, process, and practice* (9th ed.). Upper Saddle River, NJ: Pearson Education, p. 163.

5 **Answer: 4** **Rationale:** The outcome goal does not state the target time frame for when the nurse should expect to see the client behavior (*transfer*). The condition or modifier is present (*with 2 assists*). The performance criterion is "from bed to chair." **Cognitive Level:** Applying **Client Need:** Management of Care **Integrated Process:** Communication and Documentation **Content Area:** Fundamentals **Strategy:** Recall that outcome statements would include 4 essential elements (client behavior, target time, condition or modifier, and performance criteria). Analyze the goal as it is written and use the process of elimination to determine which element was

omitted. **Reference:** Berman, A., & Snyder, S. J. (2012). *Kozier & Erb's fundamentals of nursing: Concepts, process, and practice* (9th ed.). Upper Saddle River, NJ: Pearson Education, p. 225.

6 **Answer: 2** **Rationale:** The planning step of the nursing process involves formulating client goals and designing the nursing interventions required to prevent, reduce, or eliminate the client's health problems. Outcome goals are documented on the client's care plan. Assessment data is used to help identify a client's human response. Once a plan is established, the interventions are implemented, and the client outcomes are evaluated to determine the effectiveness of the interventions. **Cognitive Level:** Applying **Client Need:** Management of Care **Integrated Process:** Nursing Process: Planning **Content Area:** Fundamentals **Strategy:** The critical words are *outcome goal.* Recall which phase of the nursing process involves the formulation of outcome goals. **Reference:** Berman, A., & Snyder, S. J. (2012). *Kozier & Erb's fundamentals of nursing: Concepts, process, and practice* (9th ed.). Upper Saddle River, NJ: Pearson Education, p. 215.

7 **Answer: 2** **Rationale:** Using critical thinking skills, the nurse should try to problem solve in a situation such as this. Diluting the medication will likely prevent the "slimy" sensation the client objects to, making the medication more palatable and improving the likelihood of the client taking the medication. Critical thinking involves problem solving and omitting a dose of an essential medication may harm the client. Using threatening tactics such as this demonstrates a lack of critical thinking and problem-solving skills by the nurse. While it may ultimately be necessary to notify the provider that the client has refused an essential medication, the nurse should attempt to solve the problem before this step is taken. **Cognitive Level:** Analyzing **Client Need:** Management of Care **Integrated Process:** Nursing Process: Implementation **Content Area:** Fundamentals **Strategy:** The critical word is *first.* Recalling the definition of critical thinking will aid in the elimination of incorrect options. **Reference:** Berman, A., & Snyder, S. J. (2012). *Kozier & Erb's fundamentals of nursing: Concepts, process, and practice* (9th ed.). Upper Saddle River, NJ: Pearson Education, p. 182.

8 **Answer: 3** **Rationale:** The expert practitioner uses intuition to understand complex clinical problems and usually has been practicing at least 5 years. Novices are new practitioners that rely on rules to make clinical decisions. Competent practitioners usually have 2 to 3 years of experience and are able to analyze simple problems. A proficient nurse is able to understand the "big picture" clinically but has not yet developed sound intuition. **Cognitive Level:** Applying **Client Need:** Management of Care **Integrated Process:** Nursing Process: Assessment **Content Area:** Fundamentals **Strategy:** Specific information about Benner's model is needed to answer the question. Consider the described experience of the nurse to aid in making a selection. **Reference:** Berman, A., & Snyder, S. J. (2012). *Kozier & Erb's fundamentals of nursing: Concepts, process, and practice* (9th ed.). Upper Saddle River, NJ: Pearson Education, p. 12.

9 **Answers: 1, 5** **Rationale:** Prior to delegating any client care responsibilities, the nurse must assess the client to assure that the delegation is appropriate to his or her care. The nurse is also responsible for the outcomes of any tasks that are delegated. **Cognitive Level:** Applying **Client Need:** Management of Care **Integrated Process:** Nursing Process: Implementation **Content Area:** Fundamentals **Strategy:** The critical words are *delegating* and *must do.* Recall principles of appropriate delegation in nursing practice to select the care measures that reflect safe delegation. **Reference:** Berman, A., & Snyder, S. J. (2012). *Kozier & Erb's fundamentals of nursing: Concepts, process, and practice* (9th ed.). Upper Saddle River, NJ: Pearson Education, p. 525.

10 **Answer: 3** **Rationale:** The plan needs to be reassessed whenever goals are not met. Nursing interventions should be examined to ensure the best interventions were selected to assist the client achieve the goal. The goal may be appropriate, but the client may need more time to achieve the desired outcome, or the manner in which the nursing interventions were implemented may have interfered with achieving the outcome. It is unnecessary to notify the health care provider at this time. Failure to fully meet established goals does not indicate the client should be reassigned to another nurse. It may not be necessary to write a new nursing diagnosis. **Cognitive Level:** Applying **Client Need:** Management of Care **Integrated Process:** Nursing Process: Evaluation **Content Area:** Fundamentals **Strategy:** Recall the actions needed in the evaluation phase of the nursing process to select the correct response. **Reference:** Berman, A., & Snyder, S. J. (2012). *Kozier & Erb's fundamentals of nursing: Concepts, process, and practice* (9th ed.). Upper Saddle River, NJ: Pearson Education, p. 242.

Posttest

1 **Answer: 3** **Rationale:** In developing a plan of care, nurses engage in a partnership with the client and family. Nurses do not plan care for clients; instead they plan care with clients and families. Unless the client and family are committed to the achievement of goals, they are not likely to engage in the lifestyle changes required to meet the goals. Interventions will be most accurate and effective when carried out in partnership with the client and family. If the client and family are engaged and participate in the care-planning process, they are far more likely to comply with a medication regimen, and past adherence may not be as relevant. **Cognitive Level:** Applying **Client Need:** Management of Care **Integrated Process:** Nursing Process: Planning **Content Area:** Fundamentals **Strategy:** The critical phrases are *most important* and *developing a plan of care.*

Use knowledge of the care-planning process to make the best selection. **Reference:** Berman, A., & Snyder, S. J. (2012). *Kozier & Erb's fundamentals of nursing: Concepts, process, and practice* (9th ed.). Upper Saddle River, NJ: Pearson Education, p. 221.

2 **Answer: 3** **Rationale:** Assessment involves collecting, organizing, validating, and documenting data about a client. Observing the client's response to pain medication represents the evaluation phase. Turning the client is an activity that occurs in the implementation phase. Goal setting occurs in the planning phase. **Cognitive Level:** Applying **Client Need:** Management of Care **Integrated Process:** Nursing Process: Assessment **Content Area:** Fundamentals **Strategy:** Recall the activities that occur in the assessment phase of the nursing process to make an appropriate selection. **Reference:** Berman, A., & Snyder, S. J. (2012). *Kozier & Erb's fundamentals of nursing: Concepts, process, and practice* (9th ed.). Upper Saddle River, NJ: Pearson Education, p. 178.

3 **Answer: 1** **Rationale:** Subjective data is apparent only to the person affected and cannot be measured, seen, felt, or heard by the nurse. The client is always considered the primary source. Secondary sources of data include the family, other health personnel, and client records. **Cognitive Level:** Understanding **Client Need:** Management of Care **Integrated Process:** Nursing Process: Assessment **Content Area:** Fundamentals **Strategy:** The critical words in the question are the *client states.* **Reference:** Berman, A., & Snyder, S. J. (2012). *Kozier & Erb's fundamentals of nursing: Concepts, process, and practice* (9th ed.). Upper Saddle River, NJ: Pearson Education, p. 183.

4 **Answer: 3** **Rationale:** This is a risk diagnosis, and the diagnostic statement has 2 parts: the human response (impaired skin integrity) and the related risk factor (malnutrition). Imbalanced nutrition does not reflect the stated concern of risk for impaired skin integrity, although malnutrition may increase the client's risk for skin breakdown. No evidence was given to suggest that the client's skin integrity was actually impaired; instead, the nurse concludes the client is at risk for this problem. **Cognitive Level:** Analyzing **Client Need:** Management of Care **Integrated Process:** Nursing Process: Diagnosis **Content Area:** Fundamentals **Strategy:** The critical phrase is *at risk for skin breakdown.* Knowledge of correct nursing diagnostic terminology will assist in selecting the correct response. **Reference:** Berman, A., & Snyder, S. J. (2012). *Kozier & Erb's fundamentals of nursing: Concepts, process, and practice* (9th ed.). Upper Saddle River, NJ: Pearson Education, pp. 201–202.

5 **Answer: 2** **Rationale:** A nursing diagnosis consists of 2 parts joined by "related to." The first part (the human response) names, or labels, the problem. The second part (related factors) includes components that either contribute to or are probable etiologies of the human response. Some formats include a third part to the statement for actual (not risk) diagnoses; this third part consists of client signs or symptoms and is joined to the statement with the label "as evidenced by." Cancer is a medical diagnosis, not a nursing diagnosis. Imbalanced Nutrition is vague because the "related to" factor does not describe the etiology of the diagnosis. Impaired Physical Mobility does not provide any direction for selecting appropriate nursing interventions. It is also missing the third section of the diagnostic statement (i.e., "as evidenced by") that would specify the client's signs or symptoms that support the diagnosis. **Cognitive Level:** Applying **Client Need:** Management of Care **Integrated Process:** Communication and Documentation **Content Area:** Fundamentals **Strategy:** Recall that the diagnosis statement is an actual or potential problem that is evidenced by signs and symptoms that are related to contributing risk factors. **Reference:** Berman, A., & Snyder, S. J. (2012). *Kozier & Erb's fundamentals of nursing: Concepts, process, and practice* (9th ed.). Upper Saddle River, NJ: Pearson Education, pp. 201–202.

6 **Answers: 3, 4** **Rationale:** Outcome goals must have a specified time frame in which they are to be achieved. Having no pain is not a realistic goal for a postoperative client, and it has no specified time frame. The goal of stating pain less than or equal to 3 is worded to be specific, measurable, appropriate, realistic, and timely. The goal of pain being less than 3 by discharge meets the criteria for goal statements. Being medicated by the nurse is not a client goal; it is a nursing intervention. **Cognitive Level:** Analyzing **Client Need:** Management of Care **Integrated Process:** Communication and Documentation **Content Area:** Fundamentals **Strategy:** Recall the mnemonic SMART to recall that an outcome goal should be SMART: specific, measurable, appropriate, realistic, and timely. **Reference:** Berman, A., & Snyder, S. J. (2012). *Kozier & Erb's fundamentals of nursing: Concepts, process, and practice* (9th ed.). Upper Saddle River, NJ: Pearson Education, p. 223.

7 **Answers: 2, 5** **Rationale:** It would be appropriate to consult with the provider regarding the nurse's concern to act as a client advocate. It would be appropriate to withhold the dose until consultation can occur between the nurse and the provider. It would be unsafe to administer the dose without further investigation. Administering the dose despite concern about dosage represents unsafe nursing practice, regardless of whether the concern is charted. The nurse's license does not permit changing a medication dosage **Cognitive Level:** Applying **Client Need:** Safety and Infection Control **Integrated Process:** Nursing Process: Implementation **Content Area:** Fundamentals **Strategy:** The critical phrase is *unsafe for the client*. The nurse's first priority is client safety. Select options that maintain the safety of the client. **Reference:** Berman, A., & Snyder, S. J. (2012). *Kozier & Erb's fundamentals of nursing: Concepts, process, and practice* (9th ed.). Upper Saddle River, NJ: Pearson Education, p. 93.

8 **Answer: 1** **Rationale:** Part of the professional nurse's role is to delegate responsibility for activities while maintaining accountability. The nurse must match the needs of the client with the skills and knowledge of unlicensed assistive personnel (UAP). Generally routine tasks such as measuring vital signs can be delegated to the UAP. Assisting with an invasive procedure or adjusting the rate on an infusion pump cannot be delegated to unlicensed assistive personnel (UAP) because they are not within the legal scope of the UAP's practice. Planning and evaluation of care are always done by the registered nurse and cannot be delegated to unlicensed assistive personnel (UAP). **Cognitive Level:** Applying **Client Need:** Management of Care **Integrated Process:** Nursing Process: Implementation **Content Area:** Fundamentals **Strategy:** Recognize what is within the scope of practice of an RN, LPN, and unlicensed assistive personnel (UAP) and recall that client needs and activities delegated must be matched to the skill level of health personnel. Knowledge of the Nurse Practice Act and the institution's polices will assist the nurse in making appropriate decisions regarding delegation of care activities. **Reference:** Berman, A., & Snyder, S. J. (2012). *Kozier & Erb's fundamentals of nursing: Concepts, process, and practice* (9th ed.). Upper Saddle River, NJ: Pearson Education, p. 524.

9 **Answer: 4** **Rationale:** A change-of-shift report should include significant changes (good or bad) in a client's condition. The information should be accurate, concise, clear, and complete. The other options represent normal data and are therefore of lesser importance to convey in the change-of-shift report. **Cognitive Level:** Analyzing **Client Need:** Management of Care **Integrated Process:** Communication and Documentation **Content Area:** Fundamentals **Strategy:** Recall that communications that are clear and accurate provide the best information. Recall also that priority information in a change-of-shift report includes changes in the client's condition. **Reference:** Berman, A., & Snyder, S. J. (2012). *Kozier & Erb's fundamentals of nursing: Concepts, process, and practice* (9th ed.). Upper Saddle River, NJ: Pearson Education, p. 267.

10 **Answer: 4** **Rationale:** Evaluating is the process of comparing client responses to the outcome goals to determine whether, or to what degree, goals have been met. Diagnosing identifies health problems, risks, and strengths. Planning is the formulation of client goals and nursing strategies (interventions) required to prevent, reduce, or eliminate the client's health problems. Implementing is carrying out or delegating the nursing interventions. **Cognitive Level:** Applying **Client Need:** Management of Care **Integrated Process:** Nursing Process: Evaluation **Content Area:** Fundamentals **Strategy:** Use basic knowledge of the steps of the nursing process to identify common activities carried out in each phase. **Reference:** Berman, A., & Snyder, S. J. (2012). *Kozier & Erb's fundamentals of nursing: Concepts, process, and practice* (9th ed.). Upper Saddle River, NJ: Pearson Education, p. 178.

ANSWERS & RATIONALES

References

Berman, A., & Snyder, S. J. (2012). *Kozier & Erb's fundamentals of nursing: Concepts, process, and practice* (9th ed.). Upper Saddle River, NJ: Pearson Education, pp. 251–364.

Berman, A., Snyder, S. J., & McKinney, D. (2011). *Nursing basics for clinical practice.* Upper Saddle River, NJ: Pearson Education, Inc.

Carpenito, L. (2009). *Nursing diagnosis: Application to clinical practice* (13th ed.). Philadelphia, PA: Lippincott Williams & Wilkins.

Craven, R., & Hirnle, C. (2009). *Fundamentals of nursing: Human health and function* (6th ed.). Philadelphia: Wolters-Kluwer.

NANDA International (2012). *NANDA-I Nursing diagnoses: Definitions and classification 2012–2014.* Des Moines, IA: Wiley-Blackwell.

Potter, P., & Perry, A. (2013). *Fundamentals of nursing* (8th ed.). St. Louis, MO: Mosby, Inc.

Potter, P., Perry, A., Stockert, P., & Hall, A. (2011). *Basic nursing* (7th ed.). St. Louis, MO: Mosby, Inc.

Wilkinson, J., & Treas, L. (2011). *Fundamentals of nursing* (2nd ed.). Philadelphia, PA: F.A. Davis.

Overview of Health Assessment

2

Chapter Outline

The Health History

Preparing for the Physical Assessment

Conducting the Physical Assessment

Objectives

➤ Explain the process utilized in obtaining a health history.
➤ Identify the preparation required for physical assessment.
➤ Describe the process used to complete a physical assessment.
➤ Document health assessment findings using correct medical terminology.
➤ Identify common alterations in assessment findings characteristic of selected pathophysiologic processes.

NCLEX-RN® Test Prep

Use the accompanying online resource, NursingReviewsandRationales, to test yourself with hundreds of NCLEX®-style practice questions.

Review at a Glance

auscultation utilizes sense of hearing and a stethoscope to detect normal and abnormal sounds produced by body, including gastrointestinal tract, arteries, heart, and lungs

health history a process used by health care professionals to obtain complete relevant information about a client's physical, psychosocial, and spiritual health

inspection utilizes sense of sight to visually observe all areas of body to assess pathology, color, level of comfort, anxiety, and any visual signs that provide clues to client's health status; determining odor is also included under inspection

palpation utilizes sense of touch to examine client's body, using pressure of hands and fingers to assess masses, elevations, temperature, organ position, and any abnormal findings; palpation can be deep or light depending on area being examined; ulnar surfaces of hands and fingers are most commonly used for palpation

percussion utilizes pressure from hands and fingers to generate sounds that will elicit clues about density of underlying tissues or organs

PRETEST

1 When taking a health history, the nurse should focus on which of the following?

1. Completing the process in a timely manner
2. Using therapeutic communication skills to identify the client's health care status
3. Documenting objective data using the client's own words
4. Attempting to have no interruptions from family members who are present

2 Before palpating the abdomen during an assessment, the nurse should perform which of the following actions?

1. Put on sterile gloves.
2. Auscultate bowel sounds.
3. Elevate the client's head.
4. Percuss all 4 quadrants.

3 The nurse would attempt to gather which of the following information while obtaining a health history from a client? Select all that apply.

1. Who lives with the client and the client's support systems
2. Annual household income
3. Client's use of vitamins and herbal supplements
4. History of past illnesses and surgeries
5. Religious preference and beliefs that might relate to health care issues

4 The nurse would document which of the following in the medical record as objective data obtained during client assessment?

1. Detailed description of pain in an extremity
2. Loss of hair on lower legs bilaterally
3. Report of numbness of the right hand
4. Description of scalp itching, which occurs each evening

5 What action should the nurse take to increase the likelihood of obtaining quality data when doing a complete physical assessment?

1. Provide adequate lighting and a comfortably warm room for the interview and physical assessment.
2. Outline the process in detail prior to beginning the examination.
3. Ask all family members or significant others to wait outside the room.
4. Identify each piece of equipment used with the appropriate medical term.

6 The nurse would use which method of examination to assess for the presence of a bruit in the abdomen?

1. Auscultation
2. Percussion
3. Palpation
4. Inspection

7 In order to examine the ocular mobility of a client who recently experienced a stroke, the nurse should examine which of the following cranial nerves? Select all that apply.

1. Cranial nerves I and VII
2. Cranial nerves II and V
3. Cranial nerves III and IV
4. Cranial nerve VI
5. Cranial nerve IX

8 Which statement made by the client indicates an understanding of how the nurse will perform the Romberg test?

1. "You want me to tell you when I can no longer hear the sound from the tuning fork after you place it on my head."
2. "You want me to use my index finger to touch my nose and then your finger as quickly as possible."
3. "I am going to walk 5 or 6 steps in a straight line, placing my toes directly behind the heel of my other foot."
4. "You want me to stand with my feet together and eyes closed for a short time."

9 A client who is alert and responsive was admitted directly from the provider's office with a diagnosis of "rule out acute myocardial infarction." Of the following alterations found on the initial assessment, which is of greatest concern to the nurse?

1. Blood pressure supine is 138/76.
2. Respirations are 28 and labored.
3. Temperature is 99.8°F.
4. There are infrequent missed apical beats.

10 A nurse has conducted a physical examination on a client and notes that the thyroid gland is normal. How would the nurse document this in the medical record?

1. Thyroid slightly deviated to the left, no nodules palpated
2. Thyroid midline, smooth, with no nodules palpated
3. Thyroid midline, with parathyroid glands easily palpated bilaterally
4. Thyroid slightly deviated to the right, with pea-sized nodules at the base

➤ *See pages 54–55 for Answers and Rationales.*

I. THE HEALTH HISTORY

A. A *health history* is a collection of data about the client's present and past health status

B. Purposes of a health history
  1. To obtain all relevant information about a client's physical, psychosocial, and spiritual health in an organized manner using communication skills and interviewing techniques; a health history gathers *subjective* information
  2. An added benefit is that it provides a forum for nurse to develop a therapeutic relationship with client

C. Sources of data
  1. Primary: client, who is best source of data unless confused, too young, or too ill to participate in interview
  2. Secondary: family members, caregivers, support people; other members of health care team; old medical or other health records; and results of laboratory and diagnostic tests

D. Principles of history taking
  1. Provide privacy: draw curtains or close door to room to eliminate distractions; assure client that all information is for health records and to generate a complete picture of overall health status; immediately document data in health record for information security; do not keep any data on a loose piece of paper
   2. Maintain confidentiality: assure client that all information will remain confidential; do not discuss client or his or her family with anyone else who is not part of health team; do not discuss confidential information in corridors, on elevator, or in any public area; keep client records away from unofficial personnel
  3. Plan an appropriate time frame: may require up to 1 hour or longer; allot enough time to obtain health history; do not rush through interview because important clues

to client's health status could be missed; pace interview so as not to overtire client; if client is tired or ill, ask the most critical questions first

4. Develop trust
   a. Approach client and family in a professional manner; explain your role and rationale for the interview
   b. If interview takes place during a nonemergent situation, try to find something in common with client; this will relax the client so he or she will feel more at ease
   c. Tell client that if he or she becomes ill during interview to alert you right away
   d. Use good communication skills; listen with diligence, demonstrating active listening techniques; be aware of own nonverbal behavior; maintain good eye contact if consistent with client's cultural preference
   e. Ask appropriate follow-up questions to gather complete data
   f. Be careful with choice of words; avoid using overly technical language or excessive medical terminology; avoid overreacting to comments made by client or family
   g. Remain relaxed during interview
   h. Use touch sparingly and only as appropriate

5. Note nonverbal cues about client's demeanor, posture, and overall appearance
   a. Physical appearance: including cleanliness, body odor, personal grooming, hygiene, client's eye contact
   b. Signs of physical discomfort: diaphoresis, tremors, grimaces, and frequent changes in position
   c. Client stress: tears, skin blotching, nervous movements, inability to concentrate, arms folded, diaphoresis; if client wants to end interview, respect this request and terminate the interaction

6. Assess client's reliability
   a. Client answers questions with authority and does not change data reported
   b. Client uses proper terminology or words that indicate an understanding of health status; offers pertinent information about health status; refers to previous illnesses and their treatments; does not change the subject during discussion of an issue; is oriented to person, place, time, and event
   c. If client's family is present, they concur that data is accurate

7. Use an interpreter consistent with agency policy if nurse and client cannot communicate in the same language; an increasing number of hospitals are using special telephone numbers answered by certified interpreters

8. Conduct interview in a logical, orderly manner and focus the discussion
   a. Ask open-ended questions to determine the most important issues
   b. Ask pertinent follow-up questions; for example, if a client mentions feeling "jumpy" since beginning a medication, ask what is meant by the word *jumpy*
   c. Closed-ended questions should yield "yes/no" responses; closed-ended questions clarify previous statements made by client or family
   d. Closed-ended questions should be used when asking clients for specific additional information; for example, "Since your last heart attack have you experienced any chest pain?"

9. Clarify discrepancies: elaborate on questionable statements and use active communication skills
   a. Ask questions in a clear manner; phrase all questions after determining intellectual level of client or family; if a client does not understand a question, rephrase it or use different terms
   b. Probing questions help yield accurate information if several explanations for a symptom are offered; do not use leading questions
   c. Connect a client's explanations with symptoms; seek a logical explanation for client's descriptions and symptoms

Box 2-1	• Maintain poise and exude warmth during the history; the client and/or family may be tense and afraid.
Tips for Conducting a Successful Client Interview	• Use a nonthreatening and nonjudgmental attitude as you begin the interview. • Address the client in the manner of his or her choosing. • Be polite and respectful of the client and family. • Once the client offers the reason for his or her visit, then proceed in a logical, orderly fashion. • Pace the interview to obtain as much data as possible without overtiring the client or rushing the interview; if the interview proceeds too quickly, important information may be overlooked.

d. Provide feedback to convey to client that his or her communication is being understood; paraphrase client's descriptions to clarify accuracy of statements; summarize data collected during interview

e. Thank client and family for their assistance through this process

f. Allay client's fears and maintain open communication; be forthright with additional information

g. Confirm that client understands the next aspect of care

10. See Box 2-1 for tips on conducting a successful interview; also see Chapter 3 for further information about general communication techniques

E. Components of the health history

1. Format used may vary slightly depending on client's age, associated developmental considerations, and whether the reason for visit is routine care or to address an acute problem

2. Biographical data includes name, address, telephone number, gender, marital status, religion, occupation, health insurance information, and possibly name and contact information for primary care health care provider (physician or nurse practitioner)

3. Chief complaint: problem or reason for which client is currently seeking treatment

　a. Ask client or family to describe reason for seeking treatment

　b. Do a symptom analysis, getting data about each of the following:

　　1) Location: be as specific as possible in obtaining and recording part(s) of body involved

　　2) Quantity: sometimes referred to as *severity* or *intensity*; a numerical rating scale (0 to 10) or some type of visual analog scale is often useful in obtaining this data; frequent examples of symptoms assessed this way are pain and dyspnea

　　3) Quality: description of symptoms; various adjectives are frequently used, such as *burning*, *stabbing*, *pressure*; some disorders tend to be described in similar ways by clients, which can aid in diagnosing the current problem

　　4) Setting: location of client when symptom(s) began and a description of events going on at that time

　　5) Timing or chronology: notation of when the symptom first began; slow onset versus sudden; constant versus intermittent; whether symptom disturbs client's sleep

　　6) Aggravating or alleviating factors: factors that make symptom worse or better (such as eating, resting, use of medication, among others)

　　7) Associated factors: other symptoms that accompany the primary symptom (such as diaphoresis or shortness of breath with chest pain, as an example)

　c. Document findings verbatim using client's or family's own words

　d. Previous state of health and physical capabilities and how current symptom(s) has (have) impacted physical, emotional, and psychosocial functioning

Practice to Pass

The nurse needs to interview a client. What approaches should the nurse take to obtain information most effectively?

4. History of present illness (useful if problem has occurred more than once)
   a. When symptoms originally started
   b. How frequently exacerbations occur, and whether they are gradual or sudden in onset
   c. Client's understanding of the nature of the health problem
   d. Medications and/or other therapies used to treat problem and their degree of success (or lack of success)
5. Past health history: sometimes referred to as "past history" or "medical history"

Practice to Pass

The chief complaint of the client provides multiple clues and helps to focus the interview. What would these clues typically include?

   a. Includes other health problems that a client may have; a checklist is useful to obtain this information; focused (more detailed) assessment can be done on areas that are still currently problematic for client; it is increasingly common for clients to seek treatment for one health problem while having an active history of other health problems, called comorbidities, that require ongoing management
   b. Immunizations: includes childhood immunizations and date of last tetanus prophylaxis; may also include influenza and pneumonia vaccines
   c. Childhood illnesses: such as measles, mumps, rubella (German measles), rubeola, chickenpox, rheumatic fever, scarlet fever, streptococcal infections, or other major illnesses
   d. Prior hospitalizations: including dates, reasons (includes accidents and injuries as well as illnesses), surgical procedures, outcomes, and any complications experienced (such as reactions to anesthesia or blood products)
   e. Allergies
      1) Medication allergies: reaction and symptoms; includes prescription, over-the-counter (OTC), and herbal products
      2) Food allergies
      3) Seasonal allergies (and their treatment)
      4) Allergy to dyes used in diagnostic procedures (often determined by asking about allergy to iodine or contrast media)
   f. Pregnancy history and menstrual history as appropriate for female clients
   g. Current medications: prescribed dose, rationale and duration of drug therapy, date and time of last dose; OTC medications; herbal remedies; home remedies; complementary or adjunctive health care (if so, have client explain the remedies used and effects)
6. Family health history
   a. Includes identification of overall state of health of parents and relatives, any significant and chronic illnesses, cause of death, and age at time of death
   b. Family history is an important assessment; it can highlight genetically transmitted traits or disorders; keep in mind that ethnic background also plays a role in risk for developing certain disorders
   c. Often if a client has a strong family history for a specific disorder, the health care team is likely to focus its efforts on disease prevention and health promotion to lower client's risk in that area; for example, if a client's parent died at age 47 years from a myocardial infarction, health promotion would focus on cardiac health and healthy living
   d. Establish whether there is a history of hereditary disorders such as coronary heart disease, diabetes mellitus, stroke, high blood pressure, cancer, obesity, arthritis, bleeding disorders, or mental health disorders

Practice to Pass

The family history provides the nurse with a clear direction to follow during the health assessment. Why is the family history so significant?

7. Personal and social history: includes social data and lifestyle assessment
   a. Diet: foods eaten on a usual day; number of meals and snacks; who does the shopping and cooking; food preferences and patterns based on culture and/or religion; usual fluid intake; intake of caffeine (such as coffee, tea, cola)
   b. Activity and exercise: type, frequency and duration of exercise; ability to perform activities of daily living or ADLs (eating, bathing, elimination, dressing, grooming), ability to move about at will (locomotion)

    c. Sleep and rest: usual number of hours of sleep, sleep hygiene practices (all lights off, no television, no late-day caffeine), sleep problems, and effectiveness of any sleep aids used (prescription, OTC, or herbal)

    d. Tobacco use: number of packs per day (cigarettes) and number of years of smoking; type, frequency, and duration of use for other tobacco products

    e. Substance use: amount, frequency, and duration of alcohol or recreational drug use

    f. Living arrangements: include location, type of dwelling, number of stairs to climb, home safety information, ability to access neighborhood or community resources and services

    g. Family relationships or friendships: who is/are the support person(s) in times of need; effects of illness on client and family roles and relationships (dynamics); identification of next of kin

    h. Psychological data: major lifestyle changes or stressors experienced and how client dealt with them; client's usual coping patterns; general communication style and ability; appropriateness of verbal and nonverbal behavior; whether client is seeing a mental health professional; significance of current illness to client; effect of current illness on self-esteem or body image

    i. Occupation: presence of occupational hazards, such as exposure to carcinogens, (such as asbestos, other chemicals); distance and length of time the client commutes to work each day and associated concerns; amount of time missed from work due to illness; history of a need to change jobs in the past because of illness

    j. Travel (out of country): when, where, and amount of time; military service abroad

    k. Health resources used: current and past use of health care providers (generalists and specialists), dentists, folk healers; satisfaction with care; access to care

8. Review of systems (ROS): in a medically oriented assessment, this section includes questions about past and current health status in each system reviewed (see next); it is used to obtain subjective data; in many situations, nursing assessments use a nursing model instead of ROS to obtain this information, such as Gordon's Typology of 11 Functional Health Patterns, Orem's Self-Care Model, or Roy's Adaptation Model; health care agencies generally have a specific form to gather this data (forms based on nursing models may blend gathering of subjective data [history] and objective data [physical assessment or examination])

    a. Skin: skin disease (eczema, psoriasis, hives), changes in moles, skin dryness or moisture, itching, bruising, rashes or other lesions, changes in hair or nails, sun exposure and use of sunscreen (SPF strength, frequency of use)

    b. Head: headaches (frequency, type, and effectiveness of treatments), dizziness (vertigo) or fainting (syncope), head injury

    c. Eyes: vision problems (blurring, blind spots, reduced acuity), double vision (diplopia), glaucoma, cataracts, eye pain, redness, discharge or watering, swelling, method of vision correction being used

    d. Ears: hearing loss, hearing aid use, tinnitus, vertigo, earaches, infections, discharge, and characteristics

    e. Nose and sinuses: frequency and severity of colds, sinus pain or obstruction, discharge, nosebleeds (epistaxis), allergies, reduced sense of smell

    f. Mouth and throat: pain or lesions in mouth (or tongue), toothaches, change in sense of taste, frequency of sore throats, bleeding gums, dysphagia, hoarseness, history of tonsillectomy, frequency of dental care and presence of any dental prostheses

    g. Neck: pain, mobility, enlarged or tender lymph nodes, goiter, lumps, or other swelling

h. Breasts: history of breast disease or surgery, pain, lumps, rashes, nipple discharge, knowledge and performance of breast self-examination (BSE); date of last mammogram

i. Axilla: rash, lumps, tenderness, or swelling

j. Respiratory: history of lung disease (tuberculosis, pneumonia, asthma, chronic obstructive pulmonary disease [COPD]), shortness of breath (amount and triggering factors, such as activity level), wheezes or other noises associated with respiration, cough (frequency and characteristics), sputum production (color, amount, and if relevant, timing), pain associated with breathing, hemoptysis, and exposure to pollutants or other inhaled toxins

k. Cardiovascular: history of heart disease, murmur, hypertension, or anemia; chest pain (precordial or retrosternal, radiation, and other pain characteristics); dyspnea on exertion (specify amount); orthopnea (head elevation or number of pillows needed), paroxysmal nocturnal dyspnea (PND); edema, nocturia

l. Peripheral vascular: discoloration of extremities (especially feet and ankles; note whether associated with activity); coolness, numbness or tingling of lower limbs (note relationship to activity and time of day); history of intermittent claudication, ulcerations, thrombophlebitis, or varicose veins

m. Gastrointestinal (GI): appetite, nausea and vomiting, constipation or diarrhea, frequency of bowel movements and any recent changes, tarry or bloody stools, history of rectal conditions (such as hemorrhoids), food intolerances, dysphagia, heartburn, (frequency, triggers, and effectiveness of treatments used), pyrosis (upper-GI burning with sour eructation), indigestion, abdominal pain (with or without eating), history of GI disorder, antacid use, and prescribed diet

n. Urinary: frequency, urgency, or dysuria; nocturia (number of trips to bathroom nightly); polyuria or oliguria; characteristics of stream (narrowed, hesitancy, straining); cloudy urine or hematuria; incontinence; history of urinary disorder (renal disease or calculi, urinary tract infections); pain in back, flank, suprapubic area, or groin

o. Male genital: lumps, hernia, penile lesions or discharge, pain in testicles or penis, knowledge and performance of testicular self-examination (TSE), sexual health practices (contraceptive method and prevention of sexually transmitted infections)

p. Female genital: menstrual history (age of menarche, last monthly period, duration of cycle, premenstrual pain, intermenstrual spotting, dysmenorrhea, amenorrhea, menorrhagia), vaginal itching or discharge, age at menopause, menopausal manifestations, postmenopausal bleeding, last Pap test and gynecological exam, sexual health practices

q. Musculoskeletal: joint pain, stiffness, or swelling; history of arthritis or gout; limited movement, noise with joint movement, obvious deformity; muscle pain, weakness, or cramping; difficulty with gait or activities; back pain or stiffness, history of back pain or disease; use of mobility aids and satisfaction with ability to perform ADLs

r. Neurologic: weakness, tics or tremors, paralysis, problems with coordination, paresthesias (numbness and tingling), recent or distant memory disorder, nervousness, mood changes, history of depression or other mental health problem, hallucinations, history of stroke, fainting or blackouts, seizure disorder

s. Hematologic: easy bruising or bleeding, swollen lymph nodes, history of blood transfusion and reactions, exposure to radiation or other toxins

t. Endocrine: history of diabetes, thyroid disease, adrenal disease, abnormal hair distribution, change in skin (pigmentation, texture), excessive sweating, relationship between appetite and weight, hormone therapy

II. PREPARING FOR THE PHYSICAL ASSESSMENT

A. Purpose

1. Determines objective data (both normal and abnormal), level of a client's health, possible anomalies and whether they are life altering or life threatening, whether findings are considered normal for client, and comparison of findings with client's personal and family history

2. Regular physical assessments: evaluate client's health and offer a baseline for comparison

3. Provides health care professional with data for planning intervention

B. Equipment needed (see Box 2-2)

C. Techniques

1. Use senses of vision, hearing, smell, and touch when conducting a physical assessment; skills needed include the 4 listed next, which should be practiced until mastery occurs

2. Inspection

   a. **Inspection** is a physical assessment technique that uses observation to obtain important information about a client's state of health

   b. Ensure adequate lighting to visually inspect body without distortions or shadows; lighting can be sunlight or artificial

   c. Assess these items using skill of inspection

      1) Overall appearance

      2) Demeanor, eye contact

      3) Interactions with other health care professionals and family

      4) Skin color, hair, nail beds, skeletal deformities

      5) Clothing appropriate for weather conditions

      6) Congruence of verbal and nonverbal behavior

      7) Sense of smell: does client have a peculiar odor?

3. Palpation

   a. **Palpation** is a physical assessment technique that utilizes touch to obtain important information about a client's state of health

   b. It uses sensation of touch and pressure of hands and fingers to determine masses, elevations, temperature, organ position, and any abnormal findings

   c. The ulnar surfaces of hands and fingers are most common areas used for palpation; hands should be warm and gentle; follow standard precautions as appropriate

   d. Palpation can be light or deep depending on area of body being examined; the examiner controls amount of pressure

      1) Light palpation is 1 cm in depth

      2) Deep palpation is about 4 cm in depth; should occur after light palpation

---

Practice to Pass

The client will not remove clothing for the physical assessment. What can the nurse do to alleviate the client's discomfort?

Box 2-2			
Equipment That May Be Used for Physical Examination	Blood pressure cuff	Nasal speculum	Stethoscope
	Clean disposable gloves	Near vision charts	Tape measure
	Cotton ball	Ophthalmoscope	Thermometer
	Doppler	Otoscope	Tongue depressor or blade
	Drape	Penlight	Tuning fork
	Goniometer	Reflex hammer	Vaginal speculum
	Reflex or neurologic hammer	Skin calipers	Watch with a second hand
	Lubricant	Snellen visual acuity chart	Weight scale

Table 2-1 Percussion Notes

Tone	Quality	Pitch	Example
Tympany	Drumlike	High	Gastric bubble
Resonance	Hollow	Low	Healthy lungs
Hyperresonance	Booming	Very low	Emphysemic lung tissue
Flatness	Very dull	High	Muscle, bone
Dullness	Thudlike	Medium	Liver, spleen, heart

4. Percussion
   a. **Percussion** is a skill in which the finger of one hand touches or taps a finger of the other hand to generate vibration, which in turn produces a specific, diagnostic sound; the sound changes as practitioner moves from one area to the next
   b. To become proficient, a novice should practice this skill and listen for a change in sounds as various areas of body are percussed
   c. Sounds can be classified as tympanic, hyperresonant, resonant, dull, or flat; see Table 2-1 for further description and examples of percussion notes
5. Auscultation
   a. **Auscultation** uses sense of hearing to identify sounds produced by body; some sounds can be heard and identified without a stethoscope; others can only be identified in a quiet environment with a stethoscope
   b. Allot enough time to listen carefully to auscultated sounds; if in doubt, consult another health care professional for a second opinion
   c. Place stethoscope over bare skin to eliminate changes in sound caused by clothing
   d. Listen to sound, including duration, pitch, intensity
   e. Isolate the sounds; if client has a large amount of chest or back hair, flatten hair by wetting it to diminish extra sounds
   D. **Promoting comfort during physical assessment**
   1. Provide a comfortable room with appropriate temperature and adequate lighting
   2. Minimize distractions
   3. Ensure client privacy

IV. CONDUCTING THE PHYSICAL ASSESSMENT

A. **Vital signs**
   1. Are important indicators of a client's overall health status; compare current findings to identified norms for age and to client's previously identified baseline values
   2. Temperature: average is 37°C or 98.6°F; normal range is 35.8°C to 37.3°C or 96.4°F to 99.1°F; varies slightly depending on age, time of day, phase of menstrual cycle, exercise level, and method of measurement (rectal higher, oral or axillary lower); measure using the oral, rectal, axillary, temporal artery or otic (tympanic membrane) route
   3. Pulse: adult average is 68–78 beats per minute (bpm) with a range of 60–100; newborn average is 140 bpm (range of 120–160) and decreases with increasing age
      a. Radial: count rate, rhythm, and note amplitude
      b. Apical: listen for a full minute and compare to radial pulse; place stethoscope over chest at left fifth intercostal space (ICS), midclavicular line (apex of heart)
      c. Rhythm should be regular; if pulse is irregular, assess whether it is regularly irregular or irregularly irregular and alert appropriate health care personnel
      d. If irregular, assess for pulse deficit by measuring apical and radial rates simultaneously (requires 2 people) and note if radial rate is lower (apical and radial rates should be equal)

4. Respiration: normal adult rate is 12–20 breaths/minute; can be higher at younger age levels (e.g., 30 to 40 breaths/minute is normal in newborn); count rate, rhythm, and depth of respiration; note comfort level as client breathes; normal respirations are relaxed, silent, automatic, and regular

5. Blood pressure (BP): normal adult range is 100/60 mmHg to 120/80 mmHg; varies with age (lower pressures may be normal in childhood), gender, weight, exercise, emotion, stress, and diurnal rhythm (early morning low and late afternoon to early evening high)

    a. Select proper type and size of cuff; there are 6 sizes ranging from newborn to extra-large adult, a cone-shaped cuff for obese arm, and a thigh cuff; to insure accurate measurement of BP, the cuff selected must be 40% of client's upper arm circumference; cuff size should always be selected based on arm circumference rather than age of client

    b. Have person sit or lie down with arm supported at heart level; allow a 5-minute rest period with no activity, smoking, eating, or drinking before measuring BP

    c. Locate brachial artery by palpation (above antecubital fossa and medial to biceps tendon) for arm BP; locate popliteal artery (behind the knee) to measure thigh BP

    d. Wrap and tighten cuff around selected limb; arm is most commonly used but thigh can be used when necessary

    e. Inflate cuff by pumping the hand bulb while palpating the artery to determine when the pulse disappears; this is the expected systolic BP

    f. Deflate cuff and wait 15 to 30 seconds for venous blood to dissipate

    g. Relocate brachial pulse and place diaphragm of stethoscope over this area; inflate cuff to a point 20 to 30 mm above where the pulse disappeared to ensure measuring the true systolic pressure

    h. Watch sphygmomanometer and listen for the first sound, which indicates systolic pressure

    i. Deflate cuff slowly and listen carefully for last audible sound, which indicates diastolic pressure (range of Korotkoff sounds from tapping to silence will be heard during this process)

    j. Record systolic and diastolic BP

    k If there is a question about either of the sounds, wait 1 to 2 minutes before taking BP again to avoid falsely high diastolic readings

    l. If unable to hear, take a palpated BP by placing index finger over the brachial artery, inflating the cuff, deflating the cuff while palpating, and noting when the pulsation disappears; the systolic pressure is noted and recorded as palpated (i.e., 90/palpated)

    m. If client has diminished pulses, BP sounds may be faint; in this case or if BP cannot be palpated, use a Doppler to hear the sounds (then only a systolic pressure is noted, and it is recorded as a Doppler BP, such as 86/Doppler or 86 Doppler), or an alternate extremity with normal pulses may be used for BP assessment if available

B. Height and weight

1. Height

    a. Using a balance scale, raise headpiece on measuring pole and align it with top of head while client is shoeless, standing erect, and looking straight ahead

    b. From birth until age 2, use a horizontal measuring board to measure length; avoid using a tape measure because readings are often inaccurate; extend an infant's legs to obtain true length since infants tend to flex the legs while at rest

    c. A wall-mounted ruler can be used to measure height of small children if they have difficulty standing erect on a scale

    2. Weight

        a. Use a platform scale for adults if they can stand without assistance; electronic scales, wheelchair scales, and bed scales are also available if needed

        b. Measure infants on a platform-type balance scale, making sure that it is calibrated by noting that the beam is balanced when the weight is set to zero

    3. Use professionally authorized charts to determine if client's height and weight fall within normal limits for age; also compare readings to client's own previous measurements to detect changes

C. General appearance

    1. Includes client's grooming and attire, and personal hygiene

    2. Includes gait and posture, general body build, and behavior

D. Mental status

    1. A short mental status assessment usually is obtained in the context of the health history interview; assess client for overt signs of mental distress, crying, sullen demeanor, and comments appropriate to the situation

    2. Four key areas of functioning

        a. Appearance: as noted in previous section

        b Behavior: level of consciousness (LOC), awake, alert, aware of and responding to internal and external stimuli; lethargic and drowsy, stuporous, or unresponsive (use Glasgow Coma Scale for additional information), facial expression, speech (quality, pace, articulation of words, word choice), aphasia (receptive/Wernicke's, motor/expressive/Broca's, global, or mixed), mood and affect, apraxia (inability to carry out previously known behavior, such as tooth brushing)

        c. Cognition: orientation (to time, place, person, and events), attention span, recent memory, remote memory, new learning (4 unrelated words test), judgment

        d. Thought processes: includes thought content (logical, consistent), client's perceptions (reality based, congruent with others), and absence or presence of suicidal thoughts or ideation

        e. Remember these areas (appearance, behavior, cognition, and thought processes) by memorizing the abbreviation "A, B, C, T"

        f. The Mini-Mental State Exam (Folstein) may be used to gather this data; requires 5 to 10 minutes to administer; highest score is 30 (average people score 27)

        g. A full mental status examination may be done if indicated, and other tests can be added to gather more data when problems exist (brain lesions or stroke, aphasia, mental illness, memory changes, alcoholism, and others)

E. Integument (skin)

    1. Skin provides the first layer of protection for body, protecting against infection and trauma and preventing fluid loss

    2. It also regulates body temperature, provides sensory perception, produces vitamin D, excretes sweat and impurities, and is a barometer of emotions

    3. Inspection of skin

        a. Assess skin for color; look at entire body, including areas that are not usually exposed

        b. Daylight is the best light to detect jaundice (yellowing of skin, sclera); use good lighting for best illumination; flashlights or penlights are also very helpful for general inspection

        c. Scan body for skin color, texture, tone, distribution of lesions, skin symmetry, differences among body areas, evidence of rashes or eruptions, and hygiene

        d. Inspect body for color; compare areas that are exposed to sun and those that are not

        e. Assess moles (pigmented nevi) for defining features such as symmetry, elevation, color, and texture

	Parameter	Response	Score
Box 2-3 **Glasgow Coma Scale (Level of Consciousness)**	Eye Opening	Spontaneous	4
		To Verbal Command	3
		To Pain	2
		No Response	1
	Motor Response	To Verbal Command	6
		To Localized Pain	5
		Flexes & Withdraws	4
		Flexes Abnormally	3
		Extends Abnormally	2
		No Response	1
	Verbal Response	Oriented, Converses	5
		Disoriented, Converses	4
		Uses Inappropriate Words	3
		Incomprehensible Sounds	2
		No Response	1

Score of 15 or greater = normal response
Score of 8–14 = altered level of consciousness
Score of 7 or lower = client is comatose

Source: Teasdale G, Jennett B. *Assessment of coma and impaired consciousness*. A practical scale. Lancet 1974, 2:81-84.

    f. Normal findings: range of skin color varies from person to person, color should be uniform, sun-exposed areas will be darker, calluses appear yellow, nevi (moles) can be normal findings

    g. Abnormal findings: color changes in moles (could indicate cancer); pale, shiny skin of lower extremities (may indicate decreased peripheral circulation or diabetes mellitus); localized hemorrhages into cutaneous tissues (petechiae less than 0.5 cm in diameter or purpura greater than 0.5 cm in diameter) that appear purple-red (could indicate injury, steroid use, or vasculitis)

4. Palpation of skin

    a. Note moisture, temperature, texture, turgor, and mobility; gently pinch skin to test turgor; skin should immediately return to normal but will be altered if edema or dehydration is present

    b. Normal findings: skin should be cool to warm, dry, and smooth under normal conditions; in stressful situations, skin may feel cool and clammy; assess skin by touching bilaterally and comparing findings

    c. Abnormal findings: lesions (provide descriptions of size, shape, color, texture, elevation or depression, pedunculation, exudates, configuration, location, and distribution); edema (document site and degree of edema); edema is graded on a 0 to +4 scale (0 = no edema, +1 = depth of indentation to firm pressure is 2 mm or less, +2 = indentation of 4 mm, +3 = indentation of 6 mm, and +4 = indentation of 8 mm or more)

5. Inspection of nails

    a. Inspect nails for color, contour, texture, configuration, symmetry, and cleanliness

    b. Nails offer a quick assessment of client and cleanliness; note whether nails are clean and well-manicured, bitten down, yellow and tobacco stained; color should be pink with a brisk capillary refill (3 seconds or less) when depressed (blanch test)

      c. Normal findings: nail plate is smooth and flat or slightly convex; nail base angle is 160 degrees

      d. Abnormal findings

         1) Sudden appearance of white bands can indicate melanoma

         2) Yellow: psoriasis, fungal infections, and chronic respiratory diseases

         3) Diffuse darkening of the nail: malaria medication, candidal infection, hyperbilirubinemia, chronic trauma

         4) Green black: pseudomonas infection or nail bed trauma (subungual hematoma)

         5) White spots: cuticle manipulation or trauma

  6. Palpation of nails: should be hard and smooth with uniform thickness

      a. Squeeze nail; if it separates from nail bed can indicate psoriasis or trauma

      b. A clubbed boggy nail can indicate infection with candida or pseudomonas

F. Head and neck

  1. Inspection

      a. Head should be erect and still with symmetrical facial features

      b. Assess structure, conjunctiva, sclera, cornea, and iris of each eye

      c. Assess position, alignment, skin condition, and external meatus of ears

      d. Inspect external nose

      e. Inspect inside of mouth and throat (mucosa, tongue, teeth and gums, floor of mouth, palate, uvula)

      f. Assess for tics, spasms, lesions, and facial paralysis

      g. Neck should be symmetrical without masses

  2. Palpation: palpate from front to back assessing for smoothness and symmetry of cranium, scalp and hair; palpate temporal artery; palpate salivary glands; palpate temporomandibular joint; palpate maxillary and frontal sinuses; push on tragus of ear for tenderness; palpate thyroid gland (for size, shape, tenderness, and presence of nodules) by standing behind client and use 2 fingers of each hand on sides of trachea, then displace trachea to left and ask client to swallow (thyroid should feel smooth, small, and free of nodules); palpate for midline position of trachea

  3. Inspect and palpate cervical lymph nodes

  4. Special testing

      a. Eyes: test visual fields (confrontation), extraocular movements (EOMs), pupil size, equality, roundness, and response to light and accommodation (PERRLA); check ocular fundus (with an ophthalmoscope) for red reflex, condition of optic disc, blood vessels, and background of retina; may be documented under neurological exam

      b. Ears: use an otoscope to inspect the ear canal and tympanic membrane (should be movable, intact, and pearly white-gray in color); to visualize the adult tympanic membrane using an otoscope, pull auricle gently upward and back; in children, pull auricle gently downward to visualize tympanic membrane; use tuning fork to do the Rinne and Weber tests to check for bone and air conduction in hearing (see section on neurological exam for further information); may be documented under neurological exam

      c. Nose: use a nasal speculum to check the nasal mucosa, septum, and turbinates

G. Breasts and axillae

  1. With client in a sitting position, inspect breasts for symmetry, contour, and shape; should be rounded and generally symmetrical

  2. Look for areas of discoloration, hyperpigmentation, dimpling or retraction, swelling or edema; should be uniform in color, smooth, and elastic

  3. Detect any areas of retraction by asking client to do 3 maneuvers: raise arms above head, push hands together with elbows flexed, and press hands down on hips

4. Observe areola for size, shape, symmetry, color, general surface characteristics, lesions or masses; should be round or oval, and color may vary from person to person, from light pink to dark brown

5. Inspect nipples for size, shape, position, color, and presence of any discharge or lesions; should be round, everted, and equal in size

6. Palpate axillary, subclavicular, and supraclavicular lymph nodes using palmar surface of fingertips in these 4 areas: edge of greater pectoral muscle in anterior axillary line, thoracic wall in midaxilla, upper portion of humerus, anterior edge of latissimus dorsi muscle in posterior axillary line

7. Palpate breast for masses and tenderness, using one of 3 patterns: hands-of-the-clock, spokes-on-a-wheel, concentric circles (see Figure 2-1); there should be no masses or tenderness

8. Palpate areola and nipples for masses; there should be none

H. Chest

1. Lungs

    a. Function is to provide oxygen to blood and to assist in maintaining acid–base and water balance

    b. Use standard thoracic landmarks when performing respiratory assessment

    c. Inspection: note overall appearance, nutritional status (dyspnea can impair oral intake), ability to breathe, respirations (bradypnea, tachypnea, shortness of breath, dyspnea), contour and movement of chest (should be symmetrical); note presence of retractions and color of skin, nail beds, and lips

    d. Palpation: assess posterior aspect of chest for masses, bulges, muscle tone, subcutaneous emphysema (crepitus), and areas of tenderness

      1) Respiratory expansion: place hands on 8th to 10th ribs (posterior); place thumbs close to vertebrae; slide hand medially and grasp a small fold of skin between thumbs; ask client to take a deep breath; thumbs should move evenly away from vertebrae during inspiration; note any delay in expansion

      2) Tactile fremitus: is a palpable vibration whereby sounds generated in larynx are transmitted via patent bronchi to lung parenchyma and chest wall; to assess this, place ulnar surface of hand or balls of fingers (palmar base) on outer

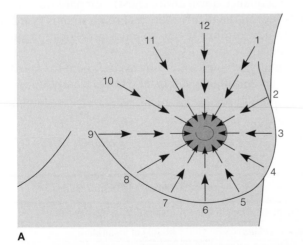
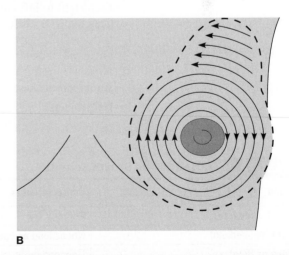

A   B

Figure 2-1

Breast Palpation. A. Hands-of-the-clock or spokes-on-a-wheel pattern, B. Concentric circle pattern.

chest wall; ask client to speak words "99" or "blue moon"; begin palpating at lung apices and work from one side to the other moving down posterior chest (but not over scapula)

   a) Vibration should be equal on both sides in any location

   b) Decreased fremitus occurs with conditions that obstruct transmission of vibrations (such as pleural effusion, pneumothorax, and others)

   c) Increased fremitus occurs with consolidation or compression of lung tissue (such as in extensive lobar pneumonia with patent bronchus)

   3) Crepitus is a palpable crackling sensation that can be felt and sometimes heard; it results from free air in subcutaneous tissues (subcutaneous emphysema) and is associated with pneumothorax

e. Percussion

   1) General procedure: have client lean forward slightly; begin by percussing over apex of left lung; then move hands systematically and compare percussion notes lobe to lobe and side to side

   2) Determine excursion: at 7th ICS, percuss downward along scapular line to diaphragm level; mark a line where resonance changes to dullness; have client take a deep breath and hold; mark a second line; the distance between them should be 3–6 cm

f. Auscultation: use flat diaphragm of stethoscope to listen systematically to posterior and anterior chest; begin posteriorly and listen from apices (at C7 level) to bases (at about T10), and laterally from axilla to 7th or 8th rib; assess actual sounds being heard with those expected in each location to determine presence of adventitious breath sounds; compare findings side to side while working downward over posterior chest

   1) Have client sit up straight and erect

   2) Trachea: listen over trachea with diaphragm of stethoscope; sounds should be bronchial

   3) Primary bronchi: listen at level of T3 to T5 to the right and left of the vertebral line for bronchovesicular sounds

   4) Lungs: begin at apex and move symmetrically from left to right, down a level, then right to left (repeat sequence down entire chest); compare sides; listen for vesicular breath sounds (normal) and adventitious breath sounds (see Table 2-2 for description of various adventitious breath sounds); note location, quality, and time of occurrence during respiratory cycle

   5) Bronchophony: assess quality of voice sounds by asking client to repeat "99"; sound should be faint or unidentifiable; if it can be heard clearly, it indicates lung density in that area

Table 2-2   Adventitious Breath Sounds

Sound	Characteristics	Timing and Occurrence
Crackles (coarse)	Popping, frying sound, moist, low pitched	Inspiration, some expiration
Crackles (medium)	Not as loud as coarse crackles	Middle of inspiration
Crackles (fine)	Noncontinuous, popping, high pitched	End of inspiration
Rhonchi or gurgles	Continuous, low pitched, prolonged	Expiration
Wheezes	Continuous, high pitched, musical	Inspiration or expiration
Pleural friction rub	Low pitched, dry, grating	Inspiration or expiration

6) Egophony: occurs over dense lung tissue; ask client to say "ee-ee-ee-ee" during auscultation; sound should be heard through stethoscope; the sound changes to a long "aaaa" sound in areas of consolidation or compression

7) Whispered pectoriloquy: have client say "1-2-3" during auscultation; the sound should be faint or muffled and almost inaudible, but will be faint yet clear and distinct with small amounts of consolidation

8) Pleural friction rub: may be heard over inflamed areas of parietal and visceral pleura; it sounds like a grating, creaking or groaning noise, and is often more noticeable on inspiration

g. Repeat the entire assessment process with anterior chest

2. Neck vessels

a. Palpate carotid arteries *one at a time* in an area medial to the sternomastoid muscle; avoid area higher in neck to prevent stimulating baroreceptors and triggering bradycardia from vagus nerve stimulation; note pulse contour and amplitude and compare findings side to side

b. Auscultate over carotid arteries for bruits using bell of stethoscope; sound should be absent; if bruit is present, note whether it sounds like a buzzing, swishing, or blowing sound; a bruit indicates turbulent blood flow from obstruction (e.g., atherosclerotic narrowing of carotid artery)

c. Assess jugular vein distention (head of bed at 30 to 45 degrees; turn head slightly away; highest pulsation should be no more than 1.5 inches above sternal notch; see Figure 2-2)

3. Heart

a. Inspection: general appearance of client and color of skin and nail beds; observe for symmetry of movement, anatomical defects, retractions, pulsations, and heaves; locate point of maximal impulse (PMI) if visible (usually at apex, 5th left ICS, midclavicular line)

b. Palpate PMI (not visible in all clients) with ball of hand, then fingertips; next assess for abnormal pulsations in sternoclavicular, aortic, pulmonic, tricuspid, and epigastric areas; palpate for thrills (over areas of turbulent blood flow)

c. Auscultate for S_1, S_2, extra heart sounds (S_3 and S_4) and murmurs; see Table 2-3 for heart sounds; place client in 3 positions for complete assessment: lying on

Practice to Pass

While performing a respiratory assessment, the nurse notes that the client has adventitious breath sounds. What would the nurse do next to complete the assessment?

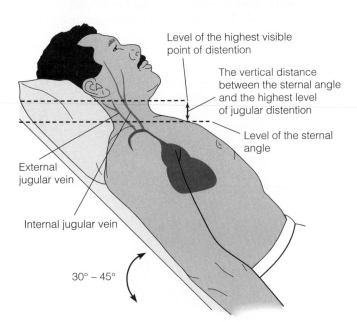

Figure 2-2

Assessment of Jugular Vein Distention (JVD)

Level of the highest visible point of distention

The vertical distance between the sternal angle and the highest level of jugular distention

Level of the sternal angle

External jugular vein

Internal jugular vein

30° – 45°

Table 2-3	Heart Sounds			
Sound	Location	Description	Character	Cardiac Manifestation
S_1	Apex	Lub	Low pitched and dull	Closure of mitral and tricuspid valves
S_2	Base	Dub	Shorter, more high pitched than S_1	Closure of pulmonic and aortic valves
S_3	Apex	"Ken-tuck-y"	Low pitched	Ventricles filling rapidly
S_4	Tricuspid or mitral areas	"Ten-nes-see"	Occurs just before S_1 after atrial contraction	Increased resistance to ventricular filling
Pericardial friction rub	Left sternal border	Grating, leathery	Muffled, high pitched, and transient	Pericardial inflammation

back with head of bed at 30 degrees, sitting up, and lying on left side; use diaphragm of stethoscope to detect higher-pitched sounds and then bell to detect lower-pitched sounds

1) Listen in a predetermined sequence; sounds are not heard over valves themselves but in the area to which blood flows distal to valve; one frequently used sequence is to listen in these areas (see Figure 2-3):

  a) Second right ICS (aortic valve area)

  b) Second left ICS (pulmonic valve area)

  c) Left lateral sternal border of 5th ICS (tricuspid valve area)

  d) Left 5th ICS, midclavicular line (mitral valve area)

2) Identify pattern of sounds heard; listen first to overall rate and rhythm; next identify S_1 and S_2 separately (one sound at a time); then listen for S_3 and/or S_4; finally, listen for murmurs

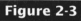

3) S_1: first heart sound, often called "lub"; heard best in pulmonic and mitral areas; indicates closure of mitral and tricuspid valves; sounds are low pitched and dull, occurring at beginning of ventricular systole

4) S_2: second heart sound, often called "dub"; heard best over aortic area at end of systole; indicates closure of pulmonic and aortic valves; is short and high pitched; a split S_2 occurs when pulmonic valve closes later than aortic valve during inspiration

Figure 2-3

Sites for auscultation of the heart

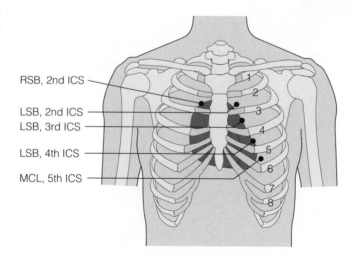

RSB, 2nd ICS
LSB, 2nd ICS
LSB, 3rd ICS
LSB, 4th ICS
MCL, 5th ICS

5) S$_3$: normal in children and clients with high cardiac output; in adults is called a ventricular gallop; is heard best over apex; is low-pitched sound that is often characterized as sounding like "Ken-tuck-y"; occurs immediately after S$_2$ heart sound in conditions when ventricles fill rapidly; is associated with congestive heart failure, pulmonary edema, atrial septal defect, and acute myocardial infarction

6) S$_4$: atrial gallop; is best heard over tricuspid or mitral areas; is often characterized as sounding like "Ten-nes-see"; occurs just before S$_1$ after atrial contraction

7) Murmurs: generally labeled as systolic or diastolic, with many variations of each; may be described by nature of sound (e.g., blowing); are typically described according to timing, loudness or intensity, pitch, pattern, quality, location, radiation, and posture (body position); Table 2-4 provides additional information about murmurs; intensity is graded on a scale of 1 to 6 and is often documented as a fraction, with 6 being the denominator (e.g., 3/6)

    a) Grade 1: very faint

    b) Grade 2: quiet

    c) Grade 3: moderately loud

    d) Grade 4: loud

    e) Grade 5: very loud, may be heard with stethoscope partly off chest

    f) Grade 6: extremely loud; may be heard with stethoscope entirely off chest

8) Pericardial friction rub: ask client to sit up, lean forward, and exhale; listen with diaphragm of stethoscope over 3rd ICS on left side of chest; if present, friction rub feels like scratching or sandpaper; client may have accompanying chest pain, pulsus paradoxus, and/or fever

Table 2-4 **Overview of Cardiac Murmurs**

Murmur	Type	Sound	Location	Pathology
Aortic stenosis	Midsystolic	Low pitched	Right SB 2nd ICS	Calcification or restricted blood flow
Pulmonic stenosis	Midsystolic	Medium pitched and harsh	Left SB 2nd to 3rd ICS	Calcified pulmonic valve with restricted right ventricular flow
Aortic insufficiency	Diastolic	High pitched, blowing decrescendo diastolic	Erb's point (left SB 3rd ICS)	Backflow of blood into pulmonic valve
Pulmonic insufficiency	Diastolic	High pitched, blowing	3rd ICS, left SB	Incomplete valve closure
Mitral stenosis	Diastolic	Low pitched, rumbling	Apex	Turbulent blood flow across stiffened valve
Mitral insufficiency	Systolic	High pitched, blowing	Apex	Regurgitation of blood into atrium
Tricuspid stenosis	Diastolic	Low rumbling	Tricuspid area, lower left SB	Calcification of tricuspid valve
Tricuspid insufficiency	Systolic	High pitched, blowing; louder during inspiration	4th ICS, left SB	Blood regurgitation into right atrium

Legend: ICS= Intercostal space; SB=sternal border

9) Percussion: can be done to locate cardiac border, where sound changes from resonance to dullness; not often performed, since chest x-ray is used to determine heart size

I. Abdomen

1. Preparation: ask client to empty bladder before beginning exam; have client lie supine with a small pillow under head; have client bend knees or place a pillow under them; expose abdomen fully; place arms at sides or across chest (not over head because it tenses abdominal muscles); warm hands and stethoscope and ensure that fingernails are short; keep room warm to prevent chilling; use distraction techniques as needed

2. Inspection: 4 quadrants for contour, symmetry, bumps, bulges, or masses; note skin color (redness, jaundice) and condition (striae, scars), umbilicus, hair distribution, and any abdominal pulsations or movements

   a. A bulge may indicate a distended bladder or hernia; look at shape and contour

   b. Midline umbilicus: to assess for umbilical hernia, have client lift arms over head; if umbilicus protrudes, hernia may be present

   c. Abdominal movements: slight, wavelike movements are normal, especially in a thin person; visible rippling waves may indicate obstruction

3. Auscultation: must auscultate before palpation and percussion to avoid increasing the frequency of bowel sounds

   a. Place diaphragm of stethoscope lightly against skin in right lower quadrant, where bowel sounds are most frequent (location of ileocecal valve)

   b. Listen in a clockwise fashion for at least 2 minutes

   c. Note character and quality; normal sounds are high pitched and gurgling at a rate of 5 to 34 times per minute

   d. Sounds are classified as normal, hypoactive (heard infrequently), hyperactive (loud high pitched, more frequent than normal)

   e. Use bell of stethoscope to detect vascular sounds over iliac, aortic, renal, and femoral arteries; listen for bruits, venous hums, and friction rubs

4. Percussion: do not percuss if abdominal aortic aneurysm is present or suspected

   a. Detects size and location of abdominal organs

   b. Percuss in all 4 quadrants

   c. Tympany: indicates an area of empty stomach or bowel or air in a cavity

   d. Dullness: is normally heard over liver (used to estimate size), kidney, full bladder, feces-filled intestines, or possibly a solid mass

5. Palpation: with warm hands, palpate lightly (about 1 cm deep with 4 fingers positioned close together) using a rotary motion in all areas to assess skin surface and superficial musculature; then repeat sequence deeply (about 4–6 cm) to determine size, shape, position, and tenderness of organs

   a. Light palpation will help detect superficial masses and fluid accumulation; a normal finding is an abdomen that is soft and nontender

   b. Deep palpation: can identify masses, tenderness, pulsations, organ enlargement (liver, spleen, kidneys)

   c. If a mass is found, note its location, size, shape, consistency (whether hard, firm, or soft), type of surface (smooth vs. nodular), mobility, pulsatility, and tenderness

   d. If a mass is noted to be pulsatile, stop palpating in that area to avoid rupture

   e. Identify rebound tenderness: if an area was tender to light palpation or if client reports pain in an area, move hand to an area away from painful site, and position hand perpendicular (at a 90-degree angle) in relation to abdomen; push down slowly and deeply and then lift up quickly; normally there is no pain or tenderness, but if present (often severe and accompanied by muscle rigidity), it indicates peritoneal inflammation, possibly appendicitis or peritonitis from another disorder

    f. Abdominal pain: indicates possible ulcers, intestinal obstruction, cholecystitis, peritonitis

    g. Ascites: use a tape measure at fullest site on abdomen, usually at or near umbilicus

    h. Inguinal area: palpate each groin for femoral pulse and inguinal nodes

J. Extremities

1. Inspect bilaterally for symmetry, skin characteristics, and distribution of hair; trophic changes (hair loss, thin shiny skin, and thickened toenails) in older adults are often due to decreased circulation from peripheral arterial disease caused by atherosclerosis

2. Palpate peripheral pulses; upper extremity pulses include radial and ulnar pulses; lower extremity pulses include the popliteal, dorsalis pedis, and posterior tibial pulses

3. Palpate skin for pretibial or other edema and to note temperature of extremities; compare side-to-side bilaterally

4. Separate toes and inspect for dryness, scaliness, maceration, or infection

K. Musculoskeletal

1. Inspect each joint for size, contour, masses, and deformity; measure any discrepancies in extremity (leg) length

2. Palpate each joint for musculature, bony articulations, and crepitation; assess for heat, swelling, or tenderness

3. Test range of motion (ROM) of joints of upper extremities (shoulders, elbows, wrists, and fingers) and lower extremities (hips, knees, ankles, and toes); describe any physical limitations; if less than full ROM is present, use a goniometer to measure joint angles more precisely

4. Note size, tone, and any involuntary movements of major muscle groups; compare findings bilaterally

5. Test strength of major muscle groups that control joints in upper and lower extremities by asking client to resist attempts to put joint through ROM; use the grading scale in Box 2-4

6. Test ROM in spine by asking client to bend forward and touch toes (flexion should be 75–90 degrees with no curvature side to side; if curvature present, suspect and further assess for scoliosis), bend sideways (35 degrees of flexion normal), bend backward (hyperextension of 30 degrees normal), and twist shoulders from one side to the other (rotation of 30 degrees bilaterally normal)

7. Straight leg raising (with knee straight) should not be painful; if it is, suspect herniated nucleus pulposus

8. Note any musculoskeletal pain that is present during assessment; pain description should be very specific

    a. Bone pain: pain unrelated to movement unless fracture is present, deep, aching, and continuous; it also causes insomnia

    b. Muscle pain: cramps or spasms with possible relationship to posture or movement; tremors, twitches, or weakness may be manifested; muscle tension may produce referred pain

Box 2-4	Grade 5: full ROM against gravity and full resistance (100% of normal, "normal")
Muscle Strength Grading Scale	Grade 4: full ROM against gravity and some resistance (75% of normal, "good")
	Grade 3: full ROM with gravity (50% of normal, "fair")
	Grade 2: full ROM with gravity eliminated; called passive ROM (25% of normal, "poor")
	Grade 1: slight contraction (10% of normal, "trace")
	Grade 0: no contraction (0% of normal, "zero")

    c. Joint pain: joint may be tender to palpation; referred pain can be present; nerve root irritation may produce radiculitis (pain is distal); mechanical joint pain is worse with movement and worsens throughout the day

L. Neurologic

  1. Assess cranial nerves; see Table 2-5 for a summary of normal and abnormal findings

    a. Olfactory nerve, cranial nerve (CN) I: not tested routinely but use items with different smells (alcohol, coffee, vanilla, peppermint, etc.) to detect abnormalities in sense of smell; test one nostril at a time if performed; sense of smell normally diminishes with aging

    b. Optic nerve, CN II: test visual acuity with Snellen chart, test visual fields by confrontation, and use an ophthalmoscope to examine fundus of eye (refer back to section on examination of head and neck)

     c. Oculomotor, trochlear, and abducens nerves (CN III, IV, VI): assess pupils for size (in mm), equality, roundness, reactivity to light, accommodation (PERRLA); assess extraocular movements by asking client to visually follow a finger through cardinal fields of gaze; observe for nystagmus (rapid back-and-forth oscillating movements of eyes in a horizontal or vertical plane, rotary direction, or combination)

Table 2-5   **Cranial Nerve Assessment**

Cranial Nerve	Assessment	Normal	Abnormal
CN I	Smell	Can identify common substances	Difficulty detecting common substances
CN II	Visual acuity	Able to read Visual fields intact	Visual field defects
CN III, IV, VI	Extraocular movements, elevation of eyelids, pupil constriction	Can elevate eyes PERRLA, eyeball movement present	Drooping of eye, ptosis, unequal pupils
CN V	Sensory: corneas, nasal and oral mucosa, facial skin Motor: jaw and chewing muscles	Sensory: able to detect both sharp and dull sensations when face touched with pointed or blunt object Motor: clenches teeth while palpating temporal and masseter muscles	Inability to feel or identify facial stimuli Muscle weakness
CN VII	Sensory: taste on anterior portion of tongue Motor: facial muscles	Sensory: can discriminate sweet, sour, and salty tastes Motor: facial symmetry present at rest and when frowning and smiling	If neurological impairment: entire side of face could be immobile
CN VIII	Hearing and equilibrium	Cochlear (hearing): cover one ear with hand and whisper into other; client can repeat what was said Vestibular (equilibrium): normal balance, absence of nystagmus	Sensorineural loss
CN IX, X	Swallowing, salivating, taste perception, voice quality	Client swallows Gag reflex present With tongue depressor against posterior pharynx, client says "ah"; movement of soft palate and uvula present	Soft palate does not rise Deviation of soft palate and uvula, no gag reflex, dysphagia, hoarseness, taste abnormalities
CN XI	Strength of sternocleidomastoid muscles and upper portion of trapezius	Client shrugs with equal strength bilaterally	Drooping shoulders, asymmetric muscle contraction
CN XII	Tongue movement in swallowing and speech	Tongue protrudes in midline; client pushes tongue against cheek while nurse offers resistance	Tongue atrophy and fasciculation, deviation

    d. Trigeminal nerve (CN V)
       1) Assess motor function by palpating temporal and masseter muscles while asking client to clench teeth and by trying to separate jaws by pushing down on chin
       2) Assess sensory function by touching client's face bilaterally in the 3 divisions of the nerve (ophthalmic, maxillary, and mandibular) and asking client to say "now" when face is touched with a wisp of cotton
       3) Test corneal reflex if necessary (may be omitted in a screening exam) by lightly touching cornea with a wisp of cotton brought in from the side of the client's face

    e. Facial nerve (CN VII): test motor function by asking client to smile, frown, close eyes tightly (while examiner tries to keep them open), lift the eyebrows, puff the cheeks, and show the teeth; test sensory function (not done routinely) by asking client to identify salty, sweet, or sour solutions applied to the tongue

    f. Acoustic or vestibulocochlear nerve (CN VIII)
       1) Use voice test (whispered words from 1–2 feet away) to determine hearing ability
       2) Do Weber test by placing a vibrating tuning fork on midline of skull and ask whether sound is heard equally, or is better in one ear than the other; test each ear separately; with conductive hearing loss, sound lateralizes to "bad" ear; with sensorineural loss, sound lateralizes to "good" ear
       3) Do Rinne test by placing a vibrating tuning fork on client's mastoid process and have client indicate when sound disappears; quickly invert tuning fork and place vibrating end near ear canal and ask client to indicate when sound disappears; normally sound is heard twice as long by air conduction (AC) as bone conduction (BC); with conductive loss, AC is equal to or less than BC; with sensorineural loss, the ratio of AC to BC is normal but is reduced overall

    g. Glossopharyngeal and vagus nerves (CN IX and X): using a tongue blade, note pharyngeal movement when client says "ahh" or yawns; watch for uvula and soft palate to rise in the midline, and for tonsillar pillars to move medially; test gag reflex by touching posterior pharyngeal wall with a tongue blade; note voice quality (should be smooth with no straining)

    h. Spinal accessory nerve (CN XI): ask client to rotate head forcibly against resistance applied to other side of chin; ask client to shrug shoulders against resistance (all findings should be equal bilaterally); examine sternomastoid and trapezius muscles for size

    i. Hypoglossal nerve (CN XII): inspect tongue; ask client to protrude tongue (should stay in midline); ask client to say words such as "light, dynamite, tight" to determine that lingual speech (the letters l, t, d, n) is clear

2. Assess motor system: inspect and palpate muscles as described in previous section

3. Assess cerebellar function
    a. Observe gait after asking client to walk 10 to 20 feet, turn, and return to starting point; efforts should be rhythmic, smooth, and without effort; step length should be about 15 inches (heel to heel); next ask client to walk heel-to-toe in a straight line (should be able to do this and maintain balance)
    b. Romberg test: ask client to stand with feet together with arms at sides; have client close eyes and hold this position for 20 seconds; client should be able to maintain posture with minimal to no swaying, but stand close by to catch client to prevent falls
    c. Other tests of cerebellar function include hopping on one leg, rapid alternating movements test (patting knees with palms of hands and then back of hands quickly) or touching each finger to thumb (one hand at a time), finger-to-finger test (touching examiner's finger and then own nose); finger-to-nose test (touching own nose with eyes closed after stretching out arm, and heel-to-shin test (placing heel of one foot on other knee and running it down leg to the heel); these movements should be done smoothly or in a straight line, depending on the test

4. Assess sensory system
   a. Requires client to be alert, cooperative, have an adequate attention span, and be in a comfortable position
   b. Test client's ability to discriminate light pain (with a sharp object such as a pin) and touch (with a dull object such as a cotton wisp or pencil eraser), to detect temperature (warm water versus cold), vibration (placement of a vibrating tuning fork on various points of body), stereognosis (recognition of objects placed in hand while eyes are closed), graphesthesia (ability to determine a number that is traced on palm of hand) with eyes closed, 2-point discrimination (ability to detect 2 separate stimuli, normally varies depending on area of the body; fingertips are most sensitive at 2 to 8 mm, and upper arms, thighs, and back are least sensitive at 40 to 75 mm)
5. Assess deep tendon reflexes using a reflex hammer
   a. Have limb relaxed and muscle partly stretched; strike reflex hammer on insertion tendon of biceps (C5 to C6), triceps (C7 to C8), brachioradialis (C5 to C6), quadriceps or "knee jerk" (L2 to L4), and Achilles or "ankle jerk" (S_1 to S_2)
   b. Reflexes are graded using the scale in Box 2-5
6. Assess superficial reflexes
   a. Abdominal (upper T8 to T10; lower T10 to T12): stroke skin with a smooth object from one side of abdomen toward midline; abdominal muscle contracts on same side as stimulus (ipsilateral response) and umbilicus deviates toward the stroke; perform at both upper and lower end of abdomen
   b. Cremasteric reflex (L1 to L2): lightly stroke inner aspect of thigh of a male client with a reflex hammer or tongue blade and watch for elevation of ipsilateral testicle
   c. Plantar reflex or Babinski reflex (L4 to S_2): use same object to stroke upward on lateral sole of foot and across ball of foot; a normal (negative) response in the adult is flexion of toes and possibly whole foot; an abnormal or positive response (that is normal in infants) is dorsiflexion of big toe and fanning of other toes
   d. Normal reflexes in infants (see Table 2-6)

M. Genitals and rectum
   1. Perianal region
      a. Put on gloves and spread buttocks to visualize site
      b. Inspect for hemorrhoids, blood, fissures, scars, lesions, rectal prolapse, discharge
      c. Palpation: lubricate a gloved index finger; ask client to take a deep breath; explain that the purpose of the exam is to palpate for rectal masses and assess stool for blood
         1) Insert finger into rectum gently and smoothly following the posterior wall of the rectum; rotate finger to follow curve of rectal wall, which should feel smooth and soft
         2) In males palpate the prostate gland on the anterior wall, noting size (should be 2.5 to 4 cm and not protrude into rectum by more than 1 cm), shape (heart shape with palpable central groove), surface (smooth), consistency (elastic or rubbery), mobility (slight), sensitivity (nontender)
         3) In females, palpate the cervix through the anterior wall; should feel like a small round mass

Practice to Pass

The neurological system controls many functions of the body. Identify them.

Box 2-5	$4+ =$ Very brisk, hyperactive with clonus (rhythmic contraction with stretching of a muscle), indicates disease
Reflex Grading Scale	$3+ =$ Brisker than usual, possibly indicates disease
	$2+ =$ Average or normal
	$1+ =$ Diminished or low normal
	$0 =$ No response

Table 2-6	Normal Reflexes in Infants
Reflex	**Description**
Rooting	Infant turns head toward side of face where cheek is touched; disappears at 3–4 months
Sucking	Infant suckles when object is placed in mouth; disappears at 10–12 months
Palmar grasp	Infant grasps finger of examiner; strongest at 1–2 months and disappears at 3–4 months
Plantar grasp	Infant's toes curl down when thumb is touched to ball of foot; present at birth and disappears at 8–10 months
Babinski	Infant's great toe dorsiflexes and other toes fan out
Tonic neck	When the infant's head is turned to one side while supine and relaxed or sleeping, the ipsilateral arm and leg extend and the opposite arm and leg flex (also called fencing position; appears by 2–3 months, decreases at 3–4 months, and disappears by 4–6 months
Moro (startle)	Infant responds to a jarring or noisy stimulus by motions that look like hugging a tree; is present at birth and disappears by 1–4 months
Placing	Infant flexes hip and knee to place foot on table when dorsal aspect of that foot is touched to underside of a table; tested while holding infant upright under arms; appears at 4 days after birth
Stepping	When infant is held upright under arms with feet on a flat surface, makes alternating regular steps; disappears before voluntary walking begins

        d. After withdrawing finger, check for stool on glove and note color and consistency (brown, soft); note presence of any frank blood and test stool for occult blood (guaiac, hematest)

    2. Male genitalia

        a. Inspection

            1) Hair distribution in pubic region

            2) Penis: assess presence of dorsal vein; retract foreskin if client uncircumcised; urethral meatus appears slitlike; note bumps, blisters, redness, lesions, and masses; assess underlying skin after moving the pubic hair

            3) Scrotum: loose, wrinkled, deeply pigmented pouch at base of penis; two compartments house testicles (oval, suspended vertically and slightly forward in the scrotum); may appear asymmetrical because the left testicle has a longer spermatic cord

        b. Palpation: use thumb and first two fingers; area is sensitive to gentle compression; penis should feel smooth, semi-firm, and nontender; testicles should feel smooth, rubbery, and movable with no nodules, lumps, swelling, soreness, masses, or lesions

    3. Female genitalia

        a. Inspect external genitalia: mons pubis, labia majora, labia minora, clitoris, vagina, urethra, and Skene's and Bartholin's glands; with gloved hands, spread labia and assess the urethral meatus; it should be a pink, slitlike opening that is midline; labia majora and minora should be moist and free from lesions; discharge should be odorless; examine vestibule for swelling, lesions, discharge, and unusual odors

        b. Palpate external genitalia: spread labia and palpate; should feel smooth

        c. Internal genitalia: vagina, uterus, ovaries, and fallopian tubes

        d. Inspect internal genitalia: need speculum, examination table, stirrups, good lighting; insert speculum after client takes a deep breath and tries to relax abdominal muscles; thin, white, odorless discharge should line the vaginal walls; assess cervix for color, position, size, shape, and discharge

        e. Palpate with lubricated index and middle fingers; note tenderness and nodules; palpate cervix; should feel smooth, firm and protrude 1.3 to 3 cm into vagina

        f. Rectovaginal palpation: with gloved lubricated finger, insert into rectum and assess for rectal sphincter, masses, tenderness, and nodules; palpate posterior wall of uterus for size, shape, tenderness, and masses

N. Postexamination responsibilities

1. Provide tissues or assist client to cleanse lubricant or secretions as needed
2. Remove drape
3. Allow client opportunity or assistance to get dressed
4. Leave client in comfortable position
5. Document data clearly, thoroughly, and immediately
   a. Compare findings to established norms and to previous findings
   b. Clearly document any risk factors to client safety that were identified in the assessment process and make sure protective measures are implemented
   c. Note specimens obtained during examination
6. Handle specimens collected during the screening in a manner consistent with standard precautions
   a. Label specimens completely and send to laboratory with requisition attached
7. Use special plastic bag with red biohazard label and follow hospital, office, or agency protocol for disposition of specimens

Case Study

A client who is a married 56-year-old female secretary has decided to retire after working for 30 years in an office located in an old warehouse in the city. She has 5 children who have moved out of the house. The youngest is preparing to leave for college in another state. The client is 5' 8" tall and weighs 184 pounds. She has smoked one pack of cigarettes per day since she was 15 years old. Her husband is a bus driver in the inner city.

She has come to the clinic to see her primary health care provider. She has had some difficulty sleeping at night and has had to use 2 pillows to breathe comfortably. She has noticed some respiratory congestion and has treated it with cough syrup. She has been afebrile but cannot seem to comfortably catch her breath. She has also noticed that her rings and shoes are a bit tight, but she attributes this to her recent weight gain. The client states, "I have not been eating much, but I seem to be gaining some weight. I no longer have the energy that I once had. Maybe I am getting old."

1. What would the nurse do first to gain the client's confidence?
2. How would the nurse approach the health history?
3. The client's symptoms "cross over" several body systems. Describe how the nurse can link the symptoms and develop appropriate nursing diagnoses.
4. The client's husband has entered the room, and he wants to take the client home. He seems angry and agitated. She begins to get dressed even though the health assessment and history are not yet completed. Describe how his agitation can impact the client's symptoms.
5. The client begins to breathe heavily and appears to be in respiratory distress. She states that she feels "one of her spells coming on." What are the next steps that the nurse should take?

For suggested responses, see pages 305–306.

POSTTEST

1 Prior to taking the health history, the nurse should first do which of the following?

1. Establish a rapport with the client.
2. Offer the client a beverage of choice.
3. Establish that insurance coverage exists.
4. Ask the client to disrobe and put on a gown.

2 The nurse would use which technique first when examining the abdomen of an infant?

1. Palpation
2. Auscultation
3. Percussion
4. Inspection

3 When assessing a client's mental status, which of the following would be key areas to include? Select all that apply.

1. The client's level of attained education
2. The client's appearance, facial expressions, mood, and affect
3. The client's gait and balance
4. The client's judgment and recent (short-term) memory
5. The presence or absence of suicidal thoughts and ideations

4 When taking a health history, which of the following is the first action the nurse should perform after the client describes the chief complaint?

1. Document verbatim what the client has said about the problem.
2. Paraphrase in the nurse's own words what the problem is.
3. Refrain from note-taking to appear focused.
4. Make a determination about the probable cause of the client's symptoms.

5 The nurse selects which piece of equipment to test for a cremasteric reflex?

1. Penlight
2. Cotton applicator
3. Neurologic hammer
4. Reflex hammer

6 The nurse preparing to assess for jugular venous distention (JVD) places the client into which position?

1. Supine with head of bed elevated 30 degrees
2. Supine with neck placed downward on chest
3. High Fowler's with head elevated upward
4. Supine with bed flat and no pillows under the head

7 The nurse selects which of the following as the highest priority nursing diagnosis for a 70-year-old male client with an absence of hair on the lower left leg?

1. Imbalanced Nutrition: Less than Body Requirements
2. Risk for Infection
3. Deficient Fluid Volume
4. Ineffective Peripheral Tissue Perfusion

8 The nurse is preparing to assess for the first time the pulse of a client who has heart disease and a history of cardiac dysrhythmias. What would be the best technique for the nurse to use?

1. Auscultate the apical pulse for one full minute while another nurse palpates the radial pulse.
2. Auscultate the apical pulse for 30 seconds and multiply the rate by 2 to obtain an accurate heart rate.
3. Auscultate the apical pulse over the second intercostal space at the midclavicular line.
4. Auscultate the apical pulse for one full minute and then palpate the radial pulse during the next minute.

9 In which position should the nurse place the client to best inspect and palpate the Bartholin glands?

1. Semi-Fowler's
2. Sim's
3. Lithotomy
4. Prone

POSTTEST

10 To adequately inspect the external ear canal of an adult client, the nurse should do which of the following prior to inserting the otoscope?

1. Require that all earrings be removed for safety purposes.
2. Pull the pinna up and back.
3. Use a cotton-tipped applicator to remove cerumen.
4. Pull the pinna down and back.

➤ *See pages 56–57 for Answers and Rationales.*

ANSWERS & RATIONALES

Pretest

1 **Answer: 2** **Rationale:** A nurse must focus on using therapeutic communication skills, which will enhance the interview. In addition, the ability to interpret nonverbal communication is paramount in achieving the goals of history taking. The time required to complete the health history is not the nurse's primary focus. The nurse must document carefully, but it is subjective data, not objective, that is recorded using the client's own words. The client can have family in the room if they do not distract the client or nurse in the interview; in many instances family members are helpful in the process. **Cognitive Level:** Applying **Client Need:** Management of Care **Integrated Process:** Communication and Documentation **Content Area:** Fundamentals **Strategy:** The critical word is *focus.* Recall that the purpose of the health history is to obtain accurate and complete information from the client; use the process of elimination to make a selection. **Reference:** Berman, A., & Snyder, S. J. (2012). *Kozier & Erb's fundamentals of nursing: Concepts, process, and practice* (9th ed.). Upper Saddle River, NJ: Pearson Education, p. 187.

2 **Answer: 2** **Rationale:** Before palpating the abdomen, the nurse should first listen to all 4 quadrants for bowel sounds. It is unnecessary to use sterile gloves unless there is an open wound or lesion. The client should be in a supine position if tolerated by the medical condition. Palpating and percussing the abdomen first can alter bowel sounds, making auscultation less reliable. **Cognitive Level:** Applying **Client Need:** Health Promotion and Maintenance **Integrated Process:** Nursing Process: Assessment **Content Area:** Fundamentals **Strategy:** The critical phrase is *before palpating.* Recalling the correct techniques for abdominal assessment will help you to choose correctly. **Reference:** Berman, A., & Snyder, S. J. (2012). *Kozier & Erb's fundamentals of nursing: Concepts, process, and practice* (9th ed.). Upper Saddle River, NJ: Pearson Education, p. 639.

3 **Answer: 1, 3, 4, 5** **Rationale:** The nurse focuses on physical, psychosocial, and spiritual concerns in obtaining information in the health history. The nurse would want to obtain information on any medications or nutritional supplements the client is using in the health history

interview. The client's past medical history is a primary focus of the health history. The nurse seeks to obtain data from the client using a holistic approach. The nurse focuses on physical, psychosocial, and spiritual concerns. Information regarding a client's personal finances is not appropriate or necessary to inquire about in the interview. **Cognitive Level:** Applying **Client Need:** Health Promotion and Maintenance **Integrated Process:** Communication and Documentation **Content Area:** Fundamentals **Strategy:** Recall the purpose of the health history and select options that collect pertinent information without unduly invading the client's privacy. **Reference:** Berman, A., & Snyder, S. J. (2012). *Kozier & Erb's fundamentals of nursing: Concepts, process, and practice* (9th ed.). Upper Saddle River, NJ: Pearson Education, p. 189.

4 **Answer: 2** **Rationale:** Objective data can be seen, heard, felt, or smelled during physical examination. The client's sensations, feelings, values, beliefs, and attitudes are regarded as subjective. Subjective data is only apparent to the person affected and can be described or verified only by that person. Itching is an examples of subjective data. **Cognitive Level:** Applying **Client Need:** Management of Care **Integrated Process:** Communication and Documentation **Content Area:** Fundamentals **Strategy:** The key term is *objective data.* Recall the criteria for objective data to make the appropriate selection. **Reference:** Berman, A., & Snyder, S. J. (2012). *Kozier & Erb's fundamentals of nursing: Concepts, process, and practice* (9th ed.). Upper Saddle River, NJ: Pearson Education, p. 183.

5 **Answer: 1** **Rationale:** A comfortable environment puts the client at ease and increases the likelihood that the nurse will be able to obtain necessary data. This approach may overwhelm the client and increase anxiety. The family may be able to provide additional data through the assessment process, and their presence may be reassuring to the client. As the nurse proceeds with the more intimate components of the assessment, the family may be asked to leave. Inform the client immediately prior to assessing each system (rather than before the examination) what is entailed to facilitate understanding. Using terminology the client can understand is always appropriate (e.g., "I am going to look in your ears now" instead of "I will examine your tympanic membrane with this otoscope"). **Cognitive Level:** Applying

Client Need: Health Promotion and Maintenance **Integrated Process:** Nursing Process: Assessment **Content Area:** Fundamentals **Strategy:** The critical words are *increase the likelihood.* Recall elements of the physical assessment process to select the best answer. **Reference:** Berman, A., & Snyder, S. J. (2012). *Kozier & Erb's fundamentals of nursing: Concepts, process, and practice* (9th ed.). Upper Saddle River, NJ: Pearson Education, p. 577.

6 **Answer: 1** **Rationale:** Auscultation uses the sense of hearing to identify sounds that are normal and abnormal during the assessment. A bruit is an abnormal sound in a blood vessel that is only detectable by listening with a stethoscope. A bruit is an abnormal sound audible only on auscultation. The turbulent blood flow that is heard as a bruit might be palpated as a thrill. A bruit cannot be seen but is heard; thus, it could not be detected on inspection. **Cognitive Level:** Applying **Client Need:** Health Promotion and Maintenance **Integrated Process:** Nursing Process: Assessment **Content Area:** Fundamentals **Strategy:** The critical word in the question is *bruit.* Use knowledge of common assessment terminology and findings to identify common alterations. **Reference:** Berman, A., & Snyder, S. J. (2012). *Kozier & Erb's fundamentals of nursing: Concepts, process, and practice* (9th ed.). Upper Saddle River, NJ: Pearson Education, p. 642.

7 **Answer: 3, 4** **Rationale:** Evaluation of ocular motility provides information about cranial nerves III, IV, and VI; their brainstem connections; and the cerebral cortex. These nerves are responsible for extraocular movements. Cranial nerve I is related to the ability to smell and cranial nerve VII controls some facial movements. Cranial nerve II is the optic nerve that controls vision (but not ocular movement), and cranial nerve V is the trigeminal nerve that controls some facial movements and sensations as well as the ability to clench the jaw muscles. Cranial nerve IX is the glossopharyngeal nerve that controls some tongue movements, swallowing, and taste. **Cognitive Level:** Analyzing **Client Need:** Health Promotion and Maintenance **Integrated Process:** Nursing Process: Assessment **Content Area:** Fundamentals **Strategy:** Recall the functions of cranial nerves to make the correct selections. **Reference:** Berman, A., & Snyder, S. J. (2012). *Kozier & Erb's fundamentals of nursing: Concepts, process, and practice* (9th ed.). Upper Saddle River, NJ: Pearson Education, p. 657.

8 **Answer: 4** **Rationale:** The Romberg test is performed to test motor function. The client is asked to stand with feet together with arms resting at the sides, and then to close the eyes. The nurse watches for the presence of swaying, which is considered normal if it is only slight. However, if the client cannot maintain foot stance, it is documented as a positive Romberg's sign. Always remember to stand close to the client during this test to prevent falls. Relating cessation of sounds would be appropriate for the Weber test. Although the finger-to-nose test is part of the neurologic exam, it is not the Romberg test. Heel-to-toe walking is also used to assess a client's balance, but it is not the Romberg test. **Cognitive Level:** Analyzing **Client Need:** Reduction of Risk Potential **Integrated Process:** Nursing Process: Assessment **Content Area:** Fundamentals **Strategy:** The critical term is *Romberg test.* Use knowledge of neurologic assessment measures to select the statement that best explains the test. **Reference:** Berman, A., & Snyder, S. J. (2012). *Kozier & Erb's fundamentals of nursing: Concepts, process, and practice* (9th ed.). Upper Saddle River, NJ: Pearson Education, p. 652.

9 **Answer: 2** **Rationale:** Using the principles of the ABCs (airway, breathing, and circulation), an alteration in respiration is always a primary concern. A disturbance in normal ventilation (normal rate = 16–20) may be occurring secondary to the medical diagnosis of myocardial infarction, but labored respirations from any source would be a cause of immediate concern. The blood pressure remains in an acceptable range. The slight temperature elevation is likely related to the overall inflammatory response of the body but is not a cause for immediate concern. Infrequent abnormalities of cardiac rhythm are common and should only be of concern when appearing frequently or with longer duration. **Cognitive Level:** Analyzing **Client Need:** Reduction of Risk Potential **Integrated Process:** Nursing Process: Diagnosis **Content Area:** Fundamentals **Strategy:** The critical phrase is *of greatest concern.* This tells you that more than one option may be partially correct and you must choose the best option. Use knowledge of normal assessment parameters and etiologies of common deviations to recognize abnormalities that would require further care. **Reference:** Berman, A., & Snyder, S. J. (2012). *Kozier & Erb's fundamentals of nursing: Concepts, process, and practice* (9th ed.). Upper Saddle River, NJ: Pearson Education, p. 624.

10 **Answer: 2** **Rationale:** The thyroid should be midline, smooth, and free of nodules. The parathyroid glands are too small to be manually palpated. The other 2 findings are abnormal. **Cognitive Level:** Applying **Client Need:** Health Promotion and Maintenance **Integrated Process:** Communication and Documentation **Content Area:** Fundamentals **Strategy:** Knowledge of normal assessment findings will allow the nurse to describe findings using appropriate terminology. **Reference:** Berman, A., & Snyder, S. J. (2012). *Kozier & Erb's fundamentals of nursing: Concepts, process, and practice* (9th ed.). Upper Saddle River, NJ: Pearson Education, p. 617.

Posttest

1 **Answer: 1** **Rationale:** In order to gain as much insight and information from the client as possible, the nurse should establish a level of trust or rapport with the client. The client will be best able to relax and answer questions if he or she is asked in a nonthreatening manner. Offering the client food and drink is not appropriate. The nurse has no need to gather information about insurance or finances since other personnel have already done this in the admissions process. The client does not need to wear an examining gown to answer questions and is not likely to be comfortable doing so. **Cognitive Level:** Applying **Client Need:** Health Promotion and Maintenance **Integrated Process:** Nursing Process: Assessment **Content Area:** Fundamentals **Strategy:** Use knowledge of basic interviewing techniques to choose the option that represents the best approach to the client. **Reference:** Berman, A., & Snyder, S. J. (2012). *Kozier & Erb's fundamentals of nursing: Concepts, process, and practice* (9th ed.). Upper Saddle River, NJ: Pearson Education, p. 188.

2 **Answer: 4** **Rationale:** During inspection, the nurse scrutinizes and evaluates by sight any clues of pathology that may be present. By first performing the other assessment techniques (auscultation, percussion, and palpation), the nurse could alter the findings. The client's age does not alter the order of the assessment. Palpating the abdomen of an infant would likely alter the results of the other modes of assessment, making them less reliable. Regardless of the client's age, inspection of the abdomen should precede auscultation. Percussing the abdomen prior to inspection could alter the findings of the assessment. **Cognitive Level:** Applying **Client Need:** Health Promotion and Maintenance **Integrated Process:** Nursing Process: Assessment **Content Area:** Fundamentals **Strategy:** The critical word in the question is *first.* Recall the correct order of abdominal assessment techniques to make the correct selection. **Reference:** Berman, A., & Snyder, S. J. (2012). *Kozier & Erb's fundamentals of nursing: Concepts, process, and practice* (9th ed.). Upper Saddle River, NJ: Pearson Education, p. 639.

3 **Answer: 2, 4, 5** **Rationale:** Four key areas of functioning to be addressed in the mental status exam are appearance, behavior, cognition, and thought processes (recall these as A, B, C, T). Judgment and recent (short-term) memory would be an important component of the mental status exam. The client's thought processes are always assessed as part of the mental status exam. Educational level is unrelated to mental status. Gait and balance are assessed as part of the neurologic exam. **Cognitive Level:** Applying **Client Need:** Health Promotion and Maintenance **Integrated Process:** Nursing Process: Assessment **Content Area:** Fundamentals **Strategy:** The core issue of the question is knowledge of the components of the mental status exam. **Reference:** Berman, A., & Snyder, S. J. (2012). *Kozier & Erb's fundamentals of nursing: Concepts, process, and practice* (9th ed.). Upper Saddle River, NJ: Pearson Education, p. 582.

4 **Answer: 1** **Rationale:** The chief complaint offers the nurse an indication of what the problem is and how health care should proceed. The nurse can continue to probe during the interview to identify contributing factors to the client's chief complaint. The client's statements must be documented using his or her own phrases and terminology. The nurse should use the client's own words to describe the complaint. This is best done at the time of

the interview to insure accuracy. The nurse should avoid the tendency to decide what the etiology of the client's symptoms is at this point in the interview. **Cognitive Level:** Applying **Client Need:** Health Promotion and Maintenance **Integrated Process:** Communication and Documentation **Content Area:** Fundamentals **Strategy:** Recall knowledge of the health history process to make the correct selection. **Reference:** Berman, A., & Snyder, S. J. (2012). *Kozier & Erb's fundamentals of nursing: Concepts, process, and practice* (9th ed.). Upper Saddle River, NJ: Pearson Education, p. 190.

5 **Answer: 2** **Rationale:** The cremasteric reflex is tested in men only. The nurse uses a cotton-tipped applicator or other smooth object to stimulate the inner thigh. The normal reaction is contraction of the cremaster muscle and elevation of the testicle on the side stimulated. A penlight would not be useful to asses this reflex. To test this reflex, the inner thigh is stroked with a soft object so a neurologic hammer would not be appropriate. A tuning fork would not be appropriate to test this reflex. **Cognitive Level:** Applying **Client Need:** Health Promotion and Maintenance **Integrated Process:** Nursing Process: Assessment **Content Area:** Fundamentals **Strategy:** The critical words are *cremasteric reflex.* Recall knowledge of reflex assessment techniques to make the correct selection. **Reference:** Berman, A., & Snyder, S. J. (2012). *Kozier & Erb's fundamentals of nursing: Concepts, process, and practice* (9th ed.). Upper Saddle River, NJ: Pearson Education, p. 663.

6 **Answer: 1** **Rationale:** To assess for jugular venous distention (which indicates fluid volume overload), the client should be lying supine with the head elevated to 30 degrees (low Fowler's). The nurse assesses the highest point of distention of the internal jugular vein in centimeters in relation to the sternal angle, the point at which the clavicles meet. The neck veins would not be easily visible with the client supine with the neck downward on the chest. High-Flower's position and flat with no pillows under the head are also incorrect positions. **Cognitive Level:** Applying **Client Need:** Health Promotion and Maintenance **Integrated Process:** Nursing Process: Assessment **Content Area:** Fundamentals **Strategy:** Recall knowledge of cardiovascular assessment techniques to select the correct response. **Reference:** Berman, A., & Snyder, S. J. (2012). *Kozier & Erb's fundamentals of nursing: Concepts, process, and practice* (9th ed.). Upper Saddle River, NJ: Pearson Education, p. 631.

7 **Answer: 4** **Rationale:** During physical assessment, the nurse inspects the client's legs for hair distribution. The most common reason for shiny skin and a complete absence of hair is poor circulation related to peripheral vascular disease (PVD). Thus, the nursing diagnosis of Ineffective Peripheral Tissue Perfusion applies. The loss of hair on the lower legs is most often related to peripheral vascular disease, not nutritional status. No information is provided to indicate hair loss has relation to an increased risk of infection. There is no apparent relationship between the described hair loss and fluid volume. **Cognitive Level:**Analyzing **Client Need:**Physiological Adaptation **Integrated Process:**Nursing Process: Assessment **Content Area:**Fundamentals **Strategy:**The critical phrase is *absence of hair on the lower left leg.* Recall common abnormalities encountered in the client assessment and their usual etiologies to make the correct selection. **Reference:**Berman, A., & Snyder, S. J. (2012). *Kozier & Erb's fundamentals of nursing: Concepts, process, and practice* (9th ed.). Upper Saddle River, NJ: Pearson Education, p. 592.

8 **Answer: 1** **Rationale:**The apical pulse should be auscultated for one full minute with the stethoscope at the fifth intercostal space in the midclavicular line (apex of the heart). While auscultating the apical pulse, the radial pulse should be palpated simultaneously to detect discrepancies caused by dysrhythmias. One radial pulse should be felt for each apical beat heard, but with some dysrhythmias, the radial pulsation is absent with early beats because of reduced stroke volume. This 2-nurse technique is the most accurate way to detect pulse deficits. The other options represent incorrect technique because of either timing or location. **Cognitive Level:** Applying **Client Need:**Health Promotion and Maintenance **Integrated Process:**Nursing Process: Assessment **Content Area:**Fundamentals **Strategy:**Use knowledge of cardiac anatomy and basic assessment techniques to select the appropriate response. **Reference:**Berman, A., & Snyder, S. J. (2012). *Kozier & Erb's fundamentals of nursing: Concepts, process, and practice* (9th ed.). Upper Saddle River, NJ: Pearson Education, pp. 553–554.

9 **Answer: 3** **Rationale:**The Bartholin glands are part of the female anatomy located on the posterior aspect of the vaginal orifice. Therefore, if the medical condition allows, having the client in a lithotomy position (on the back, knees flexed, legs apart, with feet supported on a surface or in stirrups) will provide the best opportunity for examination. The Semi-Fowler's, Sim's, and prone positions would not allow for assessment of female genitalia. **Cognitive Level:**Applying **Client Need:**Health Promotion and Maintenance **Integrated Process:**Nursing Process: Assessment **Content Area:**Fundamentals **Strategy:**The core issue of the question is knowledge of what the Bartholin glands are and then determining the proper position for physical assessment. **Reference:**Berman, A., & Snyder, S. J. (2012). *Kozier & Erb's fundamentals of nursing: Concepts, process, and practice* (9th ed.). Upper Saddle River, NJ: Pearson Education, p. 658.

10 **Answer: 2** **Rationale:**In order to facilitate visualization of the ear canal and tympanic membrane, the pinna should be pulled up and back for an adult client. If earrings are attached to the lobe, there should not be a safety issue; however, they may be removed if they are large in size or are causing the client discomfort during the examination. The nurse should not remove cerumen with an applicator because of the risk of pushing it further into the canal or rupturing the tympanic membrane. Pulling the pinna down and back would be used when examining the ears of a child not an adult. **Cognitive Level:**Applying **Client Need:** Health Promotion and Maintenance **Integrated Process:** Nursing Process: Assessment **Content Area:**Fundamentals **Strategy:**Recall of assessment techniques for the child and adult will assist in making the correct selection. **Reference:**Berman, A., & Snyder, S. J. (2012). *Kozier & Erb's fundamentals of nursing: Concepts, process, and practice* (9th ed.). Upper Saddle River, NJ: Pearson Education, p. 605.

References

Berman, A., & Snyder, S. J. (2012). *Kozier & Erb's fundamentals of nursing: Concepts, process, and practice* (9th ed.). Upper Saddle River, NJ: Pearson Education, pp. 534–667.

Berman, A. J., Snyder, S., & McKinney, D. (2011). *Nursing basics for clinical practice.* Upper Saddle River, NJ: Pearson Education, Inc.

Craven, R., & Hirnle, C. (2009). *Fundamentals of nursing: Human health and function* (6th ed.). Philadelphia, PA: Wolters-Kluwer.

Potter, P. & Perry, A. (2013). *Fundamentals of nursing* (8th ed.). St. Louis, MO: Mosby, Inc.

Potter, P. Perry, A., Stockert, P., & Hall, A. (2011). *Basic nursing* (7th ed.). St. Louis, MO: Mosby, Inc.

Seidel, H. M., Ball, J. W., Dains, J. E., Flynn, J. A., & Solomon, B. S. (2011). *Mosby's guide to physical examination* (7th ed.). St. Louis, MO: Mosby, pp. 296–330.

Wilkinson, J., & Treas, L. (2011). *Fundamentals of nursing* (2nd ed.). Philadelphia, PA: F.A. Davis.

ANSWERS & RATIONALES

3 Overview of Communication

NCLEX-RN® Test Prep

Use the accompanying online resource, NursingReviewsandRationales, to test yourself with hundreds of NCLEX®-style practice questions.

Objectives

➤ Describe the elements, levels, and forms of communication.
➤ Contrast effective and ineffective techniques of communication.
➤ Identify the purposes of maintaining a client's health care record.
➤ Explain the purpose of documentation and legal guidelines used to document a client's health care.
➤ Review various methods used by nurses to record and report a client's health care status.
➤ Identify the standards and purposes associated with client teaching and learning.
➤ Identify the basic principles of teaching and learning.
➤ Describe teaching methods used based on the client's developmental level.

Review at a Glance

affective domain learning in this domain involves feelings, emotions, interests, and attitudes

charting by exception a form of documentation in which only unanticipated client responses and events are documented; format is organized by problem (P), intervention (I), and evaluation (E)

cognitive domain learning in this domain involves processing information by listening or reading facts and descriptions; learning is a mental, intellectual, or thinking process

communication a 2-way process involving the sending and receiving of messages

critical pathways multidisciplinary guidelines for client care based on specified medical diagnoses and designed to achieve predetermined outcomes

documentation information about a client recorded in the medical record either manually or using a computer

feedback the response or message that the receiver returns to the sender during communication

focus charting a method of charting that focuses on client strengths or on problems or needs

health beliefs concepts about health that an individual believes to be true

health practice an activity that a person carries out as a result of his or her health beliefs and definition of health

Kardex the trade name for a method that makes use of a series of cards to concisely organize and record client demographic data and instructions for daily nursing care

narrative charting a descriptive record of client data and nursing interventions, written in sentences and paragraphs

nonverbal communication communication other than words, including posture, gestures, and facial expressions

problem-oriented medical record (POMR) a record in which data about the client is written and arranged according to the client's problem, rather than according to the source of the information

progress notes chart entries using a variety of methods made by all health professionals involved in a client's care, for the purpose of describing client's problems, treatments, and progress toward desired outcomes

psychomotor domain learning in this domain involves learning by doing

standards of care detailed guidelines describing the minimal nursing care that can reasonably be expected to ensure high-quality care in a defined situation

variance a deviation from expected goal achievement using a critical pathway

verbal communication communication that involves the use of words in either written or oral form

1 A nurse enters the room of a female client and asks how she is doing. The client states, "I'm a little nervous this morning." What would be the nurse's best reply?

1. "What is making you feel nervous?"
2. "You do look as if you are feeling nervous."
3. "Can I give you a backrub for your nerves?"
4. "Can you tell more about how you are feeling?"

2 A client tells the nurse that her husband has an addiction to alcohol and hasn't worked for the last 3 months. The nurse's best initial response would be which of the following?

1. "Have you tried Al-Anon meetings?"
2. "I'm really sorry to hear that."
3. "You sound worried; perhaps you should talk to the chaplain."
4. "What have you done before to cope with his problem?"

3 Which of the following care approaches would be the most appropriate for the nurse to use when caring for a client who is unresponsive and in a coma?

1. Keep radio or TV on at a moderate volume at all times.
2. Avoid verbal communication while client appears unresponsive; focus instead on gentle touch and physical care measures.
3. Speak normally and as if client can hear and understand what is being said.
4. Direct verbal communication to family members at the bedside, providing them realistic updates on client's condition.

4 Using a mannequin, a nurse has demonstrated wound care for a client. To validate client learning, which of the following would be the best nursing action at this time?

1. Complete wound care on the client, explaining the procedure while performing it.
2. Show video explaining the sterile technique to be used for the client's wound care.
3. Have client perform wound care with the nurse present to supervise.
4. Ask client to review written client education literature and perform wound care at the next scheduled time.

5 Which of the following methods would be most effective for an ambulatory care nurse to use when trying to determine the priority health-related learning needs of a client?

1. Carefully review provider's prescriptions for this client to determine what the client needs to know about medication safety.
2. Conduct a thorough nursing assessment to pinpoint the client's physiological problems.
3. Determine the amount of time required to present information on the client's medical diagnosis and treatment plan.
4. Ask client what learning needs he or she has regarding his or her current state of health.

6 An acute care nurse is preparing to discharge to home a client who needs services from a home health nurse. What discharge information is most important for the acute care nurse to give to the referral agency nurse so that a plan of care can be developed?

1. Surgical report
2. Client's current self-care abilities
3. Vital signs on discharge
4. Time of last dose for medications administered

7 Which of the following items of information would be important for the nurse to include in an inter-shift report? Select all that apply.

1. Client still needs to demonstrate that he or she can do a dressing change before being discharged.
2. Client has had family members in to visit several times today.
3. Client is on bed rest with bathroom privileges.
4. Diet was changed from NPO (nothing by mouth) to clear liquids 2 hours ago.
5. Client was transported to radiology in a wheelchair for a chest x-ray at 10 a.m.

8 Which of the following statements heard by a nurse during an intershift report provides the most useful information related to priority setting for the upcoming shift?

1. A client who had catheter removed 8 hours ago has not urinated.
2. A client is alert and oriented to person and place.
3. A client who is 3 days postoperative was experiencing incisional pain rated a 6 on a scale of 1 to 10 prior to administration of analgesic medication.
4. A client admitted for congestive heart failure has a blood pressure of 146/84.

9 The quality improvement nurse reads several nurses' notes from different records that refer to clients' moods. Examples are that the client "is in good spirits today," "feels depressed today," and "is withdrawn today." Based on these pieces of documentation, which of the following actions would be best for the quality improvement nurse to take?

1. Communicate findings to nursing administration.
2. Report findings to The Joint Commission (formerly known as JCAHO).
3. Communicate findings to the agency's Nursing Staff Development Department.
4. Do nothing, as this is acceptable documentation practice.

10 Before going off duty, a nurse reviews the notes written for a client and discovers that there has been an omission of important assessment findings. Which nursing action is most appropriate at this time?

1. Insert omitted data in the appropriate area.
2. Recopy the entire section, include missing data, and throw the original away.
3. Record the time of the entry, time of the assessment, and the missing data, and label as "late entry."
4. Verbally relay the assessment finding during intershift report and leave the record unchanged.

➤ *See pages 76–77 for Answers and Rationales.*

I. OVERVIEW OF COMMUNICATION

A. Introductory concepts

1. Effective **communication** occurs when there is an exchange of information, ideas, attitudes, and emotions; therefore, successful communication occurs when the message intended is the message received
2. Effective communication is a basic skill in providing health care to clients; nurses communicate with other health care providers and health care consumers (clients) and their support systems (family, significant others)
3. Nurses need to understand basic elements of communication that tend to promote accurate dissemination of information as well as elements that may inhibit successful communication so that clients receive effective health care
4. A therapeutic helping relationship is enhanced by nurse's ability to care for and comfort clients with an empathetic understanding and other strategies

B. Phases of therapeutic relationship

  1. Pre-interaction phase

    a. Occurs prior to initial contact with a client and is similar to the planning stage before an interview

    b. Any information that a nurse has about a client is organized and analyzed prior to contact with client; during this phase the nurse prepares for initial contact

  2. Orientation phase

    a. May also be called introductory phase or prehelping phase

    b. During this phase nurse and client get to know one another and develop a degree of trust

    c. Three processes that occur during this phase are opening the relationship, clarifying the problem, and structuring and formulating the contract

  3. Working phase

    a. Includes exploring and understanding thoughts and feelings, along with facilitating and taking action

    b. Skills required during this phase are empathetic listening and understanding, respect, genuineness, concreteness, and confrontation

    c. At the completion of this phase the client makes decisions and takes action, while the nurse provides information, collaborates, and is supportive of the client

  4. Termination phase

    a. During this phase, nurse and client have reached their goals and conclude their communication

    b. This phase may be difficult for both nurse and client; to reduce feelings of loss and ambivalence, the nurse summarizes the relationship and may make follow-up phone calls to help the client transition to independence

    c. Nurse should prepare client for termination phase early in the communication process

C. Elements of communication

  1. Sender

    a. Sometimes referred to as *encoder*; is a person or group who initiates communication in order to convey information, thoughts, ideas, or feelings to another

    b. Sender encodes information by selecting signs and symbols used in communication (language, word selection, voice intonations, gestures, etc.)

  2. Message

    a. Is the information to be communicated and includes codings (vocabulary, tone of voice, body language, and way the message is transmitted)

    b. Effective communication occurs when the message intended is the message received

  3. Channel

    a. The *channel* or *medium* or is the vehicle used to convey a message and can target any of the five senses; e.g., written documentation (sight), oral communication (hearing), and therapeutic touch

    b. It is important that nurses use the correct medium to send a message; for example, it may be necessary to write a message for a client who is hearing impaired to ensure the message intended is the message received

  4. Receiver

    a. Is the person or group that the message is intended for, also referred to as the *decoder* of the message

    b. The decoder or receiver perceives or interprets the message

  5. Environment

    a. Is the set of physical, cultural, and social conditions in which the information is transmitted

    b. This is sometimes referred to as the *context* of the communication

Practice to Pass

An unconscious client with a closed head injury has been admitted to the intensive care unit following a motor vehicle crash. How should the nurse respond to this client to promote effective communication?

6. Feedback (sometimes referred to as *response*)
   a. Requires that the receiver respond to the message communicated by the sender; the response may be verbal or nonverbal
   b. The nature of the response helps to determine whether communication was effective or ineffective

D. Levels of communication
   1. Intrapersonal: *intra-* is a prefix meaning "within"; this level of communication refers to communication that occurs within oneself and happens constantly; it involves thinking about a message before it is sent, interpreting the message, and evaluating the message (self-talk)
   2. Interpersonal: *inter-* is a prefix meaning "between"; this level of communication refers to communication occurring between people and involves the sending and receiving of a message and feedback
   3. Public communication: involves sending a message to a group of people for the dissemination of information; it generally does not require feedback

E. Forms of communication
   1. Communication occurs both verbally and nonverbally in a therapeutic relationship; purposeful communication between nurse and client is often termed *therapeutic communication*
   2. The nurse needs to be aware of the form of communication chosen to ensure the message sent is the message received
      a. For instance, if nurse's body language indicates verbal information given is not important, then client will also view it as unimportant
      b. Using a different example, if nurse invades client's territorial space, then client may not be able to focus on message sent
   3. Verbal communication: involves use of words that are either spoken or written
      a. *Therapeutic rapport*: verbal communication can be facilitated by a trusting relationship between nurse and client, in which client believes that nurse cares about client's well-being and wants to assist client in meeting health-related goals
      b. *Pacing*: rhythm and speed with which verbal message is sent can have an impact on the way that words of a message are received; the pace may indicate interest, disinterest, or anxiety, among others
      c. *Intonation*: pattern of pauses and accents or stresses when sending a message can also impact on how it is received; it can reflect an underlying mood of sender, such as anger, boredom, or excitement
      d. *Clarity and brevity*: clear and brief messages are more likely to be interpreted correctly by receiver than vague and lengthy messages; clarity of a message is influenced by congruence between content of message and nurse's body language (nonverbal behavior)
      e. *Timing and relevance*: message needs to be delivered at a time when client is interested in receiving it and content of message needs to be of interest to client at the time communication is taking place; for example, a client newly diagnosed with diabetes may not be interested in listening to information about a diabetic diet if relatives from out of state have just arrived for a visit
   4. Nonverbal communication: communication that occurs without use of words; is often referred to as body language
      a. Facial expressions: can either convey or mask emotions; cautiously interpret eye and facial movements and validate these impressions with further assessment before drawing final conclusions; some expressions are more universal, such as a smile for happiness and a frown for displeasure

      b. Eye contact: can be influenced by cultural norms; avoiding eye contact may be culturally appropriate or can indicate other feelings, such as embarrassment or lack of interest in communicating

      c. Gestures: can convey urgency of a client's message or can be a coping response when an urgent message cannot be expressed quickly enough using words; some gestures (such as a wave) have almost universal meanings while others are culture specific; gestures can also be used as signals when a client cannot communicate with words

      d. Posture and gait: can indicate a client's physical well-being, self-concept, and mood
        1) An erect posture and a steady purposeful gait generally indicate a sense of well-being
        2) Slouching or a shuffling slow gait may indicate depressed mood or being physically tired or uncomfortable
        3) A client who guards the abdomen or who is lying down with knees drawn up to the chest is most likely experiencing pain
        4) Be sure to validate with client any impressions gained from observing his or her posture and gait

      e. Territoriality and space
        1) All people, clients and nurses alike, have a physical zone around the body that is considered an extension of self and that should not be entered by others, often referred to as *personal space*
        2) The size of the space can vary considerably from culture to culture and even person to person
        3) Often other forms of body language are used as signals to indicate when someone has violated personal space (such as taking a step back or holding up a hand in front of the person)

      f. Personal appearance
        1) Can be a general indicator of self-esteem, social status, emotional status, culture, or other group association
        2) Selection of clothing is often highly personal
        3) Hygiene may be influenced by physical ability, emotional status, mental illness, energy level, and time
        4) Be careful not to judge clients on the basis of personal appearance

F. Effective communication techniques

   1. *Using silence*: allows for quiet time without conversation for several seconds or minutes to allow for reflection about a discussion that just occurred, to reduce tension, or to gather thoughts about how to proceed

   2. *Offering self*: offers nurse's presence without attaching any expectations or conditions about client's behavior during that time

   3. *Restating or paraphrasing*: ensures nurse understands the message sent; consists of verbalizing the main thought of the message sent

   4. *Clarifying*: asks for additional information to ensure understanding of the message sent; a statement like "Would you tell me more about what you have just said?" indicates that understanding the client's message is important to the nurse

   5. *Focusing*: draws client's attention to pertinent information and helps client expand on that information; this technique directs the client toward information that is important

   6. *Acknowledging*: gives nonjudgmental recognition to a client for a certain behavior or contribution, or indicates attention to and care of client

   7. *Reflecting*: redirects content of a client's message back to client for further thought or consideration

Practice to Pass

A client who has chest pain has been brought to the emergency department. The client is acutely intoxicated, angry, and belligerent. How should the nurse proceed?

8. *Giving information*: provides specific information to a client either with or without the client's request

9. *Summarizing*: may be used at the end of an interaction to identify material discussed; helps to sort out relevant information from irrelevant

G. Communication techniques to avoid

1. Self-disclosure
   a. Involves relating to a client by communicating a personal experience to the client that focuses the relationship on the nurse
   b. For instance, if a client is having difficulty adjusting to an altered body image related to an amputation, it is not helpful for the nurse to communicate how he or she would feel if faced with a similar problem
   c. A therapeutic helping relationship should be client-centered and goal-directed

2. Inattentive listening
   a. Inattentive listening blocks communication by indicating that client's needs are not important
   b. A nurse who is thinking about another client when providing care to a client will seem distracted and uncaring

3. Overuse of medical jargon
   a. Overuse of medical jargon confuses clients and indicates the nurse is not interested in ensuring health care information is understood
   b. For instance, if a nurse asks a client how many times he or she has voided and the client does not understand the word *void*, the client may not know what the appropriate response should be

4. Giving personal opinions
   a. Expressing one's opinion may give an impression that a person is closed to new ideas; in a helping relationship, clients need to manage their own lives and problems and should be assisted to formulate their own ideas and plans
   b. Giving advice needs to be avoided

5. Prying
   a. Prying or probing techniques only provide information to satisfy the nurse's curiosity
   b. If a client states that a problem was not discussed with a health care provider and the nurse asks, "Why not?" it may place the client in a defensive position
   c. Asking for information not pertinent to a client's health status actually violates the client's right to privacy

6. Changing the subject
   a. Changing the subject blocks therapeutic communication by indicating that the client should not continue to talk about the previous topic; this leads the conversation to only those areas that the nurse wants to discuss
   b. For instance, if a female client asks if her breast will be removed because of a tumor, and the nurse asks if she has had a bowel movement since admission, this implies the nurse's unwillingness to discuss the client's concern

H. Communicating with clients who have special needs

1. Difficulty hearing
   a. To ensure that effective communication occurs with a client who is hearing impaired, stand or sit near client and speak clearly and slowly using a low-pitched voice
   b. Environment should have adequate lighting and be quiet and free from distractions
   c. Use therapeutic communication techniques to ensure that the message sent is the message received
   d. It may also be necessary to use writing to enhance communication with a client who is hearing impaired

e. Avoid using a loud voice when speaking to a client who is hearing impaired; instead, speak directly into the ear that has better hearing

2. Difficulty seeing
   a. When communicating with a visually impaired client, ensure the environment has adequate light
   b. Ensure that the quality of the spoken word matches the message communicated
   c. Remember that a visually impaired client may not be able to use nonverbal cues to help interpret a message

3. Mute or unable to speak clearly
   a. When communicating with a client who is unable to speak clearly, has an artificial airway, or is mute, encourage client to write a response or use word boards or pictures to ensure effective communication
   b. Utilize the therapeutic technique of clarification or paraphrasing as needed to assist in communication

4. Cognitively impaired
   a. When communicating with a client who is cognitively impaired, use language that is simple and concise, and speak words slowly and calmly
   b. Verbalize only one thought or question at a time to allow client to focus on message
   c. Allow adequate time for client to process information
   d. Use environmental cues when possible to convey message to client; for instance, holding a toothbrush for client to see while asking if he or she would like to brush the teeth helps the client understand the message

5. Unresponsive
   a. When communicating with an unresponsive person, use touch along with the spoken word and try to elicit a response from client
   b. Asking a closed question such as, "Can you hear me?" and observing for nonverbal cues that may indicate client has received the message is one way to elicit a response
   c. Speak to client in a manner that assumes client can hear every word that is spoken; avoid having conversations about client's status or that are irrelevant to client at the bedside

6. Non–English speaking
   a. Seek an interpreter fluent in client's primary language if client does not speak English; until an interpreter is available, communicate through nonverbal means
   b. Use pictures, environmental cues, and body language to communicate with a client who speaks a different language
   c. For procedures requiring informed consent, follow agency policy to obtain an approved interpreter before explaining procedure and obtaining client's signature

Practice to Pass

A nurse needs to complete an admission assessment on a hearing-impaired client. How should the nurse proceed?

II. DOCUMENTING AND REPORTING

A. Documentation

1. The act of making an entry in a client's medical record is referred to as **documentation** or charting
2. Communicating health care information is an important aspect of providing nursing care
3. The client record (medical record or health record) provides a description of nursing and medical care received by client
4. Information should be written clearly, concisely, and accurately; it should be factual and free of personal opinions or judgments
5. The record is a written or computer-based legal documentation of a client's health status that includes client's health care problems, treatment, and responses

B. Purpose of records

1. Communication tool for health care team
   a. The record serves as a means of communication between nursing personnel and other care providers to plan a client's health care
   b. Communication among health care professionals is essential in providing care to clients and prevents fragmentation, repetition, and delays in client care

2. Legal document
   a. The record is a legal document that provides verification of the quality of care that a client receives
   b. All information in a client record is confidential and access to record is restricted to only those health professionals involved in client's care

3. Financial billing
   a. Documentation of health care received by a client is also a means for reimbursement for services provided
   b. Before a client's record can be released to insurance companies, client must authorize in writing what portions of record to release

4. Education
   a. Health care students may also use documentation for educational purposes by comparing actual cases to textbook cases
   b. Educators may use client records as a source for teaching students
   c. A review of medical records may indicate a need for continuing education for nursing staff or other health care providers
   d. It is important that records used for educational purposes protect clients' privacy at all times

5. Assessment: health records help an agency identify services utilized by clients in order to plan for staffing, educational, and fiscal needs

6. Research: the record may also provide vital statistics and data for research purposes to improve treatment protocols, identify frequency of diseases, and causes of death; client-identifying information must be removed

7. Auditing and monitoring
   a. Medical records serve as a source by which to evaluate health care received by clients to ensure quality care
   b. *Quality improvement* refers to evaluation of the level of care provided in a health care agency and can be done internally or externally
   c. These auditing procedures are completed to ensure continuity of care and that health care standards are being met by the institution; The Joint Commission (formerly known as JCAHO) is an example of an accrediting agency; **standards of care** are detailed guidelines that describe minimal nursing care needed to ensure high-quality care in a defined situation

C. Common forms used in written or electronic documentation

1. Admission nursing assessment: a comprehensive form that is organized according to a specific scheme, such as body systems, functional abilities, health problems, a nursing model, or type of unit (labor and delivery versus surgical); it may also be called an admission database or nursing history

2. Client care plans (nursing or interdisciplinary): individualized care plans or standardized care plans (plans that address usual needs of a client with an identified health problem)

3. **Kardex** or clinical worksheet: lists demographic data, including allergies, medications ordered, IV fluids ordered, currently ordered treatments and procedures, scheduled diagnostic or laboratory tests, and orders or data for meeting basic needs (diet, self-feeding ability, activity, safety, hygiene, and elimination), and possibly a problem list or plan of care; a Kardex may be electronic and it may or may not be part of the permanent client record

4. Flowsheets: forms that cluster specific data in one place for easy reference, to assess trends in data, or to document care; these include vital signs, blood glucose, intake and output, medication record, or daily nursing care; some agencies combine many of these onto one large flowsheet that is used for a 24-hour period; most flowsheets including medication administration records (MARs or EMARs) are now electronic

5. Progress notes: provide information about client progress in meeting health goals; are more fully described in a section to follow

6. Nursing discharge or referral summaries: include a concise summary of the course of hospitalization or treatment, resolved and unresolved health problems, current treatments and medications (including time of last dose), functional abilities for activities of daily living, activity restrictions, comfort level, client education completed, referrals to other health care providers, and discharge destination (home, rehabilitation facility, long-term care facility) and mode of transport (ambulatory, wheelchair, stretcher or ambulance)

D. Guidelines for legal documentation

1. Documentation is a form of verbal communication because words are used for exchange of information

2. Use words that are clear, easy to read, and complete

3. Be aware that documentation will stand alone without the benefit of nonverbal communication; avoid words with unclear meanings

4. The client's health record documents the client's health care problems, needs, and services; it truly provides a total picture of a client's health care

5. Follow these guidelines when documenting in a client's health care record:
   a. Accurate: include facts and observations rather than opinions, judgments, or interpretation of client's behavior
   b. Complete: include all relevant aspects of care, including assessments, interventions, client comments, client response to care (including nursing care, diagnostic tests, and therapeutic procedures), progress toward goal achievement, care that was omitted with reasons why and who was notified, and the substance of any communication with other disciplines
   c. Current: document as soon as care is provided whenever possible and reflect client's present condition; late entries must be so noted
   d. Organized: provide a logical flow of ideas; pieces of information that relate to each other should be grouped together; this includes proper sequencing of information and events
   e. Appropriateness: only include information that relates to client's current health care status and care being delivered; inclusion of irrelevant personal information about client can be considered an invasion of privacy (at the least) or to be libelous (at worst)
   f. Agency policies: document in a manner consistent with all agency policies, which often includes that each note contain date and time of charting; be legible; use permanent ink (if not electronic), correct spelling, approved style of documentation (see section to follow on methods of recording), and proper terminology; contain a signature (electronic documentation is automatically "signed" via user's sign-on code to computer system)

6. Pitfalls of documentation
   a. Writing illegibly: interpreting notes that are written illegibly may be difficult or impossible to do either in present time or at a later date; it is important to write carefully so everyone understands the contents of a note
   b. Leaving blank lines: provides an opportunity for someone to insert information at a later date; is generally inconsistent with health care agency policies on documentation; use a pen to draw a line through blank lines of a page and draw an "X" through blank portions of a page for the same reason

c. Altering someone else's notes: the record is a legal document and entries must not be altered once recorded; a separate entry can be made to record own observations or care if needed

d. Back-dating records: do not back-date late entries; instead include date and time of actual charting as well as date and time of original observations or care being recorded; for example, if an event that happened at 10:30 was going to be charted at 11:15 and a notation was already made at 11:00, then the entry should be made for 11:15 with the words *Addendum 10:30* at the beginning of the note

e. Correcting errors incorrectly: agency policy dictates how to correct a mistaken entry; this usually includes drawing a single line through error and writing *error* or *void* above it with nurse's initials; the purpose of a single line is to maintain legibility of words under the line

f. Inserting information between lines: should be avoided; new or omitted information should be added as an addendum note

g. Documenting for someone else: should not be done; each nurse should document own observations and care and be legally accountable for own entries

h. Expressing opinions: is not advisable; documentation should contain facts and observations; opinions that could be interpreted as negative or prejudicial could be libelous

i. Using nonmeasurable terms: tends to make documentation vague; notes should reflect clarity and brevity (use as few words as possible)

j. Failing to document communication with other health care members regarding client care: all aspects of care (including communications) that have an impact on client's health status must be documented; the familiar saying "If it wasn't documented, it wasn't done" applies to this situation as well as many others in nursing practice

E. Methods of recording

1. **Narrative charting**

   a. Is considered a source-oriented record whereby each department has a separate section in the record

   b. Provides documentation of total health status of client, including nursing interventions received, treatments performed, and client's reaction to care received

   c. Is generally written in chronological order; this format is time-consuming because a complete head-to toe-assessment is usually documented every shift

   d. Makes it sometimes difficult to focus on client's pertinent problem(s) because all routine care and normal assessment findings are integrated with documentation about problems

2. **Problem-oriented medical record (POMR)**

   a. Data is arranged according to client's problems rather than source of information

   b. Each health professional involved in client's care contributes to a given list of client problems

   c. POMR has 4 basic components, including database, problem list, plan of care, and **progress notes** (a written narrative of client progress, treatments, and other important information)

   d. Notes may be written using SOAP (subjective, objective, assessment, plan), APIE (assessment, problem, intervention, evaluation), or PIE (problem, intervention, evaluation) format

3. **Charting by exception**

   a. Charting by exception is a form of documentation whereby only exceptions to the rule are documented; notes may follow PIE format

   b. The information may be documented in narrative form, but often several standardized flowsheets are used to simplify documentation of client's health status

Practice to Pass

The nurse documents a note for one client in another client's medical record. What action should the nurse take to correct the error?

Practice to Pass

What principles of documentation should the nurse follow every time an entry is made in the client's record?

c. The PIE system eliminates the traditional care plan and incorporates an ongoing care plan into the progress notes

d. Standards of care may be preselected or preprinted and included in a client's record; these may also be individualized as needed to provide quality nursing care

4. **Focus charting**
   a. This method focuses on client needs that deviate from normal
   b. The intent of this format is to make client's needs and strengths the focus of care and results in a holistic approach for nursing
   c. Progress notes are organized into data (D), action (A), and response (R) categories

5. Critical pathways
   a. **Critical pathways** (clinical pathways, care maps) are a set of documentation forms that identify outcome criteria that certain groups are expected to achieve on each day of care
   b. Format is based on cost-effective care delivered within an established length of stay
   c. An example of an outcome criterion is that a client having a laparoscopic cholecystectomy is afebrile for first 24 hours after surgery; if this client develops a fever, this would be a **variance** or a goal not met and would be recorded as such

6. Computerized charting
   a. Computer systems are commonly used in health care facilities for maintaining client records, which often includes nursing documentation
   b. Nurses use computers to store clients' databases, add new data, create and revise care plans, document medication administration, and document overall client progress
   c. Computerization of client's medical record (also called electronic health record or EHR) has made the transfer of a client from one setting to another relatively easy
   d. Benefits of computer-driven records include legibility of records and more efficient use of nurses' time

F. **Reporting:** refers to transfer of information from nurses to nurses, or from nurses to other members of health care team; can be written or oral in form

1. Oral change-of-shift (intershift) report
   a. An oral report is given to all nurses on next shift to ensure continuity of care; may take place in a designated private area or utilize a walking rounds format
   b. The report should be organized, concise, and efficient; there are many handoff communication tools used in different facilities; a common one is the PACE tool (P = patient and problem, A = assessment and actions C = continuing treatments and changes, E = evaluation); use of a communication tool will help assure that important information is not omitted
   c. Regardless of tool used, a change of shift report should include:
      1) Demographics: client's name, age, hospital day, room number, and physician
      2) Medical diagnosis
      3) General physical and psychological condition and mental status as well as any changes in condition
      4) New physician prescriptions
      5) Scheduled diagnostic test or therapies
      6) Dietary modifications and fluid requirements
      7) Activities permitted
      8) Client teaching needs
      9) Nursing diagnoses
      10) Safety needs
      11) Other information pertinent to client's health care needs

      2. Tape-recorded intershift report

         a. Some agencies utilize a tape recorder to provide nurses with an intershift report

         b. Elements of a taped report are the same as for an oral report

         c. It is important for nurses who utilize this method to recognize that verbal communication must be accurate and detailed because oncoming nurses may not be able to ask questions, and there is minimal opportunity for feedback

         d. Procedures for maintaining confidentiality of material recorded on tape and for destroying or erasing information on tape must be followed; concerns about confidentiality are making this a less popular method in several health care agencies

      3. Written intershift report

         a. Some agencies have implemented written reports in lieu of oral or taped reports

         b. The information conveyed is the same as for other types of report

         c. Agency-specific or unit-specific forms are developed and utilized

         d. A benefit is that the nurse has immediate access to all previous written reports from the time of client admission for easy retrieval of information in an efficient manner

         e. A new report is written at end of each shift and all forms are passed on to oncoming nurse

         f. Upon discharge or transfer, shift reports are disposed of or shredded according to agency policy

      4. Bedside intershift report

         a. Report is given at client's bedside; off-going nurse and oncoming nurse meet face to face and jointly assess client and exchange information

         b. This method allows client and family to have input in the report process and interact with oncoming nurse

         c. A bedside report allows clients to be seen sooner, since the nurse assesses the client at the time of report; this has also been shown to decrease care errors

> ▶ **Practice to Pass**
>
> A nurse is preparing to give a report to staff members coming on duty. What information needs to be reported to ensure the continuity of care?

III. TEACHING AND LEARNING

    A. Assessing a client's need for health education (see Box 3-1)

    B. Purposes of client teaching

      1. Maintenance and promotion of health and illness prevention

         a. Examples include prenatal classes, immunization requirements, nutrition, exercise, and parenting

         b. Generally these programs are aimed towards groups of people with a health care need and designed to disseminate information and skills needed for clients to develop positive **health practices** (personal habits or behaviors that promote health)

      2. Restoration of health

         a. These programs are intended for clients with an active health problem and focus on cause, condition, and/or treatment

         b. An example of this type of client teaching would be insulin administration for a client that has new onset type 1 diabetes mellitus

      3. Coping with impaired functioning

         a. This type of client teaching centers around providing instruction to an individual who has not made or cannot make a complete recovery

         b. An example is a client who modifies activities of daily living because of a lower limb amputation

    ▶ **C. Domains of learning**

      1. Cognitive learning involves acquiring and using knowledge; for instance, when teaching a parenting class, a nurse provides information on developmental stages of children; applying that knowledge to toilet training a child, a parent is learning in the **cognitive domain**

Box 3-1	
Helpful Questions to Determine Client Health-Related Learning Needs	• What information does the client need to learn to effectively self-manage a health problem? What does the client already know? • Does health-related client teaching need to be individually tailored based on unique client factors such as cultural or religious practices or other health beliefs? • What is the best way to present health information so that it is understandable to the client and takes into account the client's language, emotional status, and any physical or cognitive limitations? • What does the client need to know in order to use any prescribed medications safely and effectively? How might prescribed medications interact with any other herbal or over-the-counter products that the client uses? • What information does the client need to know about general nutrition, any prescribed diet, and any possible drug-food interactions? • Does the client know what signs and symptoms indicate a need to contact the health care provider(s)? Does the client have the contact information for those health care providers? • Does the client need to learn about the use of any assistive devices (such as walker, cane, crutches, plate guard or eating utensils) to be able to function more independently after discharge? • Does the client need any modifications made to the home, such as bathroom grab bars, raised toilet seat, or ramp installation) to function more safely in the home environment? • What referrals to other disciplines or services does the client need to support self-management of health problems after discharge? (Examples include dietician, respiratory therapy, physical or occupational therapy, home health care) • To what extent does the client demonstrate understanding of any health-related information that has been taught thus far?

2. Affective learning occurs when a client changes unhealthy attitudes or feelings and values; a parent who accepts and understands that children have specific developmental stages and may not become toilet trained until after age 2 years is learning in the **affective domain**

3. Psychomotor: learning to complete a physical act is learning in the **psychomotor domain**; a client learning to self-administer injections is an example of learning in this domain

D. Factors that influence client learning

1. Motivation
   a. Motivation is a desire to learn; important to learning is that client recognizes a need to learn a new behavior
   b. Nurses can assist a client in solving problems and identifying needs that may increase his or her desire to learn

2. **Health beliefs**
   a. A client's health beliefs may or may not be congruent with the information being taught
   b. The nurse may assist a client in this way by showing a cause and effect type of relationship between negative health practices and poor health outcomes; for example, if a client believes that smoking will worsen his or her current cardiac status, client may be more likely to stop smoking
   c. Nurses need to assess a client's health care beliefs in order to develop beneficial teaching plans
   d. Be aware that a client's health care beliefs may not change, despite concentrated teaching efforts, because of multiple psychological, cultural, and environmental factors

3. Psychosocial adaptation to illness
   a. Psychosocial adaptation to illness describes the transition from a healthy independent state to an illness state
   b. Successful adaptation depends on a client's emotional makeup

    c. Recognize that a client is unlikely to learn new health-related behaviors when he or she is not ready or motivated to learn, or experiencing problems unrelated to his or her health

    d. Assess how a client is adapting on a regular basis

4. Active participation

    a. A client's active participation in the teaching–learning process makes learning more meaningful

    b. Assess a client's learning needs and involve client in the learning process to make this happen

5. Literacy level and educational level: ability of client to read materials provided and understand the spoken word

6. Developmental level

7. Individual learning style: learning is enhanced when nurse uses instructional methods that match client's preferred learning style (such as visual, auditory, kinesthetic)

E. Basic teaching principles

1. *Set priorities*: both client and nurse rank client's learning needs according to importance; it is imperative the nurse involve the client in ranking needs because learning is more likely to occur when client's perceived needs are met

2. *Use appropriate timing*: plan the period between when the client receives information and actively uses that information; for example, a client with diabetes is more likely to successfully administer insulin immediately after watching a video, rather than waiting until the next morning

3. *Organize materials*: learning occurs from simple to complex; it is important to organize material in this manner to allow learner to assimilate information more readily

4. *Promote and maintain learner attention and participation*: learning is enhanced if environment is comfortable and free from distractions, and if there is opportunity for client feedback; involve client actively in the learning process to facilitate assimilation of information; ensure client is physically comfortable to help maintain client attention; ensure that information is personally relevant to client

5. *Build on existing knowledge*: assess client's knowledge of material to be presented before beginning teaching; when nurse builds on client's existing knowledge, the material becomes more personal to client, learning is enhanced, and learner's confidence is increased

6. Select appropriate teaching methods

    a. Discussion: one-on-one formal or informal instruction allows client to set the pace of learning and engage in a verbal exchange with nurse; promotes customized learning for client

    b. Question and answer: meets needs of client for specific pieces of information as requested by client; often beneficial as a follow-up to other teaching methods

    c. Role-play, discovery: a creative strategy that allows client to simulate real-life situations and apply new knowledge or skills in an artificial or "safe" setting; helps build client's confidence in newly acquired knowledge and skills once feelings of being shy, embarrassed, or awkward are worked through

    d. Computerized instruction: allows client to be more actively engaged in learning process; allows client to regulate pace of instruction and may allow client to direct what type of material is presented next (interactive programs)

7. Use appropriate teaching aids: these are useful supplements to instruction if they are well-selected for content and client's learning style; may include visual aids (drawings, charts, models, printed materials), audiotapes, films or videotapes, programmed instruction, games, and others

Practice to Pass

A 16-year-old client is to check the blood glucose level every 8 hours after discharge from the hospital. What does the nurse have to consider when designing a teaching plan for this client?

8. Provide teaching related to developmental level
   a. Infant
      1) Topics for health promotion teaching about this age group include immunizations, infant safety, nutrition, rest and sleep patterns, and sensory stimulation
      2) Assess parents' or caregivers' learning needs and provide instruction accordingly
      3) Complete client teaching when infant is calm and happy to minimize parent or caregiver distraction
   b. Toddler
      1) Topics for health promotion teaching related to this age group include injury prevention, toilet training, dental hygiene, and appropriate play activities
      2) Toddlers fear pain and separation from parents
      3) Parent teaching for a hospitalized toddler includes participation in the care the child receives, purpose of care plans, and developmental regression that can occur as a result of hospitalization
   c. Preschooler
      1) Health promotion teaching for a preschooler includes injury prevention, dental health, nutrition, cognitive stimulation, and sleep patterns
      2) Assist a hospitalized preschooler by using visual, tactile, and auditory images to decrease fear of procedures
      3) Use of therapeutic play is also important to this age group; using dolls or puppets to demonstrate procedures before they are done is also helpful to child
   d. School-age
      1) Health promotion teaching for school-age child includes dental hygiene, safety measures, promotion of physical fitness, and hygiene measures to prevent spread of infection
      2) Nurses can assist a hospitalized school-age child by providing concrete examples and explanations of procedures to help child understand health care
      3) Encourage child to identify his or her own learning needs; forms of play may assist child to learn as well
   e. Adolescent
      1) Health promotion teaching for this age group includes the effects of drugs and alcohol, sexually transmitted infections, reducing risk of injury (e.g., motor vehicle crashes, sports), nutrition, and reducing exposure to sun
      2) Actively involving the adolescent in learning helps him or her to assimilate the information provided
      3) Client contracting and peer education also promote learning
   f. Young and middle-aged adult
      1) Health promotion teaching for this age group may include importance of routine health tests and screening, sun protection measures, importance of nutrition (especially adequate protein and calcium intake), and exercise to maintain health
      2) Evaluate client's learning needs and determine learning needs that client believes are important to maintain his or her health
   g. Older adult
      1) Health promotion teaching for this age group includes importance of exercise in maintaining joint mobility, nutritional information (including caloric and fluid requirements), and fall prevention information
      2) Ensure there is adequate lighting and use large print if necessary for client who is visually impaired
      3) If client is hearing impaired, use written teaching materials, and it may be necessary to utilize visual aids

Case Study

An 80-year-old man is being discharged from the hospital with the medical diagnosis of neurogenic bladder. His physician has ordered self-catheterization 3 times a day. He lives with his daughter but is very independent. He is also very religious and went to church daily prior to becoming ill. The daughter reported that in addition to going to church he used to volunteer at the local school, mentoring high school students for 2 hours each day. She added that since he developed the bladder problem, he has not left the house and has talked more about dying.

1. Devise a teaching plan for this client and describe how to document the client teaching provided.

2. What information is necessary to assess prior to presenting the teaching plan?

3. How might the nurse approach the client to discuss end-of-life issues and possible increasing dependency issues?

4. From the information provided, identify possible nursing diagnoses for this client and specify the supporting case study information.

5. Identify criteria that can be used to evaluate client outcomes based on the nursing diagnoses identified.

For suggested responses, see page 306.

POSTTEST

1 A nurse observes a client pacing the halls, and it appears as if the client has been crying. What is the most appropriate action by the nurse?

1. Consider the behavior as a normal reaction to illness.
2. Validate perceptions with the client.
3. Discuss the client's actions with another nurse for verification.
4. Discuss the morning schedule with the client to decrease apprehension.

2 What would be the best approach for the nurse to use when a client conveys anxiety immediately prior to surgery? Select all that apply.

1. Reassure the client of the surgeon's competency.
2. Provide teaching about the surgical procedure.
3. Explore the client's feelings with him or her.
4. Relate the nurse's personal experience of having a similar surgery.
5. Check on the client frequently until the client is transported to the operating room.

3 A nurse is preparing to complete an admission assessment on a client who is partially hearing impaired. What would be the best approach for the nurse to use?

1. Request that a family member be present.
2. Prepare written questions that cover the assessment criteria.
3. Speak slowly in a low-pitched voice while facing the client and sitting at his or her eye level.
4. Perform only the physical assessment at this time.

4 A client states, "I am so sick, I know I am going to die." The best way for the nurse to document this data would be to write which of the following statements?

1. "Client is depressed today."
2. "Client thinks he is going to die."
3. "Client is frustrated with being sick."
4. "Client states, I am so sick, I know I am going to die.'"

5 A 68-year-old female client needs to learn how to take her pulse before taking prescribed heart medication. Before beginning the client teaching, the nurse should assess which of the following about the client?

1. Cardiac status
2. Reading ability
3. Psychomotor abilities
4. Motivation to attain optimal wellness

6 A nurse can best evaluate a client's ability to carry out diabetic foot care by using which of the following methods?

1. Have the client explain how he or she would perform diabetic foot care step by step.
2. Have the client demonstrate how he or she would perform the required activities on a mannequin.
3. Have the client write down step by step how he or she would perform the activities at home.
4. Observe the client while he or she performs diabetic foot care.

7 Which of the following behaviors made by a client indicates to the nurse that learning in the cognitive domain has taken place?

1. Explaining why he is taking a new medication and how the medication works
2. Actively demonstrating a new self-care skill
3. Telling the nurse he has accepted the illness and its effects on his lifestyle
4. Reading the client education materials provided

8 Which statement would constitute a typical outcome criterion that is likely to appear on a critical pathway for a client who is postoperative for an appendectomy?

1. Administer morphine sulfate 6 mg IM q4h prn for pain.
2. Limit visitors at the bedside to immediate family.
3. Client will be afebrile within 24 hours after surgery.
4. Encourage ambulation and self-care after breakfast.

9 In order to provide optimal care to clients, the nurse would give highest priority to which information received in an intershift report?

1. Physical assessment data and client response to care
2. Client's list of active and resolved problems and associated medical treatments
3. Provider visits and new orders
4. Intake and output data and vital signs

10 Charting by exception is used by a hospital for documentation. Using this format, how would the nurse document routine morning care in the narrative notes?

1. "Morning care completed."
2. "Morning care completed; client tolerated well."
3. "Morning care completed by client."
4. Not necessary to document morning care if uneventful.

➤ *See pages 77–79 for Answers and Rationales.*

POSTTEST

ANSWERS & RATIONALES

Pretest

1 **Answer: 4** **Rationale:** Asking the client to describe feelings seeks additional information and indicates to the client that the nurse is attentive. Asking for the reason may force the client to defend herself because the client may or may not know the reason for these feelings. Stating that the client looks nervous may be interpreted as unsupportive. Providing a backrub does not allow the client to express feelings. **Cognitive Level:** Applying **Client Need:** Psychosocial Integrity **Integrated Process:** Communication and Documentation **Content Area:** Fundamentals **Strategy:** The critical words in the question are *the nurse's best reply.* Recall that the best way to obtain information related to the client's health is to have the client elaborate or clarify a statement the client made. **Reference:** Berman, A., & Snyder, S. J. (2012). *Kozier & Erb's fundamentals of nursing: Concepts, process, and practice* (9th ed.). Upper Saddle River, NJ: Pearson Education, p. 471.

2 **Answer: 4** **Rationale:** Therapeutic communication involves assessing the client's coping strengths and encouraging the client to problem solve. Asking what the client has done before focuses the client on solving her own problems and helps the nurse assess the client's coping mechanisms. This is the best first step. From there, the nurse can assist the client in problem solving. Asking about Al-Anon meetings rushes to a solution that may not be useful to the client. This type of response serves as a block to further communication. Stating one is sorry to hear the information is empathetic but does not seek further information and would likely serve as a block to communication. This response places the client's issue on hold and assumes the client would like to speak to a chaplain. **Cognitive Level:** Applying **Client Need:** Psychosocial Integrity **Integrated Process:** Communication and Documentation **Content Area:** Fundamentals **Strategy:** The critical words are *best initial response.* Use knowledge of communication techniques and the process of elimination to choose the option that gathers more information by assessing the client's ability to cope with this situation. **Reference:** Berman, A., & Snyder, S. J. (2012). *Kozier & Erb's fundamentals of nursing: Concepts, process, and practice* (9th ed.). Upper Saddle River, NJ: Pearson Education, pp. 472–473.

3 **Answer: 3** **Rationale:** Clients in coma may retain cognition and hearing even when they are unable to respond. Clients should be spoken to and cared for just as an alert, hearing client would be. Keeping radio and TV on at a moderate volume continuously does not provide meaningful stimulation in case the client is able to hear. It is helpful to provide verbal stimulation as well as gentle touch and physical care measures because it is uncertain whether a particular client who is in a coma is able to hear. Because the client may be able to hear and process what is said, discussions of the client's condition should be avoided at the bedside. **Cognitive Level:** Applying **Client Need:** Psychosocial Integrity **Integrated Process:** Caring **Content Area:** Fundamentals **Strategy:** Use knowledge of basic communication techniques to answer the question. **Reference:** Berman, A., & Snyder, S. J. (2012). *Kozier & Erb's fundamentals of nursing: Concepts, process, and practice* (9th ed.). Upper Saddle River, NJ: Pearson Education, pp. 480–482.

4 **Answer: 3** **Rationale:** Clients are more likely to successfully complete a new procedure if they can actively demonstrate the procedure immediately after instructions have been given with the nurse present the first several times. Written literature and a video do not allow for active participation; however, they can be used as supplementary learning aids. **Cognitive Level:** Applying **Client Need:** Health Promotion and Maintenance **Integrated Process:** Teaching and Learning **Content Area:** Fundamentals **Strategy:** Recall that learning is measured by a change in client behavior. Recall the most effective techniques for evaluating psychomotor skills to select the correct response. **Reference:** Berman, A., & Snyder, S. J. (2012). *Kozier & Erb's fundamentals of nursing: Concepts, process, and practice* (9th ed.). Upper Saddle River, NJ: Pearson Education, pp. 495–496.

5 **Answer: 4** **Rationale:** Learning is more likely to take place when the client's perceived needs are met. Assessing the client's needs directly identifies areas for client teaching and the client's ability to learn. The provider's prescriptions often do not address client teaching needs. A thorough nursing assessment will gather much data, but teaching needs are assessed in a focused manner. The amount of time needed to implement a teaching plan is not associated with establishing priorities. **Cognitive Level:** Applying **Client Need:** Health Promotion and Maintenance **Integrated Process:** Teaching and Learning **Content Area:** Fundamentals **Strategy:** The critical words are *most effective* and *learning needs of a client.* Recall factors that influence client learning and use the process of elimination to identify the best areas for client teaching. **Reference:** Berman, A., & Snyder, S. J. (2012). *Kozier & Erb's fundamentals of nursing: Concepts, process, and practice* (9th ed.). Upper Saddle River, NJ: Pearson Education, pp. 495–496.

6 **Answer: 2** **Rationale:** A description of the client's self-care abilities provides data to the referral nurse about information needed to continue the client's care at home. The surgical report does not have direct relevance to the client's home care needs. Vital sign information is only one parameter and would not provide enough information about the client's overall status.

Last dose of medications is important data but does not identify all of the medications the client is currently taking, which is helpful in developing a comprehensive plan of care. **Cognitive Level:** Applying **Client Need:** Health Promotion and Maintenance **Integrated Process:** Communication and Documentation **Content Area:** Fundamentals **Strategy:** Use the process of elimination and knowledge of discharge planning principles to systematically eliminate options that do not provide comprehensive or crucial information to other health care agencies or providers. **Reference:** Berman, A., & Snyder, S. J. (2012). *Kozier & Erb's fundamentals of nursing: Concepts, process, and practice* (9th ed.). Upper Saddle River, NJ: Pearson Education, p. 267.

7 **Answer: 1, 3, 4** **Rationale:** A change-of-shift report is given to ensure continuity of care and should be concise and efficient. Client learning needs are essential information so the next nurse can provide appropriate care. Permitted activities are essential information so the next nurse can provide appropriate care. Dietary modifications are essential information so the next nurse can provide appropriate care. Family visitation is not considered necessary information. Mode of transportation for a diagnostic test is not considered necessary information. **Cognitive Level:** Applying **Client Need:** Management of Care **Integrated Process:** Communication and Documentation **Content Area:** Fundamentals **Strategy:** The core issue of the question is knowledge of important information to include in an intershift report. Use knowledge of reporting guidelines and the process of elimination in selecting key information to report to the oncoming shift. **Reference:** Berman, A., & Snyder, S. J. (2012). *Kozier & Erb's fundamentals of nursing: Concepts, process, and practice* (9th ed.). Upper Saddle River, NJ: Pearson Education, p. 267.

8 **Answer: 1** **Rationale:** A client who has not urinated following catheter removal would require immediate nursing intervention, specifically assessing the client's abdominal distention, reviewing intake and output records, and possibly calling the provider for an order to do a straight catheterization. The client who is alert and oriented is not a priority since the normal orientation status indicates no threat to the health status of the client. The second priority would be the client who has incisional pain; however, since the client is 3 days postoperative, this is not as urgent a problem; the client would need to be reassessed for pain level after medication administration. The third priority would be to compare the blood pressure of the client with congestive heart failure to his or her baseline blood pressure. **Cognitive Level:** Analyzing **Client Need:** Basic Care and Comfort **Integrated Process:** Communication and Documentation **Content Area:** Fundamentals **Strategy:** The critical phrases are *most useful information* and *priority setting*. Analyze each client in the various options and choose the one that has the most critical need. **Reference:** Berman, A., & Snyder, S. J. (2012). *Kozier & Erb's fundamentals of nursing: Concepts,*

process, and practice (9th ed.). Upper Saddle River, NJ: Pearson Education, p. 267.

9 **Answer: 3** **Rationale:** The quality improvement nurse's best action is to report the findings to the Nursing Staff Development Department, which could take corrective action to improve the standards of nursing documentation in the facility. The documentation of mood reviewed by the nurse reflects that the wording of the documentation does not describe the client behavior or quote the client's original words; rather it reflects the nurse's opinion or judgment about the client status. Communicating with nursing administration would be a routine expected activity but would not directly establish a plan to improve documentation. Reporting findings to an outside agency such as The Joint Commission will not help improve the standards of nursing documentation in the facility. Doing nothing will not help improve the standards of nursing documentation in the facility. **Cognitive Level:** Analyzing **Client Need:** Management of Care **Integrated Process:** Communication and Documentation **Content Area:** Fundamentals **Strategy:** The critical words are *best and actions*. This implies that more than one option is a realistic possibility but that one option will be more effective. Use knowledge of the purpose of quality improvement to make a selection. **Reference:** Berman, A., & Snyder, S. J. (2012). *Kozier & Erb's fundamentals of nursing: Concepts, process, and practice* (9th ed.). Upper Saddle River, NJ: Pearson Education, pp. 184–185.

10 **Answer: 3** **Rationale:** Recording the time of the entry, the time of the assessment, and the missing data is an acceptable documentation practice. Inserting information in the client record is not an appropriate documentation action. Clients' records should not be recopied. Solely reporting the omission verbally is not acceptable. **Cognitive Level:** Applying **Client Need:** Management of Care **Integrated Process:** Communication and Documentation **Content Area:** Fundamentals **Strategy:** The critical phrase is *at this time*. Recall guidelines for legal documentation to aid in making a selection. **Reference:** Berman, A., & Snyder, S. J. (2012). *Kozier & Erb's fundamentals of nursing: Concepts, process, and practice* (9th ed.). Upper Saddle River, NJ: Pearson Education, pp. 263–264.

Posttest

1 **Answer: 2** **Rationale:** The nurse should validate his or her perceptions with the client to ensure the correct interpretation of the client's nonverbal behavior. Considering the behavior as a normal reaction to illness is likely a false assumption. Discussing the action with another nurse will not verify the cause of the behavior—only the client can provide this information. Discussing the morning schedule ignores the client's behavior and is not appropriate in this situation. **Cognitive Level:** Applying **Client Need:** Psychosocial Integrity **Integrated Process:** Communication and Documentation **Content Area:** Fundamentals **Strategy:** The critical phrase is *most appropriate.* Recall that client behavior, feelings, and concerns must be validated and explored by the nurse. **Reference:** Berman, A., & Snyder, S. J. (2012). *Kozier & Erb's fundamentals of nursing: Concepts, process, and practice* (9th ed.). Upper Saddle River, NJ: Pearson Education, pp. 465–466.

2 Answer: 3, 5 Rationale: Exploring the client's feelings indicates to the client that his or her feelings are important to the nurse and will provide the nurse with additional information about the client's concerns. Checking on the client frequently conveys that the nurse is concerned with the client's status. Providing reassurance about surgeon competency as an early action may dismiss the client's feelings as unimportant. Providing teaching to a client at this time is inappropriate because it may not be assimilated because of anxiety. Relating a personal experience focuses the attention on the nurse rather than the client and is rarely appropriate. **Cognitive Level:** Applying **Client Need:** Psychosocial Integrity **Integrated Process:** Caring **Content Area:** Fundamentals **Strategy:** The critical words in the question are *best approach.* Use knowledge of effective communication techniques to make a selection. **Reference:** Berman, A., & Snyder, S. J. (2012). *Kozier & Erb's fundamentals of nursing: Concepts, process, and practice* (9th ed.). Upper Saddle River, NJ: Pearson Education, p. 472.

3 Answer: 3 Rationale: For a client who is hearing impaired, speaking slowly in a low-pitched voice and facing the client will promote understanding of the message sent. Requesting that a family member be present would not be appropriate unless the nurse was unable to communicate with the client using other methods. Preparing written questions would be appropriate only if the client cannot hear at all and no other options are available to the nurse. Performing only the physical assessment will not provide enough information to effectively care for the client. **Cognitive Level:** Applying **Client Need:** Health Promotion and Maintenance **Integrated Process:** Communication and Documentation **Content Area:** Fundamentals **Strategy:** The core issue of the question is knowledge of appropriate communication techniques to use with clients who are hearing impaired. Recall that one should always face the hearing-impaired client so the client can see the facial expression of the examiner and because the client may be able to read lips. **Reference:** Berman, A., & Snyder, S. J. (2012). *Kozier & Erb's fundamentals of nursing: Concepts, process, and practice* (9th ed.). Upper Saddle River, NJ: Pearson Education, p. 480.

4 Answer: 4 Rationale: Documentation needs to be accurate and complete, and it should not express the opinions or judgment of the nurse. The best method for reporting subjective data is to use the client's own words. There is insufficient evidence given to support a claim that the client is depressed. Paraphrasing the client's statement does not reflect the client's words correctly. Stating the client is frustrated with being sick represents the nurse's interpretation of subjective data and may not be an accurate interpretation. **Cognitive Level:** Applying **Client Need:** Psychosocial Integrity **Integrated Process:** Communication and Documentation **Content Area:** Fundamentals **Strategy:** The core issue of the question is knowledge of principles of documentation. Recall that documentation must be factual and accurate. **Reference:** Berman, A., & Snyder, S. J. (2012). *Kozier & Erb's fundamentals of nursing: Concepts, process, and practice* (9th ed.). Upper Saddle River, NJ: Pearson Education, p. 266.

5 Answer: 3 Rationale: A prerequisite to learning a new psychomotor skill is that the client is able to physically perform the skill. In this case if the client doesn't have the dexterity to palpate a pulse or ability to see a clock's second hand, the client will need assistance with the skill. The client's cardiac status does not need to be assessed prior to implementing the teaching plan. It is unnecessary for the nurse to assess the client's reading ability before implementing the teaching plan. Motivation to attain better health is important but does not assume higher priority than the need to evaluate the client's ability to perform the skill. **Cognitive Level:** Applying **Client Need:** Health Promotion and Maintenance **Integrated Process:** Teaching and Learning **Content Area:** Fundamentals **Strategy:** Recall information about the 3 domains of learning (cognitive, affective, and psychomotor) and then recall that the nurse should ensure that the client has the mental and physical ability to carry out a new skill. **Reference:** Berman, A., & Snyder, S. J. (2012). *Kozier & Erb's fundamentals of nursing: Concepts, process, and practice* (9th ed.). Upper Saddle River, NJ: Pearson Education, p. 494.

6 Answer: 4 Rationale: Having the client actively demonstrate the procedure is the best way for the nurse to evaluate the client's level of skill. The other options are less effective ways for the nurse to evaluate the client's learning of diabetic foot care. **Cognitive Level:** Applying **Client Need:** Health Promotion and Maintenance **Integrated Process:** Teaching and Learning **Content Area:** Fundamentals **Strategy:** The critical phrase is *best evaluate a client's ability.* To choose the correct option, recall that the nurse needs to ensure that the client has the mental and physical ability to carry out the action. **Reference:** Berman, A., & Snyder, S. J. (2012). *Kozier & Erb's fundamentals of nursing: Concepts, process, and practice* (9th ed.). Upper Saddle River, NJ: Pearson Education, p. 514.

7 Answer: 1 Rationale: Learning in the cognitive domain involves the acquisition and use of knowledge mentally or intellectually. Demonstrating a skill is an example of learning in the psychomotor domain. Stating acceptance demonstrates learning in the affective domain, which involves changing feelings and values. Reading the materials that are provided does not guarantee that learning has taken place. **Cognitive Level:** Applying **Client Need:** Health Promotion and Maintenance **Integrated Process:** Teaching and Learning **Content Area:** Fundamentals

Strategy: Knowledge of the 3 domains of learning (cognitive, affective, and psychomotor) will allow you to accurately assess client education needs and select appropriate teaching strategies. **Reference:** Berman, A., & Snyder, S. J. (2012). *Kozier & Erb's fundamentals of nursing: Concepts, process, and practice* (9th ed.). Upper Saddle River, NJ: Pearson Education, p. 494.

8 **Answer: 3** **Rationale:** Critical pathways are documents that identify outcome criteria that a group of clients are expected to achieve on each day of hospitalization. Morphine is a medical prescription, not a client outcome criterion. Limiting visitors is a nursing intervention, not a client outcome criterion. Encouraging ambulation is a nursing intervention that might be used with a postoperative appendectomy client, but it is not an outcome criterion. **Cognitive Level:** Applying **Client Need:** Management of Care **Integrated Process:** Communication and Documentation **Content Area:** Fundamentals **Strategy:** The critical terms are *outcome criterion* and *critical pathway.* Recall that critical pathways contain outcome criteria that require documentation of variances whenever the outcomes are not met. Then recall the differences between goals or outcomes and orders or interventions to make a final selection. **Reference:** Berman, A., & Snyder, S. J. (2012). *Kozier & Erb's fundamentals of nursing: Concepts, process, and practice* (9th ed.). Upper Saddle River, NJ: Pearson Education, p. 260.

9 **Answer: 1** **Rationale:** Physical assessment data and client response to care are pieces of information that are most important in ensuring that client's health care needs are being met. The other options are useful to a nurse assuming care of a client but are more limited in the scope of information they provide (provider visits, new orders, vital signs, intake and output) or are not as relevant to the client's status in real time (resolved problems). **Cognitive Level:** Analyzing **Client Need:** Management of Care **Integrated Process:** Communication and Documentation **Content Area:** Fundamentals **Strategy:** Knowledge of reporting guidelines would assist you to be concise and still relay necessary information. **Reference:** Berman, A., & Snyder, S. J. (2012). *Kozier & Erb's fundamentals of nursing: Concepts, process, and practice* (9th ed.). Upper Saddle River, NJ: Pearson Education, p. 267.

10 **Answer: 4** **Rationale:** Charting by exception is a form of documentation in which notations are made if there was an exception to the standard of care or an unexpected response to care by the client. The other options about completing morning care are variations of normal data and are therefore not necessary to include in documentation using this format. **Cognitive Level:** Applying **Client Need:** Management of Care **Integrated Process:** Communication and Documentation **Content Area:** Fundamentals **Strategy:** The core issue of the question is knowledge of the method of charting by exception. Recall that care is documented on a flowsheet unless there is a problem or potential problem. **Reference:** Berman, A., & Snyder, S. J. (2012). *Kozier & Erb's fundamentals of nursing: Concepts, process, and practice* (9th ed.). Upper Saddle River, NJ: Pearson Education, p. 257.

References

Berman, A., & Snyder, S. J. (2012). *Kozier & Erb's fundamentals of nursing: Concepts, process, and practice* (9th ed.). Upper Saddle River, NJ: Pearson Education, pp. 267–269, 462–479, 486–510.

Berman, A. J., Snyder, S., & McKinney, D. (2011). *Nursing basics for clinical practice.* Upper Saddle River, NJ: Pearson Education, Inc.

Craven, R., & Hirnle, C. (2009). *Fundamentals of nursing: Human health and function* (6th ed.). Philadelphia, PA: Wolters-Kluwer.

Potter, P. & Perry, A. (2013). *Fundamentals of nursing* (8th ed.). St. Louis, MO: Mosby, Inc.

Potter, P. Perry, A., Stockert, P., & Hall, A. (2011). *Basic nursing* (7th ed.). St. Louis, MO: Mosby, Inc.

The Joint Commission. *Comprehensive Accreditation Manual for Hospitals: The Official Handbook.* Oak Brook, IL: Joint Commission Resources, 2012.

Wilkinson, J., & Treas, L. (2011). *Fundamentals of nursing* (2nd ed.). Philadelphia, PA: F. A. Davis.

ANSWERS & RATIONALES

Overview of Professional Standards

Chapter Outline

Overview of Nursing Leadership
and Management
Overview of Delegation

Ethics, Morals, and Values
Legal Concepts of Nursing
Practice

Roles of the Professional
Nurse

 NCLEX-RN® Test Prep

Use the accompanying online resource,
NursingReviewsandRationales, to test
yourself with hundreds of NCLEX®-style
practice questions.

Objectives

➤ Compare the concepts of leadership and management in relation
to nursing.
➤ Identify common management functions.
➤ Contrast the various models for delivery of nursing care.
➤ Identify the components of effective delegation.
➤ Describe the relationship of ethics, morals, and values to
professional nursing practice.
➤ Examine legal concepts and issues as they pertain to the health
care environment.
➤ Describe the 4 primary roles of the professional nurse.

Review at a Glance

accountability acceptance of own-ership for the results or lack of results of client care

ANA Code of Ethics for Nurses a statement of values devel-oped by the American Nurses Associa-tion to provide guidance to nurses and protection for clients and families

case manager an individual who oversees all aspects of nursing and health care; one who supervises the client's services and care rendered through communication, brokering of services, and procurement of available resources

decision making ability to sort through issues and data and develop a reasonable and prudent plan of action

that will lead to resolution of an actual or potential issue or problem

delegation a process of assigning others to complete a task or assignment; goals of delegation are to maintain seamless client care, improve skills of novice nurses, and spread tasks to appropriate personnel; complex tasks requiring specialized knowledge should not be delegated

ethics principles used by a person to make decisions and determine actions based upon moral beliefs

leadership use of a person's interpersonal skills to guide followers to achieve personal and/or organizational goals

malpractice professional failure to carry out or perform duties that results in injury to another

management ability to deploy resources to achieve an organization's goals

negligence an unintentional act or failure to act as a reasonably prudent person would act in the same or similar situation that results in injury to another; negligence can be an act of omission or commission

Nurse Practice Act determines the scope of professional nursing practice in a state and establishes guidelines whereby nurses can perform skills or services

1 The client is to undergo an invasive procedure. While giving information about the procedure, the nurse provides legal protection of a client's right to autonomy by doing which of the following?

1. Obtaining an informed consent
2. Demonstrating beneficence
3. Using the Good Samaritan law
4. Providing an advance directive

2 The unit manager is meeting with the director of nursing for the unit manager's yearly performance review. The director of nursing states that the unit manager needs to improve in leadership skills. In differentiating leadership from management, the nurse manager recognizes that which of the following will demonstrate an improvement in leadership skills?

1. Manager attends a workshop on budgeting unit resources
2. Manager applies for a higher position within the institution
3. Unit demonstrates a decreased number of staff sick calls per month
4. Manager uses interpersonal skills to encourage staff to work toward unit goals

3 Which of the following would be examples of a nurse using "expert power" to influence fellow staff members about a change in client care procedures? Select all that apply.

1. Using a sense of humor and good interpersonal skills to convince other nurses that change is needed
2. Demonstrating these new procedures to other staff members while providing client care
3. Giving less desirable assignments and longer scheduled night rotations to staff members who are reluctant to accept the change
4. Using valid and current data to speak positively to staff about advantages of the change over the current system
5. Providing information about the scientific evidence basis for new client care procedures

4 The nurse observes that which of the following nurse colleagues is maintaining client confidentiality?

1. A nurse who reads the records of clients not assigned to become more familiar with their disease processes.
2. A nurse who shares information about an interesting client with nurses from another unit who may eventually care for the client.
3. A nurse who allows the client's family to review the medical record to provide answers to questions.
4. A nurse who gives report on a client that is being transferred to another unit to the nurse that has been assigned to care for the client upon transfer.

5 The unit manager formulates rules and insists that everyone follow them. At unit meetings, the manager reads the rules to staff members with no discussion allowed. The nurse interprets that the staff is working under which type of leadership?

1. Autocratic
2. Democratic
3. Laissez-faire
4. Situational

6 A client is admitted following a medical procedure that is contrary to the nurse's personal values. Despite personal objections to the procedure, the nurse provides a high level of care to the client. In deciding to provide care based on what is right and wrong or good and bad, related to the client, the nurse's decision was generated from which of the following?

1. Laws
2. Ethics
3. The state Nurse Practice Act
4. State statutes

7 The client tells the nurse not to inform family members about the medical diagnosis or to share other details of the medical record. In meeting this request, the nurse would be upholding which of the following?

1. Informed consent
2. Confidentiality
3. Living will
4. Justice

8 Four nursing students are discussing the American Nurses Association (ANA) Code of Ethics for Nurses. The students who correctly understand the purpose of this document are the ones who conclude that the purpose of the code is to do which of the following? Select all that apply.

1. Assure the public that nurses will display ethical behaviors when providing client care.
2. Help protect the client and family.
3. Provide guidelines regarding care of individuals and for accountability to the profession and society.
4. Prevent certain individuals from practicing nursing by enforcing regulations that prohibit attainment of licensure.
5. Determine sanctions for nurses who do not uphold standards of ethical behavior.

9 The nursing unit is considering changing the mode of nursing care delivery to one that holds a nurse responsible and accountable over a 24-hour period for the care and treatment of a caseload. What care delivery system are the nursing staff considering using?

1. Primary nursing
2. Functional nursing
3. Total client care nursing
4. Team nursing

10 A nurse sees a motor vehicle crash and stops to provide first aid. The nurse would be protected by Good Samaritan laws in most states if which of the following occurred?

1. While offering assistance to the injured, the nurse asked another bystander to go for additional help.
2. The nurse attempts to perform a procedure he or she has not been trained to do against the wishes of the injury victim.
3. The nurse demanded payment for the aid rendered.
4. The nurse was grossly negligent in the care provided to the victim.

➤ *See pages 93–94 for Answers and Rationales.*

I. OVERVIEW OF NURSING LEADERSHIP AND MANAGEMENT

A. *Leadership*

1. Definition: a person's use of interpersonal skills to guide others to achieve personal goals and organizational goals; a good leader will utilize managerial skills to encourage, motivate, and create change

2. Essential leadership skills include delegation, problem-solving skills, good communication skills, decision making, confrontation and conflict resolution, time management, team building and leading, negotiation, motivation, and supervision
3. Leadership styles should be modified to meet the needs of the situation; leader should have a flexible style to maximize success; leadership styles include:
   a. Classic leadership styles
      1) Autocratic: no participation from others; the person in charge makes all decisions; there is no other input
      2) Democratic: the person in charge asks for input from group members; the group makes decisions; the leader facilitates discussion
      3) Laissez-faire: no one makes decisions; chaos can result; no goals are achieved; no direction is offered

Practice to Pass

Discuss the classic leadership style that is most useful when working with a professional staff.

4) Situational: the leader changes leadership style to meet the needs of the situation; if it is an emergent situation, the leader is more autocratic; other situations call for the group to make the decision
   b. Contemporary leadership styles
      1) Charismatic: characterized by an emotional relationship between staff followers and leader in which leader evokes strong feelings of commitment to leader's cause and beliefs (rare)
      2) Transactional: characterized by leader's engaging in a relationship or transaction with staff or followers in exchange for a resource valued by the follower (e.g., working overtime on one shift in exchange for a holiday off)
      3) Transformational: characterized by leader's ability to foster creativity, commitment, and collaboration by empowering staff or followers to share in the organization's vision and achieve goals
      4) Shared: characterized by organizational belief that many staff members are leaders and leadership emerges in response to challenges confronting a work group (e.g., shared governance)

B. *Management*
   1. Definition: ability to deploy resources to achieve an organization's goals; includes being accountable and responsible for accomplishing goals, coordinating and integrating resources, and using the management process (plan, staff, direct, organize, and control)
      a. A manager's power is vested within the position; a manager is not necessarily a leader
      b. Management skills can be learned
      c. A manager must effectively utilize resources, communicate effectively, and develop employees' skills to increase productivity and effectiveness
      d. Staff accomplishes work through mandates and protocols
      e. A manager has formal position and authority; it is an assigned role
   2. Common management processes
      a. Planning: schedules, job description, client care, staffing mixes, assignments, established goals, prognostication skills, strategic planning, contingency planning
      b. Staffing: hiring, firing, staff development, performance appraisals
      c. Organizing: daily activities, coordinate staff and work to be done, division of labor, chain of command in bureaucracy, delivery system, generating the skill mix of staff and staffing patterns
      d. Directing: leading, problem solving, decision making, work completion, meeting goals, use of communication skills
      e. Controlling: establish performance standards; determine means of measuring performance, evaluating performance, and giving feedback
      f. **Decision making**: the ability to sort through issues and data and develop a reasonable and prudent plan of action that will lead to resolution of an actual or potential issue or problem
         1) Multiple models
            a) Vroom–Yetton Expectancy Model: leader determines the amount of participation in making a decision; depends on quality and acceptance of decision; assists in determining the decision style
            b) Decision tree: problem is depicted with outlining of alternatives coupled with their potential consequences
            c) Program evaluation and review technique (PERT): is a network systems model; outlines and prioritizes activities and flow of events toward goal attainment within a set time frame

Practice to Pass

How does the management process assist in the attainment of organizational goals?

       d) Critical path method (CPM): depicts the order in which tasks are to be completed

  2) Types of power

      a) Reward: power comes with the notion that a manager or coordinator can offer a reward that the nurse wants; reward can include assignment, schedule, transfer, and promotion

      b) Coercive: power is derived from fear of repercussion

      c) Legitimate: power is vested in the position and sanctioned by the bureaucracy

      d) Expert: power comes from knowledge and skill; staff looks to gain knowledge from the expert

      e) Referent: power is based upon admiration and respect; followers are compliant because they like the person

      f) Information: power is derived from information or data that the follower desires

      g) Connection: power is generated by the leader's networking skills and links to influential people

      h) Position: power is vested within the actual job description, duties, responsibilities, authority, decision making, and ability to withhold and release resources and money

3. Quality management

  a. Refers to purposeful processes that are instituted to assure and improve quality of client care

  b. Involves input by staff nurses, managers, and administration for most optimal program outcomes

  c. Quality improvement teams may be unit based

  d. Quality programs may focus on one or more specific procedures or types of care delivery

C. Nursing care delivery models

1. Total patient care: nurse is responsible for carrying out all aspects of client care; case method; nurse gives care for entire shift; usually seen in critical care and postanesthesia care units

2. Functional: task-based nursing; clients' needs are divided into tasks and assigned to nurse and other staff, such as unlicensed assistants

3. Team nursing: nurse is either the team leader or a member of a delivery team; the team leader delegates tasks and responsibilities; the leader is the designated authority but should use democratic or participative style with team members; communication is essential for success

4. Primary: total responsibility for client care; the nurse facilitates care for client from admission to discharge; has 24-hour **accountability** and responsibility; plans, coordinates, and evaluates care for caseload of clients

5. Case management: nurse assigned as **case manager** ensures that needed services continue to be provided when client is discharged from hospital to home or other health care facility; it includes making arrangements for transfer as well

II. OVERVIEW OF DELEGATION

A. Overview of delegation

1. The process of assigning staff to complete a task or assignment

2. The goal of **delegation** is to maintain quality client care, improve the skills of novice nurses, and spread tasks to appropriate personnel

---

▶ **Practice to Pass**

What types of power does a new graduate in nursing have?

    3. Client assessment, client teaching, and complex tasks requiring specialized knowledge cannot be delegated

B. Principles and procedures used in delegation

    1. The nurse must assess the client and be sure the client is stable before delegating any task to unlicensed assistive personnel (UAP)

    2. Delegated tasks should be routine for both the client and UAP who will be performing the task

    3. Tasks to be delegated cannot require a substantial amount of scientific knowledge or skill, and task outcomes should be routine and predictable

    4. Agency policies and procedures should be followed by both the delegating nurse and the UAP to whom the task is delegated

    5. The nurse must be aware of the scope of practice and the job descriptions of anyone to whom the nurse is delegating tasks

    6. The nurse must be aware of the individual skills and abilities of UAP to whom the nurse is delegating tasks; remember, not every person may be competent in every skill in his or her job description

    7. If the nurse is not certain of a UAP's ability to perform specific tasks, the nurse should observe the UAP perform the task and demonstrate the correct technique(s) as needed

    8. Expectations must be clearly communicated, including exactly what tasks are to be performed, when they are to be done, what the expected outcomes are, who is available as a resource if needed, and what type of report is expected

    9. The nurse should create an environment of open communication; this will foster learning and improved client care

C. Obstacles to delegation

    1. Nonsupportive environment: the environment must be conducive to developing all personnel and achieving goals

    2. Limited resources: financial issues may prevent the ability to delegate; these may relate to either finances, number of qualified personnel, or necessary equipment

    3. Inexperience: a staff member's inexperience can be a hindrance to delegation; an institution can minimize this through competency-based orientation and testing; the nurse delegating the task sometimes must teach the novice the necessary skills to complete the task; with proper guidance, delegating can improve the novice's skills

    4. Fear of liability: the nurse must have the skill and knowledge to perform the task or oversee completion of the request; delegation should only be done with thorough knowledge of what needs to be done as well as appropriate supervision

    5. Fear of burdening coworkers: requesting assistance or delegating a task should be done after assessing the workload of other nurses; the assignment should not overwhelm the nurse thereby causing omissions or mistakes to occur

    6. Unwillingness of workers to accept delegated tasks: the staff should not refuse a request unless it will compromise the care of their clients

    7. Fear of failure: this can serve to motivate the nurse to learn more about the task or work toward developing the necessary skills to successfully complete the task; if the nurse is afraid of failure, these concerns must be articulated to the supervisor and assistance requested; the task or assignment should not be delegated to an unprepared nurse

D. Inappropriate delegation

    1. Underdelegation: can occur if delegator does not think that a staff member can perform an assignment and completes the assignment without delegating

        a. It is crucial to develop staff that can provide comprehensive client care

        b. If unable to perform tasks, staff development should occur to improve skills

c. Delegation should be done with caution until staff members are prepared to complete assigned skills

d. Nurses who need assistance should ask for it

2. Reverse delegation: staff requests that manager or leader completes the task because of their inability or unwillingness to do so; this can be minimized with the use of competency-based orientation programs and in-services

3. Overdelegation: tasks are delegated inappropriately; the nurse cannot successfully achieve goals if overwhelmed by numerous requests; each nurse must scrutinize the ability to take an assigned request; a good leader will balance requests after assessing needs of the unit and clients; UAP and new graduate nurses should not be assigned tasks for which they are not prepared or that are beyond their scope of practice

Practice to Pass

What should the nurse consider when delegating tasks to unlicensed assistive personnel?

III. ETHICS, MORALS, AND VALUES

A. Ethics

1. A code upon which a person bases actions and decisions
2. The process of determining right from wrong, good and bad
3. Decisions are guided by beliefs and values
4. Governs relationships with family and society
5. Are moral truths that guide thought process and actions
6. Represent the practical application of a moral philosophy

B. Ethical theories: values and behaviors are explained based on a particular viewpoint

1. Utilitarianism: what determines whether an act is *good* or *bad*, *right* or *wrong* is the outcome or consequence of that act

2. Deontology (or Kantianism): moral values are absolute and apply to all people; right is always right, and wrong is always wrong; nurses have a duty to others to behave in certain ways and to choose right actions

3. Virtue ethics: actions are chosen based on internal moral values, such as honesty, compassion, caring, responsibility, and trustworthiness; nurses make right decisions because of their moral character

Practice to Pass

How does the ANA Code of Ethics for Nurses guide nursing practice?

C. Ethical principles: guide practice and **decision making** (see Box 4-1)

D. Code of Ethics

1. The **ANA Code of Ethics for Nurses** was developed by American Nurses Association to provide guidance to the nurse and protection for the client and family (see Box 4-2)

2. The guidelines delineate values and standards for professional practice

E. Morals: a personal philosophy based on what is right or wrong, or good or bad; ethics is practical way of putting morals into practice; leads to decision making and problem solving; ethical considerations define morals essential to practice

F. Values: are personally and professionally developed and are based on philosophy and principles; values shape actions and reactions to issues and problems; provide guidance in determining actions; socialization and experiences help mold the value system

IV. LEGAL CONCEPTS OF NURSING PRACTICE

A. The practice of nursing must be done within the confines of the law; it is mandatory that nurses know the law and parameters of a nursing license

B. Legal limits of nursing: dictated by each state's board of nursing as well as state and federal laws and guidelines

1. Constitution: the law of the land; defines structure, power and limits of government, guarantees fundamental rights and liberty; other laws may not infringe on rights granted by the Constitution

Box 4-1	
Ethical Principles	

- Autonomy: consists of freedom to make decisions that will impact welfare and take action for self; is self-governing; includes 4 basic elements:
  - Respect for others
  - Ability to determine personal goals
  - Complete understanding of choice
  - Freedom to implement plan or choice
- Parentalism: is the opposite of autonomy; to act in a fatherly or motherly manner; usually restricts client's autonomy and coerces decision making; assumes that the care giver (by virtue of their knowledge and experience) knows what is best for the client; completely removes the power to make decisions from the client or client's family
- Beneficence and Nonmaleficence: to act in the best interest of others; to contribute to the well-being of others; includes client advocacy; has 3 major components:
  - To promote good (beneficence)
  - To prevent harm or evil (nonmaleficence)
  - To remove harm or evil
- Justice: fair, equitable, and appropriate treatment; resources are distributed equally to all
- Fidelity: remaining faithful to ethical principles and the ANA Code of Ethics for Nurses (see section on ANA Code of Ethics for Nurses); keeping commitments and promises
- Veracity: truth telling; compels the whole truth to be told
- Confidentiality: to maintain the privacy of the client of family; nondisclosure of data or personal information; is a component of ANA Code of Ethics for Nurses (see section on ANA Code of Ethics for Nurses)

Box 4-2	
American Nurses Association Code of Ethics for Nurses	

1. The nurse, in all professional relationships, practices with compassion and respect for the inherent dignity, worth and uniqueness of every individual, unrestricted by considerations of social or economic status, personal attributes, or the nature of health problems.
2. The nurse's primary commitment is to the patient, whether an individual, family, group, or community.
3. The nurse promotes, advocates for, and strives to protect the health, safety, and rights of the patient.
4. The nurse is responsible and accountable for individual nursing practice and determines the appropriate delegation of tasks consistent with the nurse's obligation to provide optimum patient care.
5. The nurse owes the same duties to self as to others, including the responsibility to preserve integrity and safety, to maintain competence, and to continue personal and professional growth.
6. The nurse participates in establishing, maintaining, and improving health care environments and conditions of employment conducive to the provision of quality health care and consistent with the values of the profession through individual and collective action.
7. The nurse participates in the advancement of the profession through contributions to practice, education, administration, and knowledge development.
8. The nurse collaborates with other health professionals and the public in promoting community, national, and international efforts to meet health needs.
9. The profession of nursing, as represented by associations and their members, is responsible for articulating nursing values, for maintaining the integrity of the profession and its practice, and for shaping social policy.

2. Statutory laws: laws enacted by legislative branch of government; includes licensing laws, guardianship codes, statutes of limitation, informed consent, living will legislation, protective and reporting laws; regulatory agencies are established through statutes

3. Common laws: judge-made law, derived from court decisions that establish a precedent by which other cases are judged

4. Administrative laws: laws made by administrative agencies, such as a state board of nursing

C. **Accountability:** accepting ownership for results or lack of results; there is responsibility to provide professional nursing practice for all; efforts are made to provide quality care

D. **Responsibility:** obligates a person to accomplish a task; with delegation, the responsibility must transfer also to the one assigned to complete an assignment; accountability is shared

E. **Good Samaritan laws:** designed to protect those who aid victims in emergencies

1. Statutes vary from state to state

2. It is important for each nursing professional to review that state's law

3. Situation must be an emergency; care rendered must be free of charge; provided care must be in good faith; cannot willingly or intentionally harm the victim

4. Will not protect the nurse if nurse is grossly negligent

5. Once aid is offered, must stay with victim until victim is stable or another provider with equal or greater training can take over

F. **Licensure:** a credential determined by state boards of nursing; requires completion of a nursing curriculum that leads to successful passage of a licensing examination; licensure qualifies an individual to perform designated skills and services

1. **Nurse Practice Act:** determines the scope of the professional nurse in a specific state

   a. Establishes guidelines whereby the nurse can perform skills or services

   b. The Nurse Practice Act is a set of state statutes (rules and regulations) that provide guidance to professional nurses

   c. Establishes educational, examination, and behavioral standards for nurses that protect the public

   d. To enforce these requirements, each state has a board of registration in nursing in the role of overseer

2. Liability: nurses are responsible and accountable for actions or inactions

G. **Negligence:** performance of an unintentional act or a failure to perform an act that a reasonable person would do in a similar situation that results in injury to another; the failure to act as a reasonable person; elements include:

1. Duty: the nurse has a responsibility to care for and watch over client as a component of employment; duty indicates a legal relationship between client and the nurse

2. Breech of duty: the nurse failed to complete this duty; can include acts of commission (activities the nurse did) or omission (activities the nurse failed to do)

3. Cause: there is a reasonably close causal connection between the nurse's conduct and a resulting injury

4. Injury occurred: the client has suffered physical, emotional, or financial injury; there is an actual loss or damage resulting from conduct

H. **Malpractice**

1. Negligence by a professional; professional failure to carry out or perform duties that result in the injury of another; scope of practice should be delineated in order to operate within it

2. The boundaries of malpractice are defined by statute, rules, and educational requirement

3. Malpractice is usually filed as a civil tort; a court finding of guilty usually results in restitution

4. The nurse may carry personal malpractice insurance to provide for restitution if malpractice occurs

Practice to Pass

How does the Good Samaritan law protect nurses?

5. Rarely are malpractice charges filed as criminal charges (under a finding in which a guilty verdict results in punishment, either jail or capital punishment)
6. Nursing activities to reduce risk of liability in lawsuits
   a. Practice within provisions of state Nurse Practice Act
   b. Follow ANA Code of Ethics for Nurses and standards of professional practice
   c. Treat every client with kindness and respect
   d. Maintain skills and knowledge base by completing continuing education programs
   e. Recognize personal strengths and weaknesses; seek help when facing new experiences and job requirements

Practice to Pass

How can the nurse avoid accusations of malpractice?

I. Issues in nursing practice

1. Health care provider (HCP) prescriptions
   a. Determine the prescriptive course of action; guide the course of action for client and family
   b. Includes prescriptive orders for:
      1) Medications
      2) Diet
      3) Activity level
      4) Length of stay
      5) Tests: diagnostic, blood, x-rays, procedures
   c. Nurses' actions are led by HCP prescriptions
   d. If prescriptions are inappropriate, the nurse should question and clarify them; the nurse should ensure the prescribed amount of medication is a proper dose; the nurse is responsible for knowing pharmacological principles, drug interactions, and proper dosages
      1) If an order does not seem correct, the nurse should act on the client's behalf
      2) A nurse should never give a medication that is prescribed as a toxic dose
   e. Explain prescribed procedures to client and ask for feedback
   f. HCP prescriptions should be scrutinized for legibility and accuracy; when in doubt, clarify them with the HCP

2. Informed consent: a legal protection of client rights; a client has the right to choose the type of care desired and make own decisions
   a. Informed consent is required before providing care except in an emergency situation, when the assumption exists that the client would consent if able (implied consent)
   b. The client can refuse treatment
   c. Informed consent must meet 3 requirements
      1) The individual has capacity to consent
      2) Consent is given voluntarily (freely without coercion)
      3) The individual understands the treatment and information presented
   d. Informed consent involves 2 steps
      1) Provision of information to client that includes what is being done, why it is being done, risks of a procedure, and possible alternatives to a procedure (with sufficient detail to allow client to decide whether to proceed with treatment or not); requires full disclosure
      2) Actually obtaining the consent (the person performing the procedure is required to obtain the consent)

3. Organ/tissue donation: an end-of-life issue; client must be legally dead to donate organs; a decision can be made in advance when client is alive and competent or may be made at time of death by family
   a. Transplant team harvests organs after consent is obtained
   b. Bereaved family must be approached with compassion in requesting a discussion on organ donation

    c. Goal is to assist those in need of transplant with the organ necessary to prolong life

    d. Clinical death is defined as having no brain function, no spontaneous breathing, and no response to painful stimuli; spinal reflexes may persist

4. Advance directives: a document the individual completes when competent outlining the care desired to receive in the future; advance directives are followed if client's decision-making powers are altered and they serve to provide guidance to the health care team

5. Incident reports: each agency develops a protocol for reporting unusual or adverse events involving clients; incident reports are communication tools designed to provide information to risk managers, administration, and may be used in legal cases; incident reports are used to identify problems and develop solutions to prevent the same incident from happening again

6. Risk management: goals of risk management are to protect the client and the nurse from harm, and protect the organization from liability related to harm

    a. Risk management includes:

        1) Organizational commitment to employee health and safety

        2) Comprehensive worksite risk analysis

        3) Employee participation

        4) Hazard prevention and control including waste management

    b. Guidelines are consistent with those of the Occupational Safety and Health Administration (OSHA)

7. The Joint Commission (formerly known as JCAHO) establishes guidelines for accreditation of institution or agency; health care institutions abide by standards or lose accreditation; accreditation demonstrates an acceptable level of performance

V. ROLES OF THE PROFESSIONAL NURSE

A. Direct care provider

1. The nurse provides total care for the client

2. The nurse uses the nursing process to develop an appropriate plan of care, carry it out, and evaluate its effectiveness

3. The nurse utilizes the skills of assessment, planning, intervention, and evaluation to meet client needs

4. Documentation methodically records all data acquired through interaction with client and other health care workers

5. The direct care provider may delegate some responsibilities to professional and nonprofessional personnel

B. Client advocate

1. In this role, the nurse becomes an activist speaking up for the client who cannot or will not speak for self

2. The client advocate seeks what is best for the client

3. The client advocate:

    a. Respects and upholds client's rights

    b. Ensures that client needs are met

    c. Can act as a mediator among client, family, and health care provider

    d. Provides support to the client

4. Client advocacy requires good communication skills and assertiveness on the part of the nurse

5. State Nurse Practice Acts may include nurse advocacy roles in the definition of nursing

C. *Case manager*

1. A case manager oversees all aspects of care

2. This individual attempts to procure medications and equipment, consults other disciplines, holds conferences about clients, prepares clients for discharge, and makes appropriate referrals

3. In doing these things, the case manager:
   a. Facilitates delivery of cost-efficient care
   b. Individualizes care
   c. Coordinates care
   d. Applies tools, skills, and techniques toward the desired outcome
   e. Collaborates with other health care professionals to coordinate care
   f. Monitors and evaluates options and services to meet individual and family needs

D. Client and family educator
   1. Involves instruction regarding medications, health promotion, disease prevention, and discharge
   2. Includes referring client and family to appropriate resources, literature, and websites
   3. Incorporates good communication among client, family, and health care team members

Case Study

While driving home from the hospital on a rainy evening, a registered nurse (RN) witnesses a minivan slide off the road into a tree. The nurse stops the car and runs to the mangled minivan. As the nurse looks inside the driver's window, 2 semiconscious teenagers are observed in seatbelts and are moaning for help.

1. As an RN, does the nurse have a legal obligation to stop?

2. Are Good Samaritan laws uniform from state to state?

3. If the driver and passenger are slightly injured, is the nurse bound by law to assist them?

For suggested responses, see pages 306–307.

4. If the nurse intentionally injures the victim, does the Good Samaritan law cover the nurse from liability?

5. When can the nurse leave the scene of this accident?

POSTTEST

POSTTEST

❶ Because a nurse caring for a surgical client fails to monitor the client adequately during the postoperative period according to the standard of care, the client experiences surgical complications. The nurse concludes that this action is consistent with which of the following?

1. Practicing medicine without a license
2. Malpractice for failure to observe and take appropriate action
3. A misdemeanor
4. Failure to follow the Good Samaritan law

❷ A 45-year-old male Hispanic client who speaks very little English is scheduled for surgery tomorrow. The nurse is concerned that the informed consent signed by the client on admission may not be valid for which reason?

1. The surgical consent form was not notarized.
2. It was witnessed by unlicensed personnel.
3. The client may not understand the document he signed, which outlines treatment and associated risks.
4. The client may be an undocumented immigrant.

POSTTEST

③ The new graduate nurse asks the nursing unit manager to share strategies aimed at risk management. The manager correctly recommends which of the following? Select all that apply.

1. Treat every client with kindness and respect.
2. Seek help when facing new situations if unsure about which course of action is best.
3. Observe and report suspicious behavior of colleagues.
4. Be aware of the provisions of the state's Nurse Practice Act, and function within those provisions.
5. Refuse to assist in the care of clients assigned to other nurses.

④ The clinic managers want nurses working in the unit to administer moderate sedation. To legally include this procedure in their practice, the staff nurses determine first that it is acceptable according to which source?

1. The agency's policy and procedure book
2. The nurse's liability insurance
3. Good Samaritan law
4. The state's Nurse Practice Act

⑤ A client diagnosed with early Alzheimer's disease is currently competent to make health care decisions regarding future needs. The nurse counsels the client to contact a lawyer about which of the following?

1. Advance directives
2. Temporary power of attorney
3. Self-determination
4. Informed consent

⑥ The nurse is aware that no health care provider has visited a hospitalized client for 3 consecutive days. The nurse reports this event to the nursing supervisor after determining that it is necessary to execute which nursing role?

1. Direct care provider role
2. Case manager role
3. Client educator role
4. Client advocate role

⑦ Which of the following situations observed by a nurse would be an example of overdelegation? Select all that apply.

1. A registered nurse with 3 months of experience who recently finished orientation to a hospital unit is assigned as shift charge nurse because the regular charge nurse is out ill.
2. An evening staff nurse expects the charge nurse to give report on all clients to the night shift so the nurse can leave the unit on time.
3. An experienced nursing assistant is assigned to change all the central line dressings on the unit.
4. An experienced staff nurse is assigned to orient a new graduate to the unit after the new nurse completes general orientation to the hospital.
5. A staff nurse reviews the procedure for a 24-hour urine collection with a nursing assistant who has floated to the unit for the shift.

⑧ A staff nurse is assigned responsibility for the care of an assigned client from admission to discharge. When the staff nurse is not on duty, others on the unit provide care based on instructions left by the staff nurse. The nurse understands that which care delivery system is being utilized on this unit?

1. Primary nursing
2. Team nursing
3. Case management
4. Functional nursing

9 The nurse recognizes that which of the following must be supplied to a client before an informed consent can be obtained? Select all that apply.

1. A description of the procedure to be done
2. Why the procedure is needed
3. What time the procedure will be done
4. Risks associated with the procedure
5. Possible alternative treatments that might have similar results for the client

10 A nursing student hears a client request a prescription for oral antibiotics after being diagnosed with strep throat. The provider tells the client, "oral medications will not work for your problem; an injection of antibiotics is the only way to get you well." After leaving the exam room, the provider tells the student, "This client will never take 10 days worth of antibiotics so we will just give them to her IM now and be done with it." The student understands that the provider has acted in what manner?

1. Beneficent
2. Paternalistic
3. Nonmaleficent
4. Compassionate

➤ *See pages 95–96 for Answers and Rationales.*

ANSWERS & RATIONALES

Pretest

1 **Answer: 1** **Rationale:** Informed consent provides legal protection for a client's right to autonomy and to choose his or her own medical treatment. Beneficence is the ethical term that means a person will seek to do good for others (i.e., act in the best interest of others). The Good Samaritan law protects health care providers who come to the aid of others during an emergency. Advanced directives determine the actions of the health care team when the client is unable to make decisions about their own care. **Cognitive Level:** Applying **Client Need:** Management of Care **Integrated Process:** Communication and Documentation **Content Area:** Fundamentals **Strategy:** The critical words are *right to autonomy.* Use knowledge of ethical principles to guide nursing practice and assist in making correct practice decisions. **Reference:** Berman, A., & Snyder, S. J. (2012). *Kozier & Erb's fundamentals of nursing: Concepts, process, and practice* (9th ed.). Upper Saddle River, NJ: Pearson Education, p. 85.

2 **Answer: 4** **Rationale:** Use of interpersonal skills to motivate others to achieve goals is a hallmark of leadership. Budgeting unit resources is a managerial skill, not a leadership skill. Applying for a higher position in the organization demonstrates an attempt to move to a higher level of management. The number of sick calls per month relates to many factors but could be influenced by management skills, not leadership skills. **Cognitive Level:** Applying **Client Need:** Management of Care **Integrated Process:** Nursing Process: Implementation **Content Area:** Fundamentals **Strategy:** The critical phrase is *improvement in leadership skills.* Recall basic principles of nursing leadership and management to determine which skill needs to be developed for improved performance. **Reference:** Berman, A., & Snyder, S. J. (2012). *Kozier & Erb's fundamentals of nursing: Concepts, process, and practice* (9th ed.). Upper Saddle River, NJ: Pearson Education, p. 519.

3 **Answer: 2, 4, 5** **Rationale:** Expert power has its roots in the knowledge and skill of the practitioner, which are admired and emulated by others in the group. Expert power relies on the expert skills of the practitioner to gain the admiration and confidence of the group. Referent power relies on interpersonal skills to promote change and motivate others. Coercion uses fear and threats to motivate others to do what you wish. It is not usually an effective use of power. **Cognitive Level:** Applying **Client Need:** Management of Care **Integrated Process:** Nursing Process: Implementation **Content Area:** Fundamentals **Strategy:** The critical phrase is *expert power.* Recall the types of power and their appropriate uses to make a selection. **Reference:** Berman, A., & Snyder, S. J. (2012). *Kozier & Erb's fundamentals of nursing: Concepts, process, and practice* (9th ed.). Upper Saddle River, NJ: Pearson Education, p. 521.

4 **Answer: 4** **Rationale:** The client has a right to confidentiality. Unless a nurse is assigned currently to care for an individual, the nurse should not seek or share details about a client's status. Family members would need approval from the client and the provider prior to reviewing a medical record. **Cognitive Level:** Applying **Client Need:** Management of Care **Integrated Process:**

Communication and Documentation **Content Area:** Fundamentals **Strategy:** The core issue of the question is knowledge about how to maintain client confidentiality. Recall that the American Nurses Association (ANA) Code of Ethics guides you to protect client rights and states that all client information is confidential. **Reference:** Berman, A., & Snyder, S. J. (2012). *Kozier & Erb's fundamentals of nursing: Concepts, process, and practice* (9th ed.). Upper Saddle River, NJ: Pearson Education, p. 72.

5 Answer: 1 Rationale: The unit manager allows no input from anyone else, and all decisions are made by this individual; this is consistent with autocratic leadership. Democratic leadership seeks input from those to be affected by proposed change. Laissez-faire leadership is characterized by lack of decision making; the leader allows everyone to make their own rules. In situational leadership, the individual adapts his or her style according to the needs at the time. **Cognitive Level:** Applying **Client Need:** Management of Care **Integrated Process:** Communication and Documentation **Content Area:** Fundamentals **Strategy:** Use knowledge of leadership styles to choose the option that best matches the behavior of the manager in the question. **Reference:** Berman, A., & Snyder, S. J. (2012). *Kozier & Erb's fundamentals of nursing: Concepts, process, and practice* (9th ed.). Upper Saddle River, NJ: Pearson Education, pp. 519–521.

6 Answer: 2 Rationale: Ethics is a science that deals with rights and wrongs, the "good and bad" of human decision making and behavior. Laws are considered rules of society. Laws are considered rules of society and include practice acts. Laws are considered rules of society and include statutes. **Cognitive Level:** Applying **Client Need:** Management of Care **Integrated Process:** Caring **Content Area:** Fundamentals **Strategy:** Use knowledge of how to discriminate legal from ethical matters to make an appropriate selection. **Reference:** Berman, A., & Snyder, S. J. (2012). *Kozier & Erb's fundamentals of nursing: Concepts, process, and practice* (9th ed.). Upper Saddle River, NJ: Pearson Education, pp. 57, 82–88.

7 Answer: 2 Rationale: Confidentiality protects the privacy of clients and their records. Informed consent is necessary prior to the treatment of the client but does not dictate how private information is handled. A living will is a document in which the client chooses end-of-life procedures in the event he or she becomes unable to make those decisions. Justice demands that fair and equitable treatment is given to all people and that resources are distributed equally. **Cognitive Level:** Applying **Client Need:** Management of Care **Integrated Process:** Communication and Documentation **Content Area:** Fundamentals **Strategy:** Recall the definitions of the various terms in the options and determine the one that protects client rights as outlined in this question. **Reference:** Berman, A., & Snyder, S. J. (2012). *Kozier & Erb's fundamentals of nursing: Concepts, process, and*

practice (9th ed.). Upper Saddle River, NJ: Pearson Education, p. 72.

8 Answer: 2, 3 Rationale: One of the purposes of the Code of Ethics is to provide protection to the client and family. The purpose of the American Nurses Association (ANA) Code of Ethics for Nurses is to provide guidelines regarding care and accountability. No document can assure the public that nurses will display ethical behaviors. Regulations regarding licensure are within the purview of state statutes. The Code of Ethics for Nurses does not have provisions for sanctions for individual nurses who do not uphold one of more of the statements in the Code. **Cognitive Level:** Applying **Client Need:** Management of Care **Integrated Process:** Communication and Documentation **Content Area:** Fundamentals **Strategy:** The critical phrase in the question is *the purpose of the code.* Recall that the American Nurses Association (ANA) Code of Ethics delineates the values and standards for professional nursing practice. **Reference:** Berman, A., & Snyder, S. J. (2012). *Kozier & Erb's fundamentals of nursing: Concepts, process, and practice* (9th ed.). Upper Saddle River, NJ: Pearson Education, pp. 87–88.

9 Answer: 1 Rationale: Primary nursing holds the nurse accountable for the care of a caseload of clients over a 24-hour period. Functional nursing focuses on tasks to be completed; tasks are assigned based on the provider's skill levels. With total client care nursing, the nurse provides all care for assigned clients for the duration of the work shift. Team nursing is a group of personnel that work together to provide care for a group of clients with each team member having a specific role for all clients in the group. **Cognitive Level:** Understanding **Client Need:** Management of Care **Integrated Process:** Nursing Process: Implementation **Content Area:** Fundamentals **Strategy:** The critical phrase is *accountable over a 24-hour period.* Recall the specific characteristics of various nursing care delivery systems. **Reference:** Berman, A., & Snyder, S. J. (2012). *Kozier & Erb's fundamentals of nursing: Concepts, process, and practice* (9th ed.). Upper Saddle River, NJ: Pearson Education, p. 110.

10 Answer: 1 Rationale: Remaining with a client and providing assistance after an injury is in keeping with the Good Samaritan law. Nurses should not attempt to perform procedures they are unfamiliar with against the wishes of a client. Care provided under the Good Samaritan law is not for a fee. The Good Samaritan law will not protect nurses who are negligent in care to clients. **Cognitive Level:** Applying **Client Need:** Management of Care **Integrated Process:** Caring **Content Area:** Fundamentals **Strategy:** The critical term is *Good Samaritan law.* Knowledge of this law will provide guidance for the nurse seeking to render aid in an emergency. **Reference:** Berman, A., & Snyder, S. J. (2012). *Kozier & Erb's fundamentals of nursing: Concepts, process, and practice* (9th ed.). Upper Saddle River, NJ: Pearson Education, p. 73.

ANSWERS & RATIONALES

Posttest

1 **Answer: 2** **Rationale:** Malpractice is defined as professional negligence. It occurs when a professional fails to act in a way that a reasonable, prudent person with the same experience and training would act in a similar situation. Monitoring postoperative clients is a nursing responsibility and is not related to medical practice. A misdemeanor is a criminal offense of a less serious nature. Since the nature and severity of complications are not disclosed, it is not possible to determine if the nurse's actions were criminal in nature. Good Samaritan laws protect those who help others in emergency situations; they do not apply to events that occur in a nurse's work setting. **Cognitive Level:** Applying **Client Need:** Management of Care **Integrated Process:** Nursing Process: Implementation **Content Area:** Fundamentals **Strategy:** Recall legal concepts of nursing practice to recognize which principle is related to the current situation. **Reference:** Berman, A., & Snyder, S. J. (2012). *Kozier & Erb's fundamentals of nursing: Concepts, process, and practice* (9th ed.). Upper Saddle River, NJ: Pearson Education, p. 68.

2 **Answer: 3** **Rationale:** Informed consent must always meet 3 requirements: It must be voluntary, the individual must have the capacity to consent, and the individual must understand the treatment and associated information in the consent document. Because of the language barrier, the client might not understand what he was consenting to, and if so, the document is not valid. A surgical consent document is not required to be notarized. It is not necessary for witnesses to be licensed personnel. The client's immigration status is unrelated to consent. **Cognitive Level:** Analyzing **Client Need:** Management of Care **Integrated Process:** Communication and Documentation **Content Area:** Fundamentals **Strategy:** Consider the necessary requirements to have an informed consent and use the process of elimination to make a selection. **Reference:** Berman, A., & Snyder, S. J. (2012). *Kozier & Erb's fundamentals of nursing: Concepts, process, and practice* (9th ed.). Upper Saddle River, NJ: Pearson Education, p. 59.

3 **Answer: 1, 2, 4** **Rationale:** Treating all clients with kindness and respect will reduce the nurse's risk of liability in lawsuits. Seeking assistance when confronted with new situations will reduce the nurse's risk of liability in lawsuits by helping to prevent errors in care. Practice within the provisions of the Nurse Practice Act is essential to legal nursing practice. Observing and reporting suspicious behavior is vague and does not relate directly to risk management. Refusing to help other nurses is unprofessional and at times could increase the risk of harm to clients if the unit were understaffed. **Cognitive Level:** Applying **Client Need:** Management of Care **Integrated Process:** Nursing Process: Implementation **Content Area:** Fundamentals **Strategy:** The core concept in the question is risk management. Recalling common

strategies for reducing the nurse's risk of liability in lawsuits may help prevent unnecessary involvement in legal proceedings. **Reference:** Berman, A., & Snyder, S. J. (2012). *Kozier & Erb's fundamentals of nursing: Concepts, process, and practice* (9th ed.). Upper Saddle River, NJ: Pearson Education, pp. 72–73.

4 **Answer: 4** **Rationale:** Each state has its own Nurse Practice Act that provides parameters within which nurses practice. Each state has a different interpretation of the individual acts; the Nurse Practice Act delineates the scope of practice. The agency's policy and procedures would be modified if new nursing responsibilities are assigned; however, agency policy must be consistent with the state Nurse Practice Act. Liability insurance coverage determines under what conditions the insurance company will pay a claim. Good Samaritan laws cover emergency aid rendered outside of employment. **Cognitive Level:** Applying **Client Need:** Management of Care **Integrated Process:** Communication and Documentation **Content Area:** Fundamentals **Strategy:** The critical word in the question is *first.* Nurse Practice Acts determine the scope of practice for registered nurses within each state. **Reference:** Berman, A., & Snyder, S. J. (2012). *Kozier & Erb's fundamentals of nursing: Concepts, process, and practice* (9th ed.). Upper Saddle River, NJ: Pearson Education, pp. 54–56.

5 **Answer: 1** **Rationale:** Advance directives offer guidance to the health care team when the client cannot make a decision regarding his or her own treatment. Advance directives must be written when the client is competent. The durable (not temporary) power of attorney allows a competent person the power to act on the behalf of the client in the event that the client loses decision-making capacity. The Self-Determination Act mandates that health care staff must offer the client information regarding health care decisions. Informed consent is a crucial component of health care and seeks to alert the client to all avenues of care and treatment. **Cognitive Level:** Applying **Client Need:** Management of Care **Integrated Process:** Teaching and Learning **Content Area:** Fundamentals **Strategy:** The critical phrase is *currently competent to make health care decisions regarding future needs.* Recall strategies for allowing clients to insure that their health care requests are carried out. **Reference:** Berman, A., & Snyder, S. J. (2012). *Kozier & Erb's fundamentals of nursing: Concepts, process, and practice* (9th ed.). Upper Saddle River, NJ: Pearson Education, p. 65.

6 **Answer: 4** **Rationale:** A client advocate is one who expresses and defends the cause of the client. It is the nurse's responsibility to ensure the client has access to health care services that meet health needs. A direct care provider administers nursing care such as medications and treatments. A case manager provides for continuity of care and coordination of care services. A client educator provides instruction to clients and families. **Cognitive Level:** Applying **Client Need:** Management of Care **Integrated Process:** Nursing Process:

Implementation **Content Area:** Fundamentals **Strategy:** Knowledge of basic nursing roles will assist in making the correct selection. **Reference:** Berman, A., & Snyder, S. J. (2012). *Kozier & Erb's fundamentals of nursing: Concepts, process, and practice* (9th ed.). Upper Saddle River, NJ: Pearson Education, p. 16.

7 **Answer: 1** **Rationale:** Overdelegation occurs when too much authority or accountability is transferred to the delegate as demonstrated in this example. Unlicensed assistive personnel should not be assigned tasks that are beyond their scope of practice regardless of their experience level. Reverse delegation occurs when authority is transferred to an individual of higher rank as in this example. Properly assigned staff activities are an example of appropriate delegation. It is appropriate to ensure that a delegate understands how to complete the task that is delegated. **Cognitive Level:** Understanding **Client Need:** Management of Care **Integrated Process:** Nursing Process: Implementation **Content Area:** Fundamentals **Strategy:** The core concept being tested is overdelegation. Use knowledge of this concept to select the appropriate option. **Reference:** Berman, A., & Snyder, S. J. (2012). *Kozier & Erb's fundamentals of nursing: Concepts, process, and practice* (9th ed.). Upper Saddle River, NJ: Pearson Education, p. 524.

8 **Answer: 1** **Rationale:** In primary nursing, 1 nurse is responsible for total care of a number of clients, 24 hours a day, 7 days a week. When the nurse is not present, she leaves directions for the client's care that are carried out by others on the unit. Team nursing provides nursing care to clients by a multimember nursing team led by a professional nurse. The case manager may or may not provide direct client care but coordinates health care among numerous health care workers. Functional nursing is task based and assigns different team members to complete various nursing activities, such as taking vital signs, changing dressings, or administering medications. **Cognitive Level:** Analyzing **Client Need:** Management of Care **Integrated Process:** Nursing Process: Implementation **Content Area:** Fundamentals **Strategy:** The critical phrase is *responsible for the care of a client from admission to discharge.* Use knowledge of nursing care delivery models and the process of elimination to make

a selection. **Reference:** Berman, A., & Snyder, S. J. (2012). *Kozier & Erb's fundamentals of nursing: Concepts, process, and practice* (9th ed.). Upper Saddle River, NJ: Pearson Education, p. 110.

9 **Answer: 1, 2, 4, 5** **Rationale:** Informed consent requires that the client be informed about what is to be done. Informed consent requires that the client be informed about why the procedure is needed. Informed consent requires that the client be informed about potential risks of the procedure. Informed consent requires that the client be informed about what is to be done, why it is needed, and possible treatment alternatives as well as potential risks of the procedure. It is not always possible to predict exactly when procedures will be performed, and this is not an essential element of informed consent. **Cognitive Level:** Applying **Client Need:** Management of Care **Integrated Process:** Communication and Documentation **Content Area:** Fundamentals **Strategy:** The critical words are *informed consent.* Knowledge of the elements of informed consent will aid in selecting the appropriate choices. **Reference:** Berman, A., & Snyder, S. J. (2012). *Kozier & Erb's fundamentals of nursing: Concepts, process, and practice* (9th ed.). Upper Saddle River, NJ: Pearson Education, p. 59.

10 **Answer: 2** **Rationale:** Paternalism means to act as a father to a child. It restricts the client's autonomy and generally assumes that the person making the decision knows more about what is best for the client than the client does. In this case, the provider assumed he knew what was best for the client in spite of her expressed wishes. Beneficence requires one to act in the best interest of others, to seek to do good. Nonmaleficence means to avoid doing harm to others. If acting from compassion, the provider would have considered the client's request in a desire to relieve her suffering. **Cognitive Level:** Applying **Client Need:** Management of Care **Integrated Process:** Communication and Documentation **Content Area:** Fundamentals **Strategy:** Knowledge of basic ethical concepts will guide the selection of the correct response. **Reference:** Berman, A., & Snyder, S. J. (2012). *Kozier & Erb's fundamentals of nursing: Concepts, process, and practice* (9th ed.). Upper Saddle River, NJ: Pearson Education, pp. 85–86.

References

American Nurses Association (2001). *Code for nurses with interpretative statements.* Kansas City, MO. (Classic)

Berman, A., & Snyder, S. J. (2012). *Kozier & Erb's Fundamentals of nursing: Concepts, process, and practice* (9th ed.). Upper Saddle River, NJ: Pearson Education, pp. 52–96, 519–531.

Davis, A., Fowler, M., & Aroskar, M. (2010). *Ethical dilemmas and nursing practice* (5th ed.). Upper Saddle River, NJ: Pearson Education.

Finkelman, A. (2012). *Leadership and management in nursing* (2nd ed.). Upper Saddle River, NJ: Pearson Education.

Guido, G. (2010). *Legal and ethical issues in nursing* (5th ed.). Upper Saddle River, NJ: Pearson Education.

Sullivan, E. (2009). *Effective leadership and management in nursing* (7th ed.).

Upper Saddle River, NJ: Pearson Education.

Whitehead, D., Weiss, S., & Tappen, R. (2010). *Essentials of nursing leadership and management* (5th ed.). Philadelphia, PA: F.A. Davis.

Yoder-Wise, P. (2011). *Leading and managing in nursing* (5th ed.). St. Louis, MO: Elsevier.

ANSWERS & RATIONALES

Health Promotion Throughout the Life Span

5

Objectives

➤ Analyze how body image, self-esteem, roles, and identity affect an individual's self-concept.

➤ Contrast both the concept of sexuality and health promotion activities to foster a client's sexual health.

➤ Explain growth and development changes as they occur from infancy through late adulthood.

➤ Distinguish how an individual's culture affects all aspects of life including health.

➤ Describe the various family units, theoretical frameworks, and how illness can affect family dynamics.

➤ Distinguish spirituality from religion and the relationship to health promotion.

➤ Analyze the elements of the grieving process, usual grief symptoms, and methods for health promotion related to loss and grief.

NCLEX-RN® Test Prep

Use the accompanying online resource, NursingReviewsandRationales, to test yourself with hundreds of NCLEX®-style practice questions.

Review at a Glance

body image perception of size, appearance, and function of one's body

child abuse any abuse whether physical, sexual, emotional, or neglect inflicted upon a child

colic crying that lasts 10 to 12 hours per day characterized by acute abdominal pain caused by intestinal contractions

ethnicity a demonstration of characteristics shared by a group of people belonging to the same race or national origin

ethnocentrism a belief of superiority of one's race

failure to thrive a condition that may result from an inadequate parent–child relationship characterized by feeding difficulties, irritability, and inhibited weight gain; metabolic abnormalities and malabsorption syndrome could be physiologic causes

faith absolute belief in a set of ideologies though not demonstrated logically, nor visibly apparent

health a dynamic state of being that exists on a continuum, with high-level wellness of one end, a neutral state of neither wellness nor illness in middle, and illness and death at other end

health promotion an effort to advance health that engages a person in activities to enhance wellness

health protection modification of behavior to alter or reduce effects of illness and disease

health restoration process of bringing client back to a state of homeostasis

hope thought process used by an individual in goal setting and successful attainment of these goals

identification to perceive oneself like another and mimic behavior of that person

infertility inability to conceive despite a period of unprotected intercourse for 12 months

introjection claiming attributes of others as one's own

loss absence of an object, person, body part, emotion, idea, or function that was valued

maturity a state of maximal development of physical, psychosocial, and cognitive being, enabling a person to function efficiently in environment

race a group of individuals characterized by shared biological traits inherited from a common ancestor

regressive behavior temporary return to behaviors identified with previous stages of development

religion organized expression of one's spirituality, faith, and hope

repression inhibition of experiences, thoughts, and impulses from conscious thought

self-concept complex integration of conscious and unconscious feelings, attitudes, and perception, which affects behaviors and relationships with others

self-esteem emotional evaluation of self-worth

separation anxiety fear and frustration expressed by a child when absent from parents

sexual abuse sexual behavior forced upon a vulnerable individual by a

person who has some power or control over that individual

sexual orientation feelings of erotic potential directed toward members of opposite gender or one's own gender

sexual response cycle physiological changes that occur in response to sexual arousal; 4 phases are excitement, plateau, orgasm, and resolution

spirituality belief or faith in and establishment of a relationship with a higher being; this belief includes unknown aspects of life

sudden infant death syndrome (SIDS) unexplained death of an infant less than 1 year of age

PRETEST

1 A new mother informs the nurse that a neighbor just lost a baby to sudden infant death syndrome (SIDS). She is requesting information on ways she can prevent her baby from dying of SIDS. Which response by the nurse would be best?

1. "We do not know what causes SIDS and there really is not anything you can do to prevent it."
2. "Always be sure to put your baby to sleep on her back."
3. "Breastfeeding an infant for the first 6 months of life is the best start a mother can give her baby."
4. "Always make sure your baby is on her abdomen after feeding so she will not choke if she vomits."

2 A terminally ill older adult client is being cared for by her only daughter. The daughter expresses a fear of not knowing how to care for her mother appropriately. Which nursing diagnosis is most appropriate?

1. Social Isolation
2. Powerlessness
3. Situational Low Self-Esteem
4. Ineffective Role Performance

3 When evaluating clients in a mental health clinic, one assessment the nurse makes is determining whether clients are working on appropriate psychosocial tasks as described by Erikson. Which statements by a 45-year-old client indicate that the client is working on meeting the appropriate developmental task? Select all that apply.

1. "I have a new girlfriend."
2. "My provider says I shouldn't be driving a car due to my age."
3. "I am now coaching a tee-ball team for our local baseball league."
4. "I was thinking of changing my hairstyle. What do you think?"
5. "My daughter is getting married in a month."

4 A family has a new pool, and the mother asks the pediatric nurse how to protect her 2-year-old from drowning. What would be the best response by the nurse?

1. Provide swimming lessons given by a certified instructor.
2. Place a fence around the pool.
3. Provide adult supervision at all times.
4. Purchase an approved flotation device.

5 When learning of a diagnosis of deep vein thrombosis, the client states, "If it is God's will, I will get better." What would be the highest-priority intervention by the nurse to provide culturally competent care?

1. Notify the provider immediately.
2. Convey respect for the client's belief.
3. Further assess the client's knowledge of the disease.
4. Introduce self by name and title.

6 In an effort to provide culturally competent care, the nurse would plan to provide a Chinese American male client with which of the following as the highest priority?

1. Visit from a rabbi
2. Choice of diet
3. Discharge instructions directed to female family members
4. Teaching video instead of oral and written instructions

7 A Jewish client shares with the nurse that he fears he will never walk again following back surgery. He feels his loss of health stems from punishment for past sin. The nurse concludes that what goal is of high priority for this client?

1. Restore spiritual well-being.
2. Enhance relationships with support people.
3. Walk within 3 days of surgery to facilitate coping.
4. Pray the rosary for forgiveness.

8 After a client was diagnosed with terminal liver cancer, the nurse observes that the client's family assists the client with all activities of daily living (ADLs). The nurse should communicate which rationale for self-care to the family?

1. Strengthening muscles may encourage healing of the client's cancer.
2. The client needs time alone to reason through her diagnosis.
3. A sense of loss can be lessened by retaining control in certain areas of life.
4. Increased mental activity required for self-care will enhance the client's mood.

9 The nurse is assigned to care for a client diagnosed with end-stage renal disease who has recently begun hemodialysis. The client's care plan includes a diagnosis of spiritual distress. Which comments by the client would validate that diagnosis? Select all that apply.

1. "I can't see much point in going on like this."
2. "I really hate this place. I'll be glad to get out of here and back to my own bed."
3. "Can you find a priest to come and talk to me sometime?"
4. "What kind of a God would let this happen to me?"
5. "Being in the hospital is really depressing."

10 A male client who was treated in the emergency department for chemical burns to the hands and face is admitted to the medical nursing unit. During the initial assessment, he asks the nurse to "be honest" with him about his face and tell him "how bad it looks." Which nursing diagnosis is most appropriate based on this data?

1. Ineffective Peripheral Tissue Perfusion related to burn injury
2. Deficient Fluid Volume related to traumatic event
3. Acute Pain related to traumatic event
4. Disturbed Body Image related to traumatic event

➤ *See pages 118–119 for Answers and Rationales.*

I. HEALTH PROMOTION

A. *Healthy People 2020* (*Healthy People 2020*, The U.S. Department of Health and Human Services.)
1. Is presented by *Developing Healthy People* and encompasses a vision, mission, and overarching goals for people to live longer, healthier lives
2. Identifies health improvement priorities to increase public awareness and to help public understand determinants of health, disease, and disability
3. Provides measurable objectives and goals applicable at local, state, and national levels

   4. Engages in multiple sectors to take actions to strengthen policies and improve practices that are driven by best current evidence and knowledge
   5. Overarching goals include the following:
      a. Attain a quality of life free of preventable disease, disability, injury, and premature death
      b. Achieve health equity, eliminate disparities, and improve the health of all groups
      c. Create social and physical environments that promote good health for all
      d. Promote quality of life, health development, and healthy behaviors across all life stages

B. **Definitions related to health**
   1. **Health**: a dynamic state of being that exists on a continuum, with high-level wellness at one end, a neutral state of neither wellness nor illness in middle, and illness and death at other end
   2. **Health promotion**: behavior motivated by a desire to increase well-being and actualize human health potential
   3. **Health restoration**: process of bringing client back to homeostasis
   4. **Health protection**: modification of behavior to alter or reduce effects of illness and disease

C. **Levels of prevention**
   1. Primary: consists of general health promotion activities and measures to protect against illness or infection (such as immunizations)
   2. Secondary: consists of activities designed to identify health problems early and to decrease risk of exposure to disease, so as to limit future impairment
   3. Tertiary: consists of measures aimed at returning a person to an optimum level of functioning through health restoration and rehabilitation

II. SELF-CONCEPT

A. **Self-concept**: complex integration of conscious and unconscious feelings, attitudes and perception, which affects behaviors and relationships with others

B. **Development**
   1. Erikson defined 8 psychosocial stages, also called developmental crises, which must be completed successfully in order to develop a healthy self-concept
   2. Each stage or developmental crisis builds on tasks of previous stage
   3. Erikson's psychosocial stages outline the age-associated developmental tasks assigned by Erikson (see Table 5-1)

C. **Components of self-concept**
   1. **Self-esteem**: emotional evaluation of self-worth; heavily influenced by love and approval received as an infant; how a person's standards and performances compare to others and to one's ideal self
   2. **Body image**: perception of size, appearance, and function of one's body
   3. Role Performance: how a person acts in a particular role compared to behaviors expected in that role

D. **Stressors affecting self-concept**: real or imagined factors can threaten body image, self-esteem, role, or identity
   1. Stressors affecting body image include, but are not limited to the following: amputation, disfigurement, incontinence, declining mental status, weight, and acne
   2. Self-esteem stressors include physical and emotional abuse, demotion in workplace, and lack of success in an educational setting
   3. Role stressors include death of loved one, divorce, and unrealized life goals

Table 5-1	Physical, Psychosocial, and Cognitive Development from Birth to Adolescence		
Age	**Physical Development**	**Psychosocial Development (Erikson)**	**Cognitive Development (Piaget)**
Infancy (Birth to 1 year)	Weight: Average weight at birth is 7 to 8 pounds; should triple birth weight by 1 year of age Height: 20 inches Head circumference: 33 to 35 cm Chest circumference: 30 to 33 cm Head circumference is greater than chest circumference until after 7 months of age	Trust versus Mistrust: Child learns to identify his or her physical self as separate and different from environment; development of trust is essential to self-esteem of child and is achieved through consistently having needs met	Sensorimotor period: At beginning of period (birth), child responds in a reflexive manner; by end of this period (2 years), child has ability to communicate and is mobile; at this point, child's cognitive development involves goal distinction and attainment
Toddler (1 to 3 years)	Motor skills progress from walking to running to riding a tricycle Toilet training will be accomplished Physiologic anorexia will result because metabolism slows as growth rate slows	Autonomy versus Shame and Doubt: Child learns to internalize attitudes of others towards self Toddler asserts autonomy by saying "no" frequently Separation anxiety occurs when parents are absent from child; regressive behaviors may occur (child reverts to less mature behavior by trying to return to a "safer period of time")	Sensorimotor period continues until age 2; then child begins preoperational period Logic is not well developed; child often does not understand cause-and-effect relationship Child often utilizes "magical thinking" as a way to explain world around him or her
Preschool (3 to 5 years)	Child's body build changes from short, chubby toddler to slender, long-legged preschooler Physical skills continue to develop, focusing primarily on large motor skills Child learns to climb, ride a bicycle, use utensils, and dress him- or herself	Initiative versus Guilt: Child continues learning self-esteem Failure to successfully achieve goals in this period will lead child to have feelings of guilt and poor self-esteem	Continues in preoperational period; thought process is continuing to mature but still has difficulty with causality; begins to develop intuitive thought; development of conscience is an important component of this age period
School-age (6 to 12 years)	Boys and girls remain close in size and body proportions Beginning around age 6, child loses deciduous teeth; with eruption of permanent teeth, facial proportions change	Industry versus Inferiority: Child takes pride in accomplishments Activities of this age focus on developing a sense of competence and perseverance Self-concept develops as child internalizes standards of society Child learns cooperation and becomes less self-centered	Preoperational cognitive development gives way to concrete operational thinking; child's thought process continues to mature; in learning new information, child benefits from concrete applications, which will give way to abstraction
Adolescent (13 to 18 years)	Between ages 10–18 years, males grow an average of 16 inches and gain 72 pounds, and girls grow an average of 9 inches and gain 55 pounds Primary and secondary sexual characteristics develop because of increased hormone production In males, ejaculation first occurs around age 14; menarche in females may occur between ages 8 and 16	Identity versus Role Confusion: Child establishes an identity; confidence and self-concept increases and need for independence leads adolescent to prefer spending time with peer group rather than parents	Formal operational thought process begins at 11 years and progresses through adulthood; child develops the ability to think abstractly

(continued)

Table 5-1	Physical, Psychosocial, and Cognitive Development from Birth to Adolescence (continued)		
Age	**Physical Development**	**Psychosocial Development (Erikson)**	**Cognitive Development (Piaget)**
Early adulthood (18 to 40 years)	Growth is complete, body systems function at peak efficiency Musculoskeletal system well-developed	Intimacy versus Isolation: Person is developing intimate relationships with another person or a cause, institution, or creative effort This relationship allows person to share components of personality with another and allows adjusting of behavior to behavior of another	
Middle-age (40 to 65 years)	Body changes include decreasing hormonal production Menopause (cessation of menstruation) occurs in women	Generativity versus Stagnation: Person is concerned with providing for others When successful, person will have feelings of being needed, and being vital to establishing and nurturing next generation	
Older adult (65 years to death)	Skin becomes drier, hair loses color Subcutaneous fat and muscle tissue is lost Decrease in physical strength and senses are less efficient All body organs are affected	Acceptance of self-worth, uniqueness, and death; this period is described as a coming together of all previous phases of life cycle When ego has been achieved, person will remain creative	

   4. Stressors affecting identity include physical changes experienced in aging, lack of sexual performance, and pressures exerted by peers that are inconsistent with family values

  E. **Assessment**: nurse should seek to identify behaviors suggestive of altered self-concept (see Box 5-1)

  F. **Nursing diagnoses**: Disturbed Personal Identity, Ineffective Role Performance, Chronic Low Self-Esteem, Anxiety, Disturbed Body Image, Ineffective Coping, Grieving or Complicated Grieving; Hopelessness, Readiness for Enhanced Self-Concept, Disturbed Sleep Pattern, Social Isolation, Powerlessness, Ineffective Role Performance

  G. **Planning**
   1. Nurse develops a plan of care based on assessment data gathered, including information on state of health, anxiety level, support structure, culture, and religion

Box 5-1	
Behaviors Suggestive of Altered Self-Concept	1. Overly apologetic 2. No eye contact 3. Hesitant speech 4. Excessive, inappropriate anger 5. Frequent crying 6. Demeans self 7. Unusually dependent 8. Has difficulty expressing opinions 9. Lack of interest in daily activities 10. Passive 11. Difficulty making decisions 12. Haphazard appearance

2. Goals and outcome criteria are developed with client's participation; goals would include a realistic perception of body, increased sense of self-worth, and adequate performance of roles

H. Implementation

1. To encourage an increased sense of self-concept, interventions should assist client to identify strengths and to maintain a sense of self
2. Examples of interventions for nursing diagnosis Anxiety
   a. Help client define level of anxiety
   b. Encourage verbalization of concerns
   c. Explore coping skills used in past and teach new ones as needed
   d. Decrease new stressors
   e. Alleviate pain before it progresses
   f. Teach relaxation techniques

I. Evaluation

1. Client demonstrates improved self-concept; evidence may be nonverbal cues such as resumed eye contact
2. Nurse should provide review of situation to client and reinforce change

III. SEXUAL DEVELOPMENT

A. Phases of sexual development (see Table 5-2)

B. Sexual orientation: feelings of erotic potential directed toward members of opposite gender or one's own gender

C. Sexual response cycle: physiological changes that occur in response to sexual arousal; 4 phases are excitement, plateau, orgasm, and resolution

1. Excitement is a phase of increasing sexual arousal that can last from minutes to hours
2. Plateau is a phase that lasts from 30 seconds to 3 minutes and is a period of increasing sexual tension; it is manifested by elevated heart rate and respiratory rate and increased blood pressure
3. Orgasmic phase is the climax of sexual tension that lasts only a few seconds; during this phase, the male ejaculates
4. Resolution is the phase when body returns to non-aroused state; is often accompanied by sleepiness and a feeling of relaxation

D. Sexual health

1. Sexual health is a state of physical, emotional, psychological, and social well-being according to World Health Organization
2. Is noted when sexual relationships are respectful, pleasurable, and safe
3. Is a state in which the individual:
   a. Has knowledge about sexual behavior
   b. Is able to express sexual potential
   c. Is able to make autonomous decisions
   d. Understands sexual pleasure in relation to physical, psychological, cognitive, and spiritual well-being
   e. Expresses emotions related to sexuality
   f. Makes reproductive choices
   g. Gains access to health care related to sexuality

E. Alterations in sexual health

1. Infertility: inability to conceive despite a period of unprotected intercourse for 12 months
   a. Primary infertility refers to a couple that has never conceived
   b. Secondary infertility refers to a couple that has conceived before but is unable to do so at this time

---

Practice to Pass

The nurse is caring for a 30-year-old female client who is postoperative following a mastectomy. Following assessment, the nurse has chosen the nursing diagnosis Situational Low Self-Esteem related to loss of body part. What client outcomes are appropriate for this diagnosis?

Table 5-2	Sexual Development	
Phases	**Age**	**Characteristics**
Infancy	Birth–18 months	Gender is assigned; genitals sensitive; males may have erections; females have vaginal lubrication
Preschool	1–5 years	Identifies gender; labels body parts correctly; parent of opposite sex is focus of love
Childhood	6–12 years	Becomes curious about sex roles and reproduction; friends are usually of same sex
Adolescence	12–18 years	Sex characteristics develop; friendships may include opposite sex; may engage in masturbation and sexual activity
Adulthood	18–65 years	Establishes family, to include sexual activity, values, and family roles; between ages 40 and 65, hormone production decreases leading to climacteric in both sexes
Older adulthood	65 years–death	Frequency of sexual activity decreases; men and women experience altered sexual functioning

2. **Sexual abuse**: sexual behavior forced upon another person; the behavior varies from inappropriate touching to rape; abuser can be of either gender although male perpetrators are more common; the abused can be an adult or a child but often is a person with less power than the abuser; the impact of sexual abuse can be long lasting
3. Sexual dysfunction: change in sexual functioning altering the normal sexual pattern; males may have erectile dysfunction; females may have orgasmic dysfunction or dyspareunia (painful intercourse); sexual dysfunction can arise from many factors, including prescribed medications, drug categories that may contribute to dysfunction include the following:
   a. Antihypertensives: may decrease sexual desire and cause erectile dysfunction
   b. Antidepressants: may decrease sexual desire or cause erectile or orgasmic dysfunction
   c. Antihistamines: may cause decreased vaginal lubrication and sexual desire
   d. Anticholinergics: may decrease sexual response
   e. Sedatives or tranquilizers: in large doses may decrease sexual desire or cause orgasmic dysfunction and impotence
   f. Ethyl alcohol: in moderate amounts increases sexual functioning, while chronic use may cause decreased sexual desire, female orgasmic dysfunction, and impotence
   g. Barbiturates: increase sexual pleasure in low dose, while chronic use decreases desire and causes sexual dysfunction
   h. Diuretics: decrease vaginal lubrication and sexual desire and cause erectile dysfunction
   i. Opioid analgesics and other narcotics: inhibit sexual desire and response
4. Sexual desire disorders
   a. Sexual aversion: sexual abuse or rape as a child can result in a severe aversion to, or a distaste for, sexual activity
   b. Diminished sexual desire: is a state of being disinterested in sex related to decreased satisfaction with sexual partner
F. **Common nursing diagnoses related to change in sexuality**: Ineffective Sexuality Pattern; Disturbed Body Image; Fear; Anxiety; Pain; Deficient Knowledge; Decisional Conflict; Rape-Trauma Syndrome; Disturbed Self-Esteem; Sexual Dysfunction
G. **Health promotion for sexual functioning**
   1. Client teaching is important to prevent sexual difficulties and to assist in behavior change needed to restore sexual health
      a. Subject matter for client teaching is chosen according to client age; for instance, women over 50 need information about comfort measures to reduce symptoms of

Practice to Pass

Outline an appropriate teaching plan for a 20-year-old male who has significant risk factors for testicular cancer.

menopause while priority information for women 20 years of age would be contraception and prevention of sexually transmitted infections (STIs)

    b. Because sexual matters usually involve intimate content, nurse provides client privacy to facilitate a proper learning environment

2. Sexual health promotion in acute care includes early disease detection, prompt intervention, prevention of complications and disabilities (such as teaching self-examination of breasts and testicles), STI prevention, and contraceptive use

3. Sexual health promotion in restorative care assists client in rehabilitation to optimum level of functioning; most likely includes both partners; specific teaching includes dealing with impotence, orgasmic dysfunction, and infertility

IV. GROWTH AND DEVELOPMENT

A. General information relative to growth and development (refer back to Table 5-1)

  1. Growth refers to an increase in size of body

  2. Development describes an increase in function and capability of body; principles of development include the following:

    a. Cephalocaudal development refers to head to tail maturation; child will develop control of head before learning control of legs

    b. Proximodistal development describes development of trunk prior to development in extremities

  3. Cognitive development of child is described by Piaget's theory; unlike Erikson's theory which goes throughout life, Piaget's theory describes development from birth to end of adolescence

B. Infancy (birth to 1 year)

  1. Physical development: significant physical change occurs in weight, length, head circumference, refinement of sight, hearing, smell, taste and touch, reflexes, and motor skills; develop from turning head side-to-side to walking alone and feeding self

  2. Psychosocial development: trust versus mistrust (refer again to Table 5-1)

  3. Cognitive/intellectual development: Piaget outlines cognitive development as progressing from reflexive action to goal distinction and attainment

  4. Health promotion: major health concerns

    a. **Failure to thrive** is a condition that may result from an inadequate parent–child relationship and is characterized by feeding difficulties, irritability, and inhibited weight gain; this impaired parent–infant relationship must be differentiated from physiologic causes of failure to thrive, which include inadequate feeding and malabsorption syndromes

    b. **Colic** is acute abdominal pain lasting 10–12 hours per day caused by intestinal contractions; it typically occurs in first 3 months of life; cause is unknown, but result is an infant who cries for long periods; prolonged crying upsets caregiver and caregiver distress may then contribute to infant's emotional distress

      1) Possible causes include allergy to infant formula, rapid feeding, and swallowing air

      2) Treatment to reduce colic may include changing formula, changing nipples, and increased burping; cuddling and swaddling may be of benefit; caregivers need reassurance that colic will end at approximately 3 months of age

    c. **Sudden infant death syndrome (SIDS)** is unexplained death of an infant under 1 year of age; although an autopsy is performed, no reason for death can be found

      1) SIDS occurs more frequently in males, preterm infants, and those with family history of SIDS

      2) Parents need to know that there was nothing they could have done to predict infant's death

      3) Studies have shown that putting infant to sleep on his or her back reduces risk of SIDS

         d. Child abuse can include any abuse whether it is physical, sexual, emotional, or neglectful in nature

           1) Symptoms will depend upon type of abuse

              a) Physical abuse can be manifested by bruises, burns, and fractures; the history of the injury does not match physical findings; for instance, the history states the child fell off a porch, but the fracture is a spiral fracture, which occurs with twisting of a limb

              b) Sexual abuse may be discovered when a child is found to have an STI

              c) Neglect may be noted when child is severely undernourished without physical cause

              d) Emotional abuse is harder to identify but may be observed if abuser is verbally abusing child; at other times it may be quite difficult to detect

           2) Take the history without comment; make no accusations to parents; note if child is improperly dressed for weather; teachers may report a sudden change in behavior or school performance

           3) Nurses have a responsibility to report suspected abuse to authorities using processes outlined in agency policy; failure to report suspected abuse can lead to nurse's liability; possible abuse reported in good faith will not lead to legal repercussions

      5. Screening and assessment

         a. Health care examinations should be done at 2 weeks and at 2, 4, 6, and 12 months

         b. Immunizations are high priority (see Table 5-3)

         c. Assess for safety issues such as risks for falls, burns, motor vehicle crashes, drowning, poisoning, choking, suffocation, and strangulation

Table 5-3	Immunization Schedule for Ages 0 to 11 Years, 2011
Vaccine	**Recommended Age**
Hepatitis B (Hep B)	First dose at birth prior to hospital discharge; second dose at 1–2 months; third dose after 24 weeks of age If mother is hepatitis B surface antigen (HBsAg)-positive, administer 0.5 mL of Hepatitis B immune globulin within 12 hours of birth
Rotavirus (Rota)	First dose at 2 months; second dose at 4 months; third dose at 6 months
Diphtheria, tetanus, pertussis (DTaP)	First dose at 2 months; second dose at 4 months; third dose at 6 months; fourth dose at 15–18 months; fifth dose at 4–6 years; tetanus booster at 11–15 years, and every 5–10 years thereafter
H. influenza type B (Hib)	First dose at 2 months; second dose at 4 months; third dose at 6 months; fourth dose at 12–18 months
Inactivated polio (IPV)	First dose at 2 months; second dose at 4 months; third dose at 6–18 months, fourth dose at 4–6 years
Pneumococcal conjugate (PCV)	First dose at 2 months, second dose at 4 months, third dose at 6 months; fourth dose at 12–15 months
Measles, mumps, rubella (MMR)	First dose 12–18 months; second dose 4–6 years
Varicella	First dose 12–15 months; second dose 4–6 years
Hepatitis A (HepA)	In selected areas 2–18 years
Human papillomavirus (HPV)	First dose females age 11–12 years; second and third doses 2 and 6 months later
Influenza	Yearly for children age 6 months through 18 years
Meningococcal (MCV4 or MPSV4)	Age 11 years (MCV4) and age 2 or older (MPSV4) if high risk

        d. Assess feeding method techniques and schedule

        e. Developmental assessment includes physical, psychosocial, and cognitive areas

C. Early childhood: toddlers (1 to 3 years) and preschool children (4 to 5 years)

  1. Physical development

    a. Motor skills in toddlers progress from walking to running to riding a tricycle; preschool child runs well, jumps, balances on toes, and dresses self

    b. Toilet training may begin after child can walk well, pull clothing up and down, recognize urge for elimination and control that urge until in proper setting

    c. Toddler often experiences physiologic anorexia caused by a slowing of metabolism to accommodate moderate growth rate

    d. Growth in preschool child is greater in height than weight

  2. Psychosocial development

    a. Toddler: autonomy versus shame and doubt (refer again to Table 5-1)

    b. **Separation anxiety** occurs when parents are absent from child and is expressed by fear and frustration

      1) It is also called toddler hospitalization reaction and consists of 3 stages

        a) Protest: child is angry, screams and hollers; may bite or kick when health care personnel try to console child; some children remain in this phase throughout hospitalization, while others quickly move into next phase

        b) Despair: child mourns loss of parent or caregiver; may continue to refuse to eat and have difficulty sleeping; may draw up into a fetal position and avoid contact with health care personnel; often cries softly

        c) Denial: in third phase, child is often thought to have recovered or adapted to separation; this is incorrect, and child may have severe difficulty resulting from separation; in this phase, child appears happy and plays, eats, and sleeps without difficulty; when parents visit, child may ignore them

      2) Support both child and parents or caregivers when separation occurs; nursing activities include the following:

        a) Provide physical comfort to child

        b) Remind child that the parents or caregivers love him or her and will return

        c) Encourage parents or caregivers to visit or stay with child as appropriate

        d) Encourage parents or caregivers to leave an article of clothing or a possession with child

    c. **Regressive behavior** such as bed wetting or "baby talk" may occur when child feels threatened; during these periods, child attempts to return to a safer period of development; regression is common during and after a hospitalization; provide emotional support and allow child to exhibit regressive behavior

    d. Preschool children: initiative versus guilt (refer to Table 5-1); preschooler learns **identification** (ability to perceive oneself like another and mimic behavior of that person); he or she also has **introjection** (claiming attributes of others as one's own); imagination is an important part of child's play life; **repression** (inhibition of experiences, thoughts, and impulses from conscious thought) is also expected at this stage

  3. Cognitive and intellectual development: at age 2 years, child enters preoperational period; logic is not well developed; child often does not understand cause-and-effect relationships; child often utilizes "magical thinking" as a way to explain the world

  4. Health promotion: major health concerns for toddler and preschooler include the following:

    a. Accidents, including motor vehicle crashes, drowning, burns, poisoning, and falls; accidents are leading cause of mortality in toddlers and are common in preschoolers as well

    b. Respiratory tract and ear infections are common to toddlers and preschoolers

     5. Screening and assessment

       a. Health care examinations for toddler should be scheduled at 15 and 18 months of age and then as needed; toddlers should visit dentist by age 3; preschoolers should have exams every 1–2 years

       b. Immunizations (see Table 5-3)

       c. Discuss safety issues and methods to use to avoid accidents

       d. Developmental assessment includes physical, psychosocial, and cognitive areas; the Denver Developmental Screening Tool (Denver II) can be used by nurse to evaluate development

D. School age (6 to 12 years)

     1. Physical development

       a. Deciduous teeth are lost and permanent teeth begin to erupt, which changes physical appearance of child's face

       b. Weight gain occurs rapidly and is usually related to preadolescent growth spurts; females' growth spurt in height begins some years prior to males'

       c. Preadolescence begins about age 10 for females and age 12 for males; endocrine functions increase leading to increased perspiration and active sebaceous glands

     2. Psychosocial development

       a. Industry versus inferiority: self-concept develops as school-age child internalizes standards of society (refer to Table 5-1)

       b. School-age children learn cooperation and to become less self-centered through peer interaction; parental relationships contribute more to self-esteem than peer groups

     3. Cognitive and intellectual development: child develops an understanding of logical reasoning, money, time, and day of the week; self-motivation develops

     4. Health promotion

       a. Major health concerns: communicable diseases, parasitic infestations, homicide, and violence

       b. Screening and assessment

         1) Annual health care examinations

         2) Immunizations (refer to Table 5-3)

         3) Teach sports safety, emphasizing personal responsibility

         4) Developmental assessment includes physical, psychosocial, and cognitive areas

E. Adolescence (12 to 18 years)

     1. Physical development: between the ages of 10 and 18, males grow an average of 16 inches and gain 72 pounds; during this same period, females grow an average of 9 inches and gain 55 pounds

     2. Psychosocial development: the adolescent seeks to establish identity; appearance and perception of others is important; when valued, loved, and accepted by family and peers, confidence and self-concept increases; the need for independence leads the adolescent to prefer spending time with the peer group rather than parents

     3. Psychosexual development: increased hormone production leads to the development of primary (maturation of reproductive organs) and secondary sexual characteristics (pubic hair growth, breast development, voice changes); in males, ejaculation first occurs around age 14; in females, menarche may occur between ages 8 and 16; intimacy with a partner lays a foundation for commitment necessary for adult relationships; sexual experimentation may occur

     4. Health promotion

       a. Major health concerns: alcohol and/or drug abuse, motor vehicle crashes and other types of accidents, suicide, homicide, heart disease, depression

       b. Screening and assessment

         1) Health care examination as necessary

         2) Immunizations (refer to Table 5-3)

        3) Offer education concerning contraception, STIs, and emotional issues

        4) Offer safety assessment and teaching concerning motor vehicles, sports, and substance abuse

        5) Assess for nutritional alterations such as anorexia nervosa, bulimia, or obesity

        6) Developmental assessment includes physical and psychosocial areas

F. Early adult (20 to 40 years)

  1. Physical development: body systems function at peak efficiency; weight changes occur from influences of diet and exercise

  2. Psychosocial development: in early adulthood **maturity** develops; maturity is a state of maximal development of physical, psychosocial, and cognitive being, enabling a person to function efficiently in the environment; important lifestyle decisions are made such as education, occupation, marriage, children, and social responsibility

  3. Psychosexual development: sexual activity increases; lifestyle choices are established based on adopted values

  4. Health promotion

    a. Major health concerns: accidents, suicide, hypertension, substance abuse, STIs, domestic abuse, and malignancies

    b. Screening and assessment

        1) Health care examination should be done every 1–3 years for females; every 5 years for males

        2) Dental checkups are recommended every 6 months; vision and hearing assessments should be done as needed

        3) Females should have a Papanicolaou (Pap) smear yearly, breast self-examination (BSE) should be done monthly, and clinical breast exam should be done every 1–3 years

        4) Males should perform testicular self-examination (TSE) monthly

        5) Screening for cardiac disease should be done as needed

        6) Teach motor vehicle safety, sun protection, and occupational safety

G. Middle adulthood (40 to 65 years)

  1. Physical development: the hair thins and grays; skin turgor declines; fat is redistributed to abdominal area; loss of height occurs because of thinning of intervertebral discs; blood vessels thicken and lose elasticity; visual acuity decreases; males are more prone to decline in auditory acuity; metabolism slows; constipation is common because of a decrease in intestinal tone

  2. Psychosocial development: concerns relate to guiding the next generation through acts of service such as church, social, or political work; value of intellectual abilities surpasses physical attractiveness; individuals with difficulty in psychosocial development often demonstrate self-centeredness

  3. Psychosexual development: a decrease in hormone production produces menopause in females 40 to 55 years (including stages of perimenopause, menopause, and postmenopause) and the climacteric in males; couples may focus more on quality of sexual encounters rather than frequency

  4. Health promotion

    a. Major health concerns: accidents, cancer, cardiac disease, obesity, alcoholism, mental health changes

    b. Screening and assessment

        1) Health care examinations for females should be done yearly; for males they should be scheduled every 2–3 years

        2) Regular dental examinations should continue

        3) Continue BSE and TSE monthly

        4) Screen for cardiac disease and for colorectal, breast, cervical, uterine, and prostate cancers

       5) Discuss safety hazards in home, workplace, and in a motor vehicle

       6) Begin yearly mammograms at age 40

       7) Discuss initial screening colonoscopy at age 50 then every 10 years if no pathology is noted

       8) Note that screening for osteoporosis begins at age 50

H. Late adulthood (over 65 years)

  1. Physical development

    a. Integumentary changes include dryness, pallor, wrinkling, age spots, decreased perspiration, and thinning of hair

    b. Neuromuscular changes include loss of height, osteoporosis, joint stiffness, and impaired balance

    c. Sensory changes include loss of visual and auditory acuity, decreased sense of taste and smell, and increased sensitivity to pain, touch, and temperature

    d. Pulmonary changes include decreased lung expansion and possible dyspnea

    e. Cardiovascular changes include increased blood pressure and decreased cardiac output

    f. Gastrointestinal changes include delayed swallowing, increased indigestion, and constipation

    g. Urinary changes include urgency and frequency, and impaired renal function

    h. Genital changes include male prostate enlargement and atrophy of reproductive organs in the female

  2. Psychosocial development: issues may include retirement, economic change, relocation, maintaining independence, and experiences of grief

  3. Psychosexual development: lessening sexual activity

  4. Health promotion

    a. Major health concerns: accidents, arthritis, cardiac disease, pulmonary disease, pharmaceutical misuse, alcoholism, dementia, and abuse

    b. Screening and assessment

       1) Health examinations should continue as they did during middle adulthood

       2) Explore safety issues such as fall prevention

       3) Encourage older adults to have lower intake of calories including adequate roughage and to maintain moderate exercise as able

       4) Assess for cognitive impairment and abuse

V. CULTURE AND HEALTH PROMOTION

A. Four basic characteristics of culture

  1. Learned from birth by family and peers through language (both nonverbal and verbal) and socialization

  2. Values, beliefs, patterns of behavior, language, food, dress, and other factors are shared by members of same cultural group

  3. Common cultural aspects are influenced by specific conditions such as environment, technology, and resources

  4. Culture is dynamic and ever-changing as members' needs change

B. Culturally based characteristics

  1. Space and distance: culture defines relationship of body to objects and other individuals; e.g., some cultures may view being in close proximity to others as impolite

  2. Eye contact: a form of nonverbal communication with specific meaning for the culture; e.g., Americans view eye contact as a demonstration of self-confidence and interest, while Navajo Indians consider eye contact a sign of disrespect

  3. Time: the past, the present and the future are defined and emphasized by a culture; e.g., Irish Americans value their heritage and tend to be past oriented, whereas

Native Americans are more often present oriented, viewing time casually and accomplishing work as the need arises; Americans tend to be future oriented, planning tasks to accomplish goals

4. Touch: may be interpreted as casual or intimate; Hispanics value close relationships that include physical touching; in the Hmong culture, the head is never touched by anyone other than an elder

5. Observance of holidays: these are specific to culture and are valued differently; a significant winter holiday for many Christians is Christmas, while Hanukkah is the valued holiday for those of Jewish culture

6. Diet: culture dictates staple foods, food preparation, presentation of food, behaviors related to diet, and use of foods as cures for illness; rice is a staple food for Asians, and pasta is plentiful in diet of many Italians

C. Cultural assessment

1. Is a systematic review of cultural beliefs and practices of individuals, groups, or communities

2. To evaluate culture, ask questions and address items such as the following:
    a. Where were you born? Your mother? Your father? Your grandparents?
    b. What is necessary to maintain health? Certain foods? Certain behaviors? Certain religious practices?
    c. Where do you think illness originates? What aspects of illness concern you?
    d. What difficulties arise when you are ill? For your family? Related to your employment?
    e. Describe how you seek to restore your health when ill.
    f. Whom do you seek assistance from when ill?
    g. Are there remedies used for illness? Describe these.
    h. What role do women have in health practices? During illness?
    i. What role do men have in health practices? During illness?
    j. Please list any other practices important to your culture that are important to you.

D. Ethnicity

1. A demonstration of characteristics shared by a group of people belonging to same race or national origin

2. **Race**: a group of individuals characterized by shared biological traits inherited from a common ancestor
    a. Races may be discriminated against as a result of **ethnocentrism**: a belief of superiority of one's race; federal, state, and local laws govern discrimination based on race
    b. Economic status may be related to race and also be a result of discrimination and lack of opportunities
    c. Political campaigns and practices may target specific racial issues

VI. OVERVIEW OF THE FAMILY

A. Family diversity: definitions of family as the basic unit of society have broadened to include varying forms of family

1. Nuclear family: consists of parents and children and includes first-marriage families, blended or stepparent families, and adoptive families

2. Binuclear family: a post-divorce family in which children are part of 2 nuclear families with varying amounts of time spent in each family

3. Intergenerational family: includes more than one generation of family living together, such as older parents (grandparents)

4. Extended family: consists of parents, children, grandparents, aunts, and uncles

5. Single-parent family: consists of one male or female parent and children

Practice to Pass

In order to communicate with a Russian client, an interpreter is necessary. List the characteristics of an ideal interpreter. Discuss key points in working with an interpreter.

6. Cohabiting family: unrelated individuals or families that live under the same roof

7. Gay or lesbian family: same-sex adults living together with the same goals of caring and commitment as heterosexual adults

B. **Frameworks used for understanding family**

1. General systems theory: family is a dynamic system with identifiable parts that interact; this system is composed of matter (people), energy, and communication (interactions with members and with those outside family); a family is an open system continually interacting with and influenced by community

2. Structural-functional theory: this theory defines 2 aspects of family, structure and function; structure is the constantly evolving members and their relationships; functions of family include assigning purpose, providing affiliation, socializing members, and providing care

3. Developmental theory: families (like individuals) progress through stages of development; families must create an environment that encourages progression through these stages

4. Nursing theories can be adapted to assist with health promotion activities conducted by the nurse

   a. In Betty Neuman's systems model, a client or family would be considered an open system surrounded by 3 levels of boundaries, which, when activated, protect the entity; health promotion would focus on strengthening these boundaries

   b. Sr. Callista Roy defines an adaptive system in which client and family interacts with environment to meet needs; these needs can by physiologic, self-concept, role function, or interdependence; nurses can facilitate interactions that promote health

   c. Imogene King developed a nursing theory that assists in defining social system in which a family functions; goal attainment occurs through transactions; transactions may include bargaining, negotiating, and common frames of references; nurses can facilitate a family's transactions and therefore goal attainment

C. **Illness impacts the family in a variety of ways**

1. Anxiety, stress, and/or depression may occur as members consider outcomes of an illness; the degree of anxiety, stress, and/or depression experienced is related to coping skills utilized

2. Careers of family members may be affected if increased demands on their time interfere with work schedules; anxiety, stress, and/or depression may also interfere with job performance; financial strain may occur with extended absences from work

3. Roles may change within a family during illness, particularly if a matriarch or patriarch is ill and children must become caregivers

4. Caregiver strain occurs as an illness becomes lengthy and additional responsibilities are assumed

D. **Family assessment**

1. Family structure: type of family, number of members, age of members, gender of members

2. Family roles: responsibilities of each family member

3. Physical health status: illness, health promotion, illness care, genetic predisposition to disease

4. Patterns of communication and intimacy

5. Family values: religion, cultural traditions, education

6. Coping: emotion support, stress, financial needs

E. **Common nursing diagnoses**: Ineffective Family Processes; Disabled Family Coping; Compromised Family Coping; Readiness for Enhanced Family Coping; Impaired Home Maintenance; Interrupted Family Processes

VII. SPIRITUALITY

A. **Spirituality** is belief or faith in and establishment of a relationship with a higher being; this belief includes unknown aspects of life; these beliefs bring meaning, purpose, and hope; faith provides inner strength

1. **Faith**: absolute belief in a set of ideologies that are not demonstrated logically or visibly apparent; strength and trust are derived from faith
2. **Hope**: thought process used by an individual in goal setting and successful attainment of these goals; hope is enhanced through inner strength, relationships, and faith in God; an absence of hope leads to despair
3. **Religion**: organized expression of one's spirituality, faith, and hope

B. **Promotion of spiritual health**

1. Definition: spiritual health is a state of wellness encompassing personal fulfillment and fulfillment in life and with others; characterized by expression of peace, love, and joy; a defined life purpose; and existence within a set of values as outlined by one's community and oneself
2. Nursing interventions
   a. Encourage hope in these ways: assisting client to recall past experiences where hope was used while in crisis; goal revision to emphasize small steps of progress; defining important, future events such as trips or family celebrations in which client can anticipate; providing reading material or companionship to encourage client; and support of religious practices
   b. Encourage evaluating a crisis with clarity; give factual information about client's state of health; refer client as necessary to members of health care team; encourage a trusting relationship where emotions and fears can be expressed
   c. Assist with suffering by encouraging client to interpret suffering; listen and be available; assist client in discovering positive aspects of suffering

> **Practice to Pass**
>
> How can the nurse assess spiritual development of the preschooler?

Table 5-4	Religious Beliefs about Health
Religion	**Belief About Health**
Christianity	Prayer for healing is appropriate; rosary may be used Catholic and Eastern Orthodox Christians may request a priest to administer sacrament of communion, reconciliation, or anointing (sacrament of the sick) Pictures of saints and angels may provide comfort
Judaism	Dietary restrictions: milk and meat are not mixed; nonkosher products include predatory fowl, shellfish, and pork Prayer for healing is appropriate Artificial insemination, autopsy, use of birth control, use of blood and blood products, medications, and surgery are permitted Euthanasia is prohibited
Hinduism	Characterized by a belief that for every action there is a corresponding reaction, therefore illness is caused by previous actions, even those in another life Eating meat is prohibited Medications, surgery, organ donation, and use of blood or blood products are acceptable
Jehovah's Witness	Abortion, artificial insemination, use of blood or blood products, and organ donations are forbidden Healing prayer may be requested Reading of Scripture may provide comfort
Islam	Allah is God; practice the Five Pillars of Islam; pork and alcohol are prohibited; strong views on health; fasting during Ramadan; follow customs for birth and death; men of the family provide consent to care

C. **Spiritual distress**
 1. May occur in acute illness, chronic illness, terminal illness, or near-death experience
 2. Characteristics of spiritual distress
  a. Questioning of belief of life, death, and suffering
  b. Losing hope and developing feelings of discouragement or despair
  c. Doubting or abandoning religious practices
  d. Requesting spiritual assistance
D. **Religious beliefs about health (see Table 5-4)**
E. **Religious rituals related to birth and death (see Table 5-5)**

VIII. LOSS AND GRIEF

A. *Loss*
 1. Absence of an object, person, body part, emotion, idea, or function that was valued
 2. Actual versus perceived loss: actual losses are identified and verified by others while a perceived loss cannot be verified by others; for example, loss of a home caused by fire is an actual loss while loss of companionship following a move to a distance city is a perceived loss
 3. Maturational versus situational loss: maturational losses occur during normal development while situational losses occur without expectation; for example, parental sorrow produced from a child going away to college is a maturational loss while the death of the same child would be a situational loss
 4. Death, the ultimate loss: death results in a loss for the dying person as well as for those left behind; can be viewed as a time of growth for all who experience it (see Table 5-6 for an overview of the concept of death by age)
B. **Grieving process (see Table 5-7)**
C. **Anticipatory grief**: expression of symptoms of grief prior to actual loss; grief period following the loss may be shortened and intensity lessened because of previous expression of grief; for example, a child told that a family move is expected may grieve about losing friends prior to actually leaving
D. **Complications of bereavement**
 1. Chronic grief: symptoms of grief occur beyond expected time frame and severity of symptoms is greater; depression may result
 2. Delayed grief: when symptoms of grief are not expressed and are suppressed, a delayed grief reaction occurs; nurse should discuss normal process of grieving with client and give permission to express these symptoms

Practice to Pass

A parent is caring for her terminally ill child at home. She asks the nurse, "How will I know when death is near?" What should be the nurse's response?

Table 5-5	Religious Rituals Related to Birth and Death	
Religion	**Birth Rituals**	**Death Rituals**
Judaism	Males are circumcised on eighth day following birth Females are named in synagogue on Sabbath following birth	When death is likely, no new heroic measures are taken Euthanasia is prohibited
Islam	After birth, a prayer is recited in child's ear Child is named on seventh day following birth Tuft of hair is shaved from head on seventh day following birth	Request that following death, head be turned to Mecca Ritual bath following death
Christianity	Baptism is done after birth to document that child was born into a Christian family Baptism is done at birth of a seriously ill child; family or nurse may perform baptism	Speaking of afterlife is comforting as client is dying

Table 5-6 **Development of the Concept of Death**

Age	Beliefs and Attitudes
Infancy to 5 years	Does not understand concept of death Infant's sense of separation forms basis for later understanding of loss and death Believes death is reversible, a temporary departure, or sleep Emphasizes immobility and inactivity as attributes of death
5 to 9 years	Understands that death is final Believes own death can be avoided Associates death with aggression or violence Believes wishes or unrelated actions can be responsible for death
9 to 12 years	Understands death as an inevitable end of life Begins to understand own mortality, expressed as interest in afterlife or as fear of death
12 to 18 years	Fears a lingering death May fantasize that death can be defied, acting out defiance through reckless behaviors (e.g., dangerous driving, substance abuse) Seldom thinks about death, but views it in religious and philosophic terms May seem to reach "adult" perception of death but still be emotionally unable to accept it May still hold concepts from previous developmental stages
18 to 45 years	Has attitude toward death influenced by religious and cultural beliefs
45 to 65 years	Accepts own mortality Encounters death of parents and some peers Experiences peaks of death anxiety Death anxiety diminishes with emotional well-being
65+ years	Fears prolonged illness Encounters death of family members and peers Sees death as having multiple meanings (e.g., freedom from pain, reunion with already deceased family members)

Table 5-7 **Theories of Grief, Dying, and Mourning**

Bowlby's Three Phases of Grief	*Protest*: lack of acceptance concerning loss; characterized by anger, ambivalence, and crying *Despair*: denial and acceptance occur simultaneously causing disorganized behavior; characterized by crying and sadness *Detachment*: loss is realized; characterized by hopefulness, accurately defining the relationship with the lost individual, and energy to move forward in life
Kübler-Ross's Five Stages of Grieving	*Denial*: characterized by shock and disbelief; serves as a buffer to mobilized defense mechanisms *Anger*: resistance to loss occurs; anger is typically directed toward others *Bargaining*: deals are sought with God or other higher power in an effort to postpone loss *Depression*: loss is realized; may talk openly or withdraw *Acceptance*: recognition of the loss occurs; disinterest may occur; future thinking may occur
Worden's Four Tasks of Mourning	1. Accept reality of loss; the loss is accepted 2. Experience pain of grief; healthy behaviors are accomplished to assist in grieving process 3. Adjust to environment without the deceased; tasks are accomplished to reorient the environment (e.g., remove clothes of deceased from closet) 4. Emotionally relocate deceased and move forward with life; correctly align past and present, and look toward future

E. **Symptoms of normal grief**
  1. Feelings include sadness, exhaustion, numbness, helplessness, loneliness, disorganization, preoccupation with lost object or person, anxiety, depression
  2. Thought patterns include fear, guilt, denial, ambivalence, anger
  3. Physical sensations include nausea, vomiting, anorexia, weight loss or gain, constipation or diarrhea, diminished hearing or sight, chest pain, shortness of breath, tachycardia
  4. Behaviors include crying, difficulty carrying out activities of daily living, and insomnia

F. **Nursing interventions to assist client and significant others through end-of-life stages**
  1. Provide client with physical support to relieve pain, with an intent to enhance dying process
  2. Provide emotional support for all individuals experiencing grief; acknowledge their grief
  3. Provide information on community resources, such as grief counselors and not-for-profit agencies that assist in grief support
  4. Explore and implement ethnic, cultural, and religious practices related to end-of-life care
  5. Implement therapeutic communication skills to assist clients in their journey through the grief process
  6. Do not offer false hope; only the client and family really know how they are feeling
  7. Encourage client and family to express their grief
  8. Educate client and family about the grief process

Case Study

A client is an 82-year-old Polish female who states that her religion is Catholic. She has right-sided heart failure and receives weekly visits from a home health nurse. The client states she is a burden to everyone and wishes it was not against her religious beliefs to commit suicide.

1. What spiritual assessment data should the nurse obtain?

2. What spiritual nursing diagnosis might be appropriate?

3. State the expected outcomes for this nursing diagnosis.

4. What interventions are appropriate to help this client?

5. How would the nurse evaluate the stated outcomes?

For suggested responses, see page 307.

POSTTEST

1 The nurse is caring for a male client who has recently had his left leg amputated. Which assessment should the nurse make related to subjective data regarding the client's body image?

1. Client's feelings regarding surgery
2. Strength of femoral pulses bilaterally
3. Client's description of his personality
4. Status of wound healing

2 A nurse is admitting a client who became ill while visiting in the United States. The nurse is unfamiliar with the cultural practices and health beliefs of the client's home country. Which of the following questions would be appropriate to ask in the admission assessment? Select all that apply.

1. "Are there remedies you have used for this illness before coming to the hospital?"
2. "Who do you usually see for help or care when you are ill?"
3. "What do you believe is causing your current illness?"
4. "What has influenced you to choose that type of clothing?"
5. "Can you tell me about your usual diet?"

3 A client reports a decrease in sexual desire. The nurse should examine the client's medication list for which of the following medications? Select all that apply.

1. Azithromycin (Zithromax)
2. Propranolol (Inderal)
3. Ascorbic acid (vitamin C)
4. Warfarin (Coumadin)
5. Sertraline (Zoloft)

4 The nurse is interviewing an adolescent client. The nurse can best facilitate communication with the client by making which statement?

1. "If you read the pamphlet, you'll know all you need to know."
2. "We can talk about this with your mother."
3. "Tell me about how you feel. You said you were depressed."
4. "Tell me about the last time you had sexual intercourse."

5 Several parents have asked the pediatric nurse to assess whether their toddlers are ready for toilet training. The nurse concludes that which toddlers demonstrate readiness for toilet training? Select all that apply.

1. One who can dress and undress self.
2. One who pulls to a standing position and says "pee" when urinating.
3. One who needs assistance with removing clothes.
4. One who crawls well and cries loudly after urination.
5. One who walks well.

6 A 4-year-old Mexican American child has recently been diagnosed with leukemia. When considering the client's culture, the nurse would employ which of the following as the most appropriate intervention?

1. Limit all visitors, including extended family.
2. Encourage visits from extended as well as immediate family.
3. Restrict any visits from alternative healers.
4. Make diet selections for the child and family.

7 Before acting upon the perceived nonverbal behavior of a client from Italy, the nurse should do which of the following?

1. Validate his or her perception.
2. Use a translator.
3. Get another nurse to assess the client.
4. Form a nursing diagnosis.

8 An older adult client expresses difficulty sleeping because her spirit is disturbed due to "sin in my life." The nurse should select which of the following as the priority intervention?

1. Call the chaplain and schedule a visit.
2. Ascertain what religious practice is appropriate to the client.
3. Pray immediately with the client.
4. Administer sleep medications as ordered.

POSTTEST

9 A client who is in the final stage of cancer is depressed and distant. The client asks the nurse, "Why is God punishing me?" What would be the most appropriate action for the nurse to take?

1. Be available to the client.
2. Share personal religious belief with the client.
3. Tell the client to pray for answers.
4. Call the provider for antianxiety medication orders.

10 A nurse finds multiple bruises in various stages of healing and signs of old injuries during an infant assessment. The nurse suspects the child may be the victim of abuse. Which action would be most important for the nurse to take?

1. Investigate the mother's feelings toward the infant.
2. Refer the child to a center for abused children.
3. Document objective findings and report suspected abuse as outlined in agency policy.
4. Make a note on the chart so the child will be assessed carefully on future visits.

➤ *See pages 120–121 for Answers and Rationales.*

ANSWERS & RATIONALES

Pretest

1 **Answer: 2** **Rationale:** Babies placed on their backs to sleep have a lower incidence of sudden infant death syndrome (SIDS) than those placed on their abdomens. Studies have shown the incidence of sudden infant death syndrome (SIDS) is increased when a baby is placed on his or her stomach for sleep. Breastfeeding has many health benefits for the newborn and does not increase the risk of sudden infant death syndrome (SIDS). Vomiting and aspiration is not the cause of sudden infant death syndrome (SIDS). SIDS occurs when the infant reinhales previously exhaled carbon dioxide as a result of the nose and mouth being close to the sheets, which prevents inhalation of oxygen. **Cognitive Level:** Applying **Client Need:** Health Promotion and Maintenance **Integrated Process:** Teaching and Learning **Content Area:** Maternal-Newborn **Strategy:** The critical words are *prevent* and *SIDS.* Use knowledge of major health concerns of infants to select the response that represents sound parent teaching. **Reference:** Berman, A., & Snyder, S. J. (2012). *Kozier & Erb's fundamentals of nursing: Concepts, process, and practice* (9th ed.). Upper Saddle River, NJ: Pearson Education, p. 378.

2 **Answer: 4** **Rationale:** As the primary caregiver of her mother, this role is new in her life and she states she does not know how to implement her responsibilities effectively. The client's daughter is not experiencing social isolation; she is having difficulty with her role as the caregiver. The client's daughter may feel powerless, but her ineffective role performance is the primary concern. There is no indication that the client's daughter is experiencing low self-esteem. **Cognitive Level:** Analyzing **Client Need:** Health Promotion and Maintenance **Integrated Process:** Nursing Process: Diagnosis **Content Area:** Foundational Sciences **Strategy:** The core issue of the question is

knowledge of various psychosocial nursing diagnoses. Use this information and the process of elimination to make a selection. **Reference:** Berman, A., & Snyder, S. J. (2012). *Kozier & Erb's fundamentals of nursing: Concepts, process, and practice* (9th ed.). Upper Saddle River, NJ: Pearson Education, p. 211.

3 **Answer: 3, 5** **Rationale:** Mentoring the next generation is a psychosocial task of the middle adult. Middle adults experience changes as their children also age and progress developmentally. Having a new girlfriend is not a psychosocial task of the middle adult. An older adult may be limited in the act of driving, but it is not a psychosocial task of the middle adult. Changing a hairstyle is not a psychosocial development task. **Cognitive Level:** Analyzing **Client Need:** Health Promotion and Maintenance **Integrated Process:** Nursing Process: Evaluation **Content Area:** Fundamentals **Strategy:** Recall that the psychosocial tasks of the middle adult include establishing a steady income, developing leisure, assisting adolescent children to become adults, and enjoying spouse and caring for aged parents. **Reference:** Berman, A., & Snyder, S. J. (2012). *Kozier & Erb's fundamentals of nursing: Concepts, process, and practice* (9th ed.). Upper Saddle River, NJ: Pearson Education, pp. 406–407.

4 **Answer: 3** **Rationale:** Adult supervision around a pool of water is the most important action to prevent drowning. Providing swimming lessons is important to the swimmer's skill in the water but this is not the best response. Placing a fence around the pool will help prevent unauthorized access but will not provide the most effective prevention against drowning. Approved flotation devices assist in keeping swimmers above water but will not be as effective as adult supervision. **Cognitive Level:** Applying **Client Need:** Safety and Infection Control **Integrated Process:** Teaching and Learning **Content Area:** Fundamentals **Strategy:** The critical phrase is *protect her*

2-year-old from drowning. Use knowledge of major health concerns for children in the toddler years to select the option that provides appropriate safety information and guidance to parents. **Reference:** Berman, A., & Snyder, S. J. (2012). *Kozier & Erb's fundamentals of nursing: Concepts, process, and practice* (9th ed.). Upper Saddle River, NJ: Pearson Education, p. 386.

5 **Answer: 2** **Rationale:** Conveying respect for the client's belief is a primary nursing responsibility. The nurse's responsibility is to assess the client's statement. This would only be reported to the health care provider if the client refuses prescribed treatment. Further assessment of the client's knowledge of the disease is important but should take place only after the assessment of culture and spirituality. Introducing self by name and title is important, but this is not the priority of care. **Cognitive Level:** Applying **Client Need:** Psychosocial Integrity **Integrated Process:** Caring **Content Area:** Fundamentals **Strategy:** Awareness of nursing interventions to promote spiritual health will assist you in selecting the option that aids in establishing a positive relationship with the client. Recall that religion may provide a framework for a client's health beliefs. **Reference:** Berman, A., & Snyder, S. J. (2012). *Kozier & Erb's fundamentals of nursing: Concepts, process, and practice* (9th ed.). Upper Saddle River, NJ: Pearson Education, p. 1061.

6 **Answer: 2** **Rationale:** Dietary choices are important aspects of culturally competent care. A Chinese American client likely will not practice the Jewish faith indicative of needing a Rabbi. The Chinese culture tends to be male dominated, and discharge instructions are more likely to be given to the eldest son. A teaching video may or may not be effective, while verbal instructions allow for discussion and exchange of questions and answers. **Cognitive Level:** Applying **Client Need:** Psychosocial Integrity **Integrated Process:** Nursing Process: Planning **Content Area:** Fundamentals **Strategy:** The critical terms in the question are *culturally competent* and *Chinese American.* Knowledge of culturally based characteristics will direct you to select actions that will be useful to clients from a specified culture. **Reference:** Berman, A., & Snyder, S. J. (2012). *Kozier & Erb's fundamentals of nursing: Concepts, process, and practice* (9th ed.). Upper Saddle River, NJ: Pearson Education, p. 513.

7 **Answer: 1** **Rationale:** It is vitally important that the client's spiritual well-being is restored. Relationships from supportive people are important but are not the highest priority. Encouraging the client to walk within 3 days will not facilitate coping if the client is experiencing spiritual distress. Praying the rosary is a practice in the Catholic faith, not Judaism. **Cognitive Level:** Analyzing **Client Need:** Psychosocial Integrity **Integrated Process:** Nursing Process: Planning **Content Area:** Fundamentals **Strategy:** Critical phrases in this question are *punishment for past sin* and *goal.* Use knowledge of spirituality to assist in setting appropriate goals for client outcomes. **Reference:** Berman, A., & Snyder, S. J.

(2012). *Kozier & Erb's fundamentals of nursing: Concepts, process, and practice* (9th ed.). Upper Saddle River, NJ: Pearson Education, p. 1067.

8 **Answer: 3** **Rationale:** Performing activities of daily living (ADLs) enhances control of one's life after surgery and can enhance the client's ability to deal with a terminal diagnosis. Performing activities of daily living (ADLs) will not strengthen muscles and increase healing. Encouraging self-care will have no effect on reasoning and coping with a diagnosis of cancer. Performing activities of daily living (ADLs) may enhance the client's mood but is not the priority in dealing with a terminal illness. **Cognitive Level:** Applying **Client Need:** Psychosocial Integrity **Integrated Process:** Teaching and Learning **Content Area:** Fundamentals **Strategy:** Use awareness of the stages of grief to enable you to select the option that best provides guidance to family members in time of loss. **Reference:** Berman, A., & Snyder, S. J. (2012). *Kozier & Erb's fundamentals of nursing: Concepts, process, and practice* (9th ed.). Upper Saddle River, NJ: Pearson Education, p. 1110.

9 **Answer: 1, 3, 4** **Rationale:** Not seeing "much point in going on" indicates the client is depressed and needs to discuss his options with someone. Asking for a priest is a valid request to help the client understand the effect his end-stage renal disease has on his spirituality and ultimate end-of-life care. Questioning God's will is indicative of spiritual distress. Stating dissatisfaction with being hospitalized and wishing to go home does not indicate spiritual distress. Stating that being hospitalized is depressing reflects state of mind but not spiritual distress. **Cognitive Level:** Applying **Client Need:** Psychosocial Integrity **Integrated Process:** Nursing Process: Diagnosis **Content Area:** Fundamentals **Strategy:** Critical words in the question are *spiritual distress* and *validate diagnosis.* Recall the characteristics of spiritual distress to make an accurate diagnosis. **Reference:** Berman, A., & Snyder, S. J. (2012). *Kozier & Erb's fundamentals of nursing: Concepts, process, and practice* (9th ed.). Upper Saddle River, NJ: Pearson Education, p. 1066.

10 **Answer: 4** **Rationale:** The client states his concern about the appearance of his face, and disfigurement can result in a body image disturbance. The question by the client does not indicate ineffective tissue perfusion. The client's communication is not pertinent to fluid volume deficit. The client has not stated he is in pain. **Cognitive Level:** Analyzing **Client Need:** Psychosocial Integrity **Integrated Process:** Nursing Process: Diagnosis **Content Area:** Fundamentals **Strategy:** The critical term is *most appropriate.* Assessment of body image changes is important in providing holistic care for this client. Remember body image is the perception of the physical self. **Reference:** Berman, A., & Snyder, S. J. (2012). *Kozier & Erb's fundamentals of nursing: Concepts, process, and practice* (9th ed.). Upper Saddle River, NJ: Pearson Education, p. 1027.

ANSWERS & RATIONALES

Posttest

1 **Answer: 1** **Rationale:** To assess body image, the nurse must gather information about the client's perception of his or her body. The client's description of personality is not related to body image. Assessing femoral pulses and wound healing constitutes objective data. **Cognitive Level:** Applying **Client Need:** Psychosocial Integrity **Integrated Process:** Nursing Process: Assessment **Content Area:** Fundamentals **Strategy:** The critical words in the question are *subjective data* and *body image*. Remember, whenever asked for subjective data you are looking for client perceptions, opinions, or concerns. **Reference:** Berman, A., & Snyder, S. J. (2012). *Kozier & Erb's fundamentals of nursing: Concepts, process, and practice* (9th ed.). Upper Saddle River, NJ: Pearson Education, p. 1027.

2 **Answer: 1, 2, 3, 5** **Rationale:** Understanding remedies already utilized may impact the care to be provided. Understanding the client's health care practices will help in providing culturally sensitive care. A cultural assessment should include the person's beliefs regarding the origin of illness. Understanding what foods, activities, and sites visited may assist in narrowing down a cause of the illness. Assessing the client's dietary intake will allow the nurse to determine if the illness is food related and provides a basis for providing culturally sensitive care. The person's reason for dressing in a particular manner is not relevant, and the question may be viewed as rude or intrusive. **Cognitive Level:** Analyzing **Client Need:** Psychosocial Integrity **Integrated Process:** Nursing Process: Assessment **Content Area:** Fundamentals **Strategy:** Awareness of cultural influences on health care beliefs and practices will enable you to assess a client's needs for culturally competent care. **Reference:** Berman, A., & Snyder, S. J. (2012). *Kozier & Erb's fundamentals of nursing: Concepts, process, and practice* (9th ed.). Upper Saddle River, NJ: Pearson Education, p. 303.

3 **Answer: 2, 5** **Rationale:** Antihypertensives, narcotics, diuretics, antipsychotics, antidepressants, antihistamines, and other medications decrease sexual desire. Propranolol (Inderal) is an antihypertensive while sertraline (Zoloft) is an antidepressant. Azithromycin (Zithromax) is an antibiotic. Ascorbic acid (vitamin C) is a water-soluble vitamin. Warfarin (Coumadin) is an anticoagulant. **Cognitive Level:** Applying **Client Need:** Pharmacological and Parenteral Therapies **Integrated Process:** Teaching and Learning **Content Area:** Fundamentals **Strategy:** The critical phrase is *decrease in sexual desire*. Recall common side effects of frequently prescribed groups of medications to assist you in eliminating the incorrect options. **Reference:** Berman, A., & Snyder, S. J. (2012). *Kozier & Erb's fundamentals of nursing: Concepts, process, and practice* (9th ed.). Upper Saddle River, NJ: Pearson Education, p. 1046.

4 **Answer: 3** **Rationale:** Requesting that the client tell the nurse how he or she feels will enhance communication by affirming the client's feelings. Adolescents will feel more willing to discuss private issues if parents are not present and if they understand that their concerns are common with other teens. Questions should be sensitively worded rather than intrusive. Written instructions should supplement teaching rather than being the primary vehicle for teaching. **Cognitive Level:** Applying **Client Need:** Psychosocial Integrity **Integrated Process:** Communication and Documentation **Content Area:** Fundamentals **Strategy:** The critical phrase is *facilitate communication* and *adolescent*. Use knowledge of psychosocial development throughout the life span to choose the option that allows effective communication with adolescents. **Reference:** Berman, A., & Snyder, S. J. (2012). *Kozier & Erb's fundamentals of nursing: Concepts, process, and practice* (9th ed.). Upper Saddle River, NJ: Pearson Education, pp. 472–473.

5 **Answer: 1, 5** **Rationale:** Developmental readiness for toilet training is demonstrated by standing and walking well, dressing self, recognizing the need for elimination, and having the physical ability to delay elimination. Lack of these abilities can indicate that the toddler needs additional time before attempting toilet training. **Cognitive Level:** Analyzing **Client Need:** Health Promotion and Maintenance **Integrated Process:** Teaching and Learning **Content Area:** Fundamentals **Strategy:** The critical term in the question is *demonstrates readiness*. Use knowledge of the sequence of physical development in early childhood to select the option that has the greatest likelihood for success. **Reference:** Berman, A., & Snyder, S. J. (2012). *Kozier & Erb's fundamentals of nursing: Concepts, process, and practice* (9th ed.). Upper Saddle River, NJ: Pearson Education, p. 1308.

6 **Answer: 2** **Rationale:** The extended family is considered a source of strength, support, and emotional stability for the Mexican American family. Alternative healers and specific foods also may be important to the state of health, so these should not be restricted or limited. **Cognitive Level:** Applying **Client Need:** Psychosocial Integrity **Integrated Process:** Caring **Content Area:** Fundamentals **Strategy:** Key words are *Mexican American* and *considering the client's culture*. Use knowledge of family roles within different cultures to assist you in selecting culturally competent interventions for this client. **Reference:** Berman, A., & Snyder, S. J. (2012). *Kozier & Erb's fundamentals of nursing: Concepts, process, and practice* (9th ed.). Upper Saddle River, NJ: Pearson Education, pp. 383–384.

7 **Answer: 1** **Rationale:** Nonverbal behavior may have varied meaning among different cultures; therefore, the nurse must validate meaning. There is insufficient information to determine the need for a translator. Another nurse's assessment is not necessary. The development of a nursing diagnosis is premature because the nurse has insufficient data. **Cognitive Level:** Analyzing **Client Need:** Psychosocial Integrity **Integrated Process:** Communication and Documentation **Content Area:** Fundamentals

Strategy: Recall that the Italian culture may utilize nonverbal communication and behavior and therefore you need to select the option that seeks to interpret that behavior. **Reference:** Berman, A., & Snyder, S. J. (2012). *Kozier & Erb's fundamentals of nursing: Concepts, process, and practice* (9th ed.). Upper Saddle River, NJ: Pearson Education, pp. 472–473.

8 **Answer: 2** **Rationale:** Assessing the religious practice will enable the nurse to obtain spiritual care that is most appropriate for the client. The client may or may not want a visit from the chaplain, as the chaplain may or may not be of the same religious denomination as the client. Also, the nurse would not act without verifying that this is acceptable to the client. The client may or may not be comfortable with prayer and it may not provide the best choice to deal with the client's spiritual distress. Administering sleep aids would not be the priority intervention to address the concern expressed by the client, which is consistent with spiritual distress. **Cognitive Level:** Analyzing **Client Need:** Psychosocial Integrity **Integrated Process:** Communication and Documentation **Content Area:** Fundamentals **Strategy:** Recall common nursing interventions to promote spiritual health and use the process of elimination to select actions that aid in identifying and helping clients meet their spiritual needs. **Reference:** Berman, A., & Snyder, S. J. (2012). *Kozier & Erb's fundamentals of nursing: Concepts, process, and practice* (9th ed.). Upper Saddle River, NJ: Pearson Education, pp. 1065–1066.

9 **Answer: 1** **Rationale:** Attention to the client's needs is the priority nursing intervention at this time. The nurse should offer self to the client by being physically present and attentive, and listening to the client's feelings and concerns. The nurse's personal religious beliefs are not central to the plan of care. Stating the client should pray for answers does not assist the client to cope with end-of-life issues. The administration of antianxiety medications does not address the statement made by the client. **Cognitive Level:** Applying **Client Need:** Psychosocial Integrity **Integrated Process:** Nursing Process: Implementation **Content Area:** Fundamentals **Strategy:** Recall that the nurse should be present to the client and aid the client in achieving spiritually deserved outcomes. **Reference:** Berman, A., & Snyder, S. J. (2012). *Kozier & Erb's fundamentals of nursing: Concepts, process, and practice* (9th ed.). Upper Saddle River, NJ: Pearson Education, p. 1067.

10 **Answer: 3** **Rationale:** Assessment and documentation of objective findings are key to legal standards and to standards of nursing practice. The mother's feelings about the child are not the central concern, since she may not be the abuser. Focusing on the mother may also prevent nursing care from being administered in a timely manner. The nurse would be able to refer the client only after a thorough assessment. Assessments upon future visits do not assist the child now and may place the child at risk for further injury. **Cognitive Level:** Analyzing **Client Need:** Psychosocial Integrity **Integrated Process:** Communication and Documentation **Content Area:** Fundamentals **Strategy:** The critical terms are *nurse suspects* and *victim of abuse.* Recall common patterns of child abuse to aid in identifying possible victims and reporting concerns. **Reference:** Berman, A., & Snyder, S. J. (2012). *Kozier & Erb's fundamentals of nursing: Concepts, process, and practice* (9th ed.). Upper Saddle River, NJ: Pearson Education, p. 378.

References

Ball, J. & Bindler, R. (2010). *Child health nursing: Partnering with children and families.* (2nd ed.). Upper Saddle River, NJ: Pearson Education.

Berman, A., & Snyder, S. J. (2012). *Kozier & Erb's fundamentals of nursing: Concepts, process, and practice* (9th ed.). Upper Saddle River, NJ: Pearson Education.

Carpenito, L. J. (2011). *Nursing diagnosis: Application to clinical practice* (13th ed.). Philadelphia, PA: Lippincott Williams & Wilkins.

Centers for Disease Control and Prevention (2012). *Recommended immunization schedule for persons aged 0 through 6 years—United States, 2012.* Retrieved February 16, 2012 from www.cdc.gov/vaccines/recs/schedules/downloads/child/0-6yrs-schedule-bw.pdf

D'Amico, D. & Barbarito, C. (2012). *Health & physical assessment in nursing* (2nd ed.). Upper Saddle River, NJ: Pearson Education.

Davidson, M., London, M., & Ladewig, P. (2012). *Maternal-newborn nursing and women's health across the lifespan* (9th ed.). Upper Saddle River, NJ: Pearson Education.

LeMone, P., Burke, K., & Bauldoff, G. (2012). *Medical-surgical nursing: Critical thinking in patient care* (5th ed.). Upper Saddle River, NJ: Pearson Education.

Murray, R. B., Zentner, J. P., & Yakimo, R. (2009). *Health promotion strategies through the life span.* (8th ed.). Upper Saddle River, NJ: Pearson Education.

Pender, N., Murdaugh, C., & Parsons, M. (2011). *Health promotion in nursing practice* (6th ed.). Upper Saddle River, NJ: Pearson Education, pp. 14–36, 66–94, 113–191.

Spector, R. (2009). *Cultural diversity in health and illness* (7th ed.). Upper Saddle River, NJ: Pearson Education.

U. S. Dept. of Health and Human Services. Office of Disease Prevention and Health Promotion. (2010). *Healthy people 2020.* Washington, DC: Author.

ANSWERS & RATIONALES

6

Overview of Skills Necessary for Safe Practice

Chapter Outline

Principles of Asepsis and
    Infection Control
Medical Asepsis versus
    Surgical Asepsis

Overview of Vital Signs
Overview of Body Mechanics

Overview of Cardiopulmonary
    Resuscitation

 NCLEX-RN® Test Prep

Use the accompanying online resource,
NursingReviewsandRationales, to test
yourself with hundreds of NCLEX®-style
practice questions.

Objectives

➤ Analyze the infectious process, modes of transmission, risk factors,
  and diagnostic tests used to detect infection and inflammation.
➤ Compare and contrast medical and surgical asepsis and the
  principles associated with each.
➤ Examine the significance of and techniques for measuring vital signs.
➤ Examine the scientific principles and guidelines for use of proper
  body mechanics.
➤ Analyze the procedures used to provide basic life support for both
  the adult and child client.

Review at a Glance

aerobic requiring oxygen to live
afebrile a condition in which body
temperature is not elevated
anaerobic an ability to live without
oxygen
apnea absence of breathing
blood pressure force of blood
against an arterial wall
body mechanics efficient use of
body as a machine and as a means of
locomotion
bradycardia slow heart rate, less
than 60 beats per minute
bradypnea slow respiratory rate
diastolic pressure least amount of
pressure exerted on arterial walls, which
occurs when heart is at rest between
ventricular contractions

dyspnea difficulty breathing
endogenous infection one in
which the causative organism comes
from client's own microorganisms
eupnea normal respiration
exogenous infection an infection
in which the causative organism is found
outside host
febrile a condition in which body
temperature is elevated
**health care–associated
infection** an infection that occurs as
a result of being treated in a health care
organization
hypertension blood pressure elevated above upper limit of normal
hypotension blood pressure below
lower limit of normal

iatrogenic infection an infection
that occurs as a result of a treatment or
diagnostic procedure
infection a disease state resulting
from pathogens in or on body
medical asepsis practice designed
to reduce number and transfer of pathogens; synonym for clean technique
orthostatic hypotension a temporary fall in blood pressure associated
with assuming an upright position;
synonym for *postural hypotension*
pathogen a disease-producing
organism
pulse a wave produced in the wall of
an artery with each beat of the heart
pulse deficit an apical rate greater
than the radial rate

surgical asepsis a set of practices that render and keep objects and areas free from all microorganisms; synonym for sterile technique

systolic pressure highest point of pressure on arterial walls when ventricles contract

tachycardia elevated heart rate above 100 beats per minute in an adult

tachypnea elevated respiratory rate

PRETEST

1 A client has been identified as having a very virulent bacterial infection that is spread through close physical contact. To decrease the chance of spreading this organism, the nurse would implement which infection control precautions?

1. Airborne precautions
2. Droplet precautions
3. Contact precautions
4. Protective isolation

2 A nurse needs to make rounds on 4 clients who are stable. Using the principle of medical sepsis, which client should be seen first?

1. A postsurgical cardiac client who has hypostatic pneumonia.
2. A client who has a draining wound.
3. A client who is severely neutropenic.
4. A child who has chicken pox.

3 A client develops a bloodstream infection from a central venous access device that has been in place for several months. The culture reports indicate that the infection is endogenous. The nurse concludes that which of the following would be a potential source of the infectious organism?

1. Hands of a caregiver
2. Client's skin flora
3. Airborne bacteria from another client
4. Bacteria from contaminated IV fluids

4 The nurse needs to bathe a client who has an infection spread by droplets, and the client has been placed on droplet precautions. Prior to reporting to work, the nurse's hands were scratched by a pet cat. The nurse puts on which of the following pieces of protective equipment before caring for this client? Select all that apply.

1. Mask
2. Gown
3. Goggles
4. Gloves
5. Head cover (cap)

5 A nurse is preparing to take vital signs on an alert client admitted to the hospital with dehydration secondary to vomiting and diarrhea. What is the best method to assess this client's body temperature?

1. Oral
2. Axillary
3. Rectal
4. Heat-sensitive tape

6 A nursing intershift report has indicated that a client's pulse volume is described as 1. After receiving the report, the initial action of the nurse should be to do which of the following?

1. Notify provider.
2. Assess client right away.
3. Document that pulse volume is normal.
4. Change the client's position.

7 A client is lying in bed with 2 blankets. The nurse assesses the client's temperature, which is 100.4°F. The client's skin is flushed. What would be the most appropriate action by the nurse at this time?

1. Place ice bags on the client's skin.
2. Remove blankets and offer fluids.
3. Increase the client's activity.
4. Decrease the client's oral fluid intake.

8 The home care nurse is assessing a client's vital signs. Which of the following findings would be of greatest concern to the nurse taking a client's pulse?

1. Mild tachycardia in a febrile client
2. Mild bradycardia in a young, otherwise healthy male who is asleep
3. Eighteen-month-old with a heart rate of 120 beats/minute
4. Pulse deficit with an apical rate of 88 beats/minute and a peripheral pulse of 72

9 While eating in a restaurant, a nurse notices a male patron choking on food. The individual is coughing loudly, his face is red, and he is unable to answer questions. Which of the following actions should the nurse take?

1. Place arms around the choking individual's waist and exert fist pressure on the abdomen.
2. Lay the individual on the floor and straddle the individual's legs to position self for the Heimlich maneuver.
3. Stand by and further observe the individual's response.
4. Slap the choking individual firmly on the back 3 times before attempting chests thrusts.

10 A nurse is evaluating a nurse orientee's performance during a mock code blue. The nurse concludes that chest compressions for the adult receiving CPR are adequate when the orientee depresses the sternum to a depth of a minimum of how many inches? Provide a numeric answer.

_____ inches

➤ *See pages 145–147 for Answers and Rationales.*

I. PRINCIPLES OF ASEPSIS AND INFECTION CONTROL

A. Chain of infection

1. Chain of infection refers to those elements that must be present to cause an infection from a microorganism (see Figure 6-1)
2. Basic to the principle of infection control is to interrupt this chain so that an **infection** from a microorganism does not occur in clients

3. *Etiologic agent*: a microorganism that is capable of causing infection if found in sufficient numbers in a susceptible host, and is able to live in host's body
   a. Are referred to as an infectious agent or a **pathogen**
   b. Examples of infectious agents or pathogens are bacteria, viruses, yeast, fungi, and protozoa
   c. In order for an infectious agent to produce an infection, the following circumstances must apply:
      1) Organism needs to be virulent
      2) Length of exposure needs to be sufficient
      3) Host must be susceptible
   d. If pathogen does not produce symptoms in host, the infection is called asymptomatic or subclinical; an opportunistic pathogen only causes an infection in a susceptible host
   e. A local infection is an infection that is limited to a certain area of body
   f. A systemic infection occurs when microorganisms spread to different parts of body
   g. Colonization refers to a microorganism in body that becomes resident flora that grows and reproduces but does not produce disease
4. *Mode of transmission*: microorganism must have a means of transmission to get from one location to another; called direct and indirect (see next section)

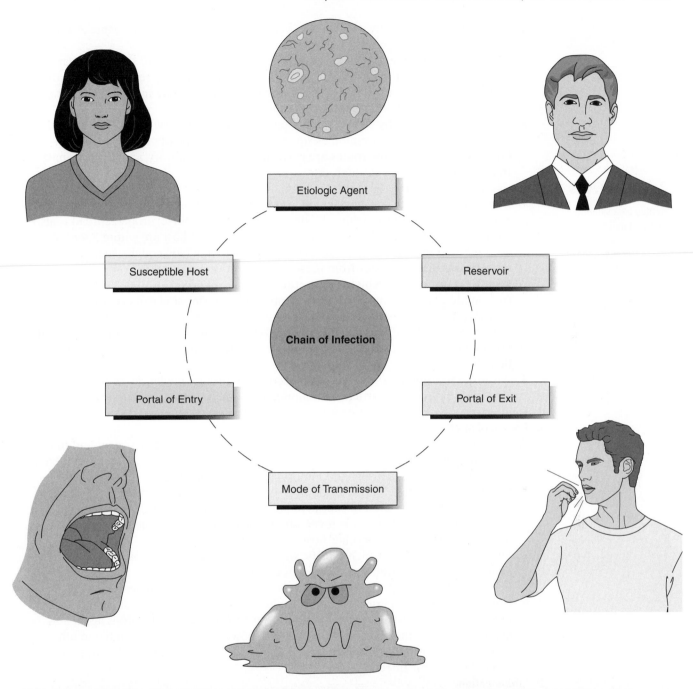

Figure 6-1

Chain of Infection

Berman, Audrey J.; Snyder, Shirlee, *Kozier & Erb's Fundamentals of Nursing*, 9th Ed. © 2012. Reprinted and Electronically reproduced by permission of Pearson Education, Inc., Upper Saddle River, New Jersey.

5. *Susceptible host*: describes a host (human or animal) with inadequate resistance against a particular pathogen to prevent disease or infection from occurring when exposed to pathogen; in humans this may occur if client's resistance is low because of poor nutrition, lack of rest, lack of exercise, or a coexisting illness that weakens host

6. *Portal of entry*: means by which a pathogen enters a host; can be the same as the portal of exit (see information that follows)

7. *Reservoir*: environment in which a microorganism lives to ensure survival; it can be a person, animal, arthropod, plant, soil, or a combination of these things; reservoirs that support organisms that are pathogenic to humans include inanimate objects, food and water, and other humans and animals

8. *Portal of exit*: means by which a pathogen escapes from reservoir and can cause disease; there is usually a common escape route for each type of microorganism; in humans, common escape routes are gastrointestinal, respiratory, and genitourinary tracts, and may also be through skin

B. Modes of transmission

1. Direct transmission: way in which microorganisms are transferred from person to person through biting, touching, kissing, or sexual intercourse; droplet spread is also a form of direct contact but can occur only if source and host are within 3 feet of each other; transmission by droplet can occur when a person coughs, sneezes, spits, or talks; it is direct transfer from person to person

2. Indirect transmission: vehicle-borne transmission can occur through fomites (inanimate objects or materials) or vector-borne transmission can occur through vectors (animal or insect, flying or crawling); fomites or vectors act as a vehicle for transmission; examples of fomites are handkerchiefs, toys, cooking utensils, surgical instruments or dressings, water, and food; examples of vectors are flies, mosquitoes, fleas, bats, cows, and cats

3. Airborne transmission: involves droplets or dust; droplet nuclei can remain in air for long periods and dust particles containing infectious agents can become airborne, infecting a susceptible host generally through respiratory tract

C. Course of infection

1. Incubation: time interval between initial contact with an infectious agent and first signs or symptoms of host infection; incubation period varies for different pathogens; microorganisms are growing and multiplying during this stage

2. Prodromal stage: time period from onset of nonspecific symptoms to appearance of specific symptoms related to causative pathogen; symptoms range from being fatigued to having a low-grade fever with malaise; during this phase it is still possible to transmit pathogen to another host

3. Full stage: time during which specific signs and symptoms of infectious agent are evident; this is also referred to as acute stage; during this stage, it may be possible to transmit infectious agent to another, depending on agent's virulence

4. Convalescence: time period during which host returns to pre-illness state; also called recovery period; host defense mechanisms have responded to infectious agent and manifestations of disease disappear; the host, however, is more vulnerable to other pathogens at this time; an appropriate nursing diagnostic label related to this process would be Risk for Infection

D. Inflammation

1. Definition: protective response of body tissues to injury or infection; inflammatory response is a physiological reaction to injury or infection; it may be acute or chronic

2. Body's response

    a. Inflammatory response begins with vasoconstriction and is followed by a brief increase in vascular permeability; blood vessels dilate, allowing plasma to escape into injured tissue

    b. White blood cells (neutrophils, monocytes, and macrophages) migrate to area of injury and attack and ingest invaders (phagocytosis); this process is responsible for signs of inflammation

Practice to Pass

Identify assessment data that indicate a client may have increased susceptibility to infections.

    c. Redness occurs when blood accumulates in dilated capillaries; warmth occurs as a result of heat from increased blood in area; swelling occurs from fluid accumulation; and pain occurs from pressure or injury to local nerves

E. Immune response

  1. Involves specific reactions in body to antigens or foreign material

  2. This specific response is body's attempt to protect itself, and involves activating 2 types of lymphocytes, the T-lymphocytes and B-lymphocytes

  3. Cell-mediated immunity: T-lymphocytes are responsible for cellular immunity

    a. When fungi, protozoa, bacteria, and some viruses activate T-lymphocytes, they enter circulation from lymph tissue and seek out antigen

    b. Once antigen is found they produce proteins (lymphokines) that increase migration of phagocytes to area and keep them there to eradicate antigen

    c. After antigen is gone, lymphokines disappear

    d. Some T-lymphocytes remain and keep a memory of the antigen and are reactivated if antigen appears again

  4. Humoral response: ability of body to develop a specific antibody to a specific antigen (antigen–antibody response)

    a. B-lymphocytes provide humoral immunity by producing antibodies that convey specific resistance to many bacterial and viral infections

    b. Active immunity is produced when immune system is activated either naturally or artificially

      1) Natural immunity involves acquisition of immunity through developing the disease

      2) Active immunity can also be produced through immunizations, which introduce into the body weakened or killed antigens (artificially acquired immunity)

      3) Passive immunity does not require a host to develop antibodies, rather it is transferred to host; passive immunity occurs when a mother passes antibodies to a newborn or when a person is given antibodies in the form of immune globulins from an animal or person who has had the disease; this type of immunity only offers temporary protection from the antigen

F. Health care–associated infection

  1. **Health care–associated infections** are those that are experienced as a result of a health care delivery system

  2. Clients become exposed to an infectious agent while in a health care agency even if infection may not be apparent at the time

  3. **Iatrogenic infection**: these health care–associated infections are directly related to client's treatment or diagnostic procedures; an example is a bacterial infection that results from an intravenous line or *Pseudomonas aeruginosa* pneumonia as a result of respiratory suctioning

  4. **Exogenous infection**: these health care–associated infections are a result of health care facility's environment or personnel; an example would be an upper respiratory infection resulting from contact with a caregiver who has an upper respiratory infection

  5. **Endogenous infection**: can occur from clients themselves or from reactivation of a previous dormant organism such as tuberculosis; an example of endogenous infection would be a vaginal yeast infection arising in a woman receiving antibiotic therapy; yeast organisms are always present in vagina, but with elimination of normal bacterial flora, yeast flourish

G. Factors increasing susceptibility to infection

  1. Age: young infants and older adults are at greater risk of infection because of reduced defense mechanisms

    a. Young infants have reduced defenses related to immature immune systems

      b. In older adults, physiological changes occur in body that make them more susceptible to infectious disease; some of these changes are as follows:

        1) Altered immune function (specifically, decreased phagocytosis by neutrophils and by macrophages)

        2) Decreased bladder muscle tone resulting in urinary retention

        3) Diminished cough reflex, loss of elastic recoil by lungs leading to reduced ability to evacuate normal secretions

        4) Gastrointestinal changes resulting in decreased swallowing ability and delayed gastric emptying

2. Heredity: some people have a genetic predisposition or susceptibility to some infectious diseases

3. Cultural practices: health care beliefs and practices, as well as nutritional and hygiene practices, can influence a person's susceptibility to infectious disease

4. Inadequate nutrition: nutritional practices that do not supply body with basic components necessary to synthesize proteins affect the way a body's immune system can respond to a pathogen

5. Stress: physical and emotional stressors affect body's ability to protect against invading pathogens; stressors affect body by elevating blood cortisone levels; if elevation of serum cortisone is prolonged, it decreases the anti-inflammatory response and depletes energy stores, thus increasing risk for infection

6. Rest, exercise, and personal health habits: altered rest and exercise patterns decrease body's protective mechanisms and may cause physical stress to body, resulting in an increased risk of infection; personal health habits such as poor nutrition and unhealthy lifestyle habits increase risk of infections over time by altering body's response to pathogens

7. Inadequate defenses: any physiological abnormality or lifestyle habit can influence normal defense mechanisms in body, making client more susceptible to infection; the immune system functions throughout the body and depends on the following:

    a. Intact skin and mucous membranes

    b. Adequate blood cell production and differentiation

    c. A functional lymphatic system and spleen

    d. An ability to differentiate foreign tissue and pathogens from normal body tissue and flora; in autoimmune disease, the body has difficulty recognizing its own tissue and cells; people with autoimmune disease are at increased risk of infection because of their immune system deficiencies

8. Environmental: an environment that exposes individuals to an increased number of toxins or pathogens also increases risk for infection; pathogens grow well in warm moist areas with oxygen (**aerobic**) or without oxygen (**anaerobic**) depending on microorganism

9. Immunization history: inadequately immunized people have an increased risk of infection specifically for those diseases for which vaccines have been developed

10. Medications and medical therapies: examples of therapies and medications that increase risk for infection include radiation treatment, antineoplastic drugs, anti-inflammatory drugs, and surgery

H. Diagnostic tests used to screen for infection

1. Signs and symptoms of localized infection are associated with the area infected; for instance, symptoms of a local infection on skin or mucous membranes are localized swelling, redness, pain, and warmth

2. Symptoms of systemic infection include fever, increased pulse and respirations, lethargy, anorexia, and enlarged lymph nodes

3. Certain diagnostic tests are ordered to confirm presence of an infection (see Table 6-1)

Table 6-1	Diagnostic Tests Related to the Infectious Process	
Test	**Normal Values/Conventional Units**	**Purpose/Indication**
White blood cell count (WBC)	4,500 to 11,000/mm³	A nonspecific blood test that indicates a response to either an infectious agent or to therapy; an elevation can indicate infection, tissue necrosis, stress, or neoplastic changes in bone marrow; an abnormally low count may also signal an increased risk for infection
WBC count with differential	Total neutrophils: 50–70% Bands: 0–5% Lymphocytes: 25–45% Monocytes: 2–6% Eosinophils: 1–3% Basophils: 0.4–1.0%	The total WBC is differentiated according to the various leukocytes; elevation of immature neutrophils (granulocytes or bands) indicates a bacterial infection (shift to the left); eosinophil elevation indicates an allergic disorder or a parasitic infestation; lymphocytes are elevated in viral or chronic infections; monocytes are elevated in viral infections and chronic inflammatory disorders; basophils are elevated in acute or severe infection
Erythrocyte sedimentation rate (ESR)	Male: 40–54% Female: 38–47%	ESR measures the rate at which red blood cells settle in unclotted blood; marked elevation of the ESR may occur in acute or severe bacterial infections; ESR can also provide information about the course of an infectious disease and the client's response to treatment
Culture and sensitivity (C&S)	Dependent upon source; findings will indicate organism present as well as antibiotics to which the organism is sensitive	Cultures are obtained from body fluids (urine, blood, wound exudate, cerebrospinal fluid); tissue cells are differentiated from microorganisms; stains are added to identify the organism structure; gram stains can broadly classify the organism; this information is useful for prescribing antibiotic therapy before sensitivity results are completed

II. MEDICAL ASEPSIS VERSUS SURGICAL ASEPSIS

A. Medical asepsis: a clean technique that involves health care practices that limit the number of pathogens present that could cause infections; application of barrier techniques to break the infectious cycle is a major nursing responsibility

1. Centers for Disease Control guidelines (see Box 6-1); CDC has designated two tiers of precautions:
   a. Standard precautions are standards used for all clients regardless of medical diagnosis
   b. Transmission-based precautions are used for suspected and documented infections; isolation procedures or precautions are practices that health care personnel use to prevent spread of microorganisms and are based on CDC recommendations; in some cases where client's immune system is altered (leukopenia or low white blood cell count [WBC]), protective isolation practices are used to protect client from microorganisms

2. Standard precautions: include specific behaviors and use of personal protective equipment by health care workers to protect themselves from acquiring pathogens from clients in their care and to protect clients from any pathogens the health care worker may have; generally no special technique is involved in removal of equipment unless there is a reason to suspect garments or hands of health care worker may become soiled; hands are always washed after removal of equipment

   a. Handwashing or hand hygiene: should occur before health care workers handle food, before and after eating, before and after each client contact, and after removing gloves; hand hygiene is considered the first line of defense against the spread of microorganisms and should be done frequently
   b. Gloves: are worn by health care workers to protect hands when likely to be in contact with any body fluids or secretions (blood, urine, feces, sputum, mucous membranes, and non-intact skin) or when any condition exists that may cause

transfer of endogenous microorganisms to client; for example, microorganisms on health care worker's hands may infect a client's non-intact skin; gloves also reduce risk of transmitting microorganisms from one client to another; assess whether client has a latex allergy; clients and staff with latex allergies should be provided latex-free supplies (such as gloves) and equipment

---

Box 6-1

Summary of CDC Guidelines

Standard Precautions

- Perform hand hygiene between client contact and after removing gloves using non-microbial soap or hand rub for routine handwashing. Use antimicrobial soap if hands may be contaminated with body secretions or a specific infectious disease is present.
- Wear clean gloves and appropriate type of personal protective equipment (such as gowns, face protection) when contact with various body secretions is expected.
- Change gloves between tasks on the same client.
- Handle used client equipment and soiled linen carefully to prevent the spread of microorganisms and follow procedures for cleaning equipment that is obviously contaminated with body fluids.
- Do not recap used needles. Place used needles and sharps in a puncture-resistant container.
- Clients who are likely to contaminate their environment should be placed in private rooms.
- Ensure that environmental controls such as room cleaning and disinfection procedures are followed.

Transmission-Based Precautions

- Are recommended in addition to Standard Precautions to prevent the spread of microorganisms based on route of transfer.

Airborne Precautions

- Used for clients with infections spread through the air (tuberculosis, varicella, rubeola).
- Provide a private room with monitored negative air pressure, 6 to 12 air changes per hour with air discharged to the outside or through a filter system, in relation to surrounding areas.
- Keep client in the room with door closed.
- Use respiratory protective equipment (N95) when entering room for clients with tuberculosis and if health care worker is not immune to varicella or rubeola.
- Transport client out of room, if required, wearing a surgical mask.

Droplet Precautions

- Used for clients with an infection that is spread by large-particle droplets (rubella, mumps, diphtheria, and adenovirus infection in children).
- Place client in a private room if possible or with other clients with same infection (cohorting).
- Wear respiratory protective equipment when providing care or if within 3 feet of client.
- Visitors should wear respiratory protective equipment if within 3 feet of client.
- Transport client after giving client a surgical mask to wear.

Contact Precautions

- Used for clients with an infection that is spread by direct or indirect contact or who are colonized with microorganisms like methicillin-resistant staphylococcus aureus (MRSA), or vancomycin-resistant enterococcus (VRE).
- Provide a private room or place with other clients who have the same microorganisms.
- Wear gloves when entering the room. Remove gloves in client's room and wash hands with an antiseptic or antimicrobial agent.
- Wear personal protective equipment when in contact with infected body secretions.
- Limit movement of the client outside the room.

Source: Centers for Disease Control

    c. Gowns: clean gowns or disposable waterproof gowns are worn when there is a risk of health care worker's clothing becoming soiled from client's body secretions

    d. Masks: are worn when there is a risk of infection from airborne route, droplet contact, or by splatters of body secretions; there are different types of masks depending on suspected pathogen; single-use disposable masks should be discarded when becoming wet or soiled, and generally are effective during client care procedures; particulate respiratory masks are used for disease spread by airborne transmission such as tuberculosis

    e. Protective eyewear: eyeglasses, goggles, or face shields are used if there is a risk of body secretions being splattered on face or in eyes

3. Soiled equipment and supplies: each health care facility has policies related to disposal and decontamination of reusable supplies and equipment; health care workers should follow agency policies and apply general principles of medical asepsis

    a. Sharps: needles, syringes, and sharps (lancets, razors, scalpels, broken glass) are placed into a puncture-resistant container; needles should never be detached from the syringe or re-capped before disposal

    b. Dishes: if client has a condition where there is a high risk of transmission of pathogens, most agencies use disposable dishes; handling of nondisposable dishes is minimized after client's meals by using trays to transport dirty dishes from client rooms

    c. Separate glass and metal that can be sterilized; rubber and plastic products must be cleaned by gas sterilization

    d. Trash: garbage and soiled disposable equipment are placed in a plastic bag that lines waste container

        1) If articles are contaminated, they are placed in a bag that is impervious to microorganisms before removal

        2) Articles that have infective material on them such as blood, pus, body fluid, or respiratory secretions are handled according to CDC's bloodborne pathogen guidelines

        3) If facility does not have impervious bags, it is necessary to double-bag soiled equipment before removing it from client's room

        4) Health care workers and clients should never retrieve articles from any waste container

    e. Thermometers: most agencies use disposable thermometers that are disposed of in client's waste container; nondisposable thermometers are disinfected after use

    f. Linen: all soiled linen should be handled as little as possible; it should be placed in a linen bag and closed prior to removal from client's room; laundry bags that are impervious to microorganisms are used by most agencies

4. Laboratory specimens: are placed in a leak-proof container with a secure lid; many agencies also require that they be placed in a sealed plastic bag labeled with a "biohazard" logo for transport to the laboratory; avoid contaminating the outside of the container

 5. Transporting persons with infections: when transporting a client with an infection, take precautions to prevent spread of pathogens; for instance, if a client has a respiratory infection a mask may be needed for transport; notify the receiving department of the situation

 6. Routine cleaning: all health care facilities have procedures for routine cleaning of clients' rooms

    a. Generally all equipment is disinfected before a new client is admitted to room; this includes bed, bathroom, tables, trays, telephones, call lights, remote controls, and any medical equipment kept in room

---

Practice to Pass

What information should the nurse provide to parents of a chronically ill child to reduce the risk of infection while promoting normal growth and development?

       b. Care is taken to prevent spread of organisms from one client to another by use of barriers

       c. Blood pressure cuffs do not require special precautions unless they are contaminated; follow agency policy for decontamination of the cuff; nondisposable thermometers are disinfected after each use

B. Surgical asepsis

      1. General principle: **surgical asepsis** involves those techniques that keep objects and areas free from all microorganisms, and are used for certain diagnostic procedures, and in operating rooms and labor and delivery areas (see Table 6-2); surgical aseptic (sterile) technique is indicated for procedures that require penetration of a client's skin such as with injections and IV catheter insertion

      2. Sterilization, disinfection, and cleaning: these procedures interrupt chain of infection and are used in health care facilities and by health care workers to reduce spread of infectious organisms

       a. Sterilization: kills all microorganisms, including spores and viruses; 4 commonly used methods are moist heat, gas, boiling water, and radiation; follow agency policies because method of sterilization is associated with type of object to be sterilized

       b. Disinfection: takes place through use of chemicals on objects; these chemicals may be toxic to tissues and are both bactericidal and bacteriostatic; when disinfecting articles, follow agency policies and manufacturer's recommendations for the disinfectant used; it is important that the disinfectant come in contact with the surface of the object and be exposed for the recommended time

       c. Cleaning: reduces the growth of microorganisms but does not totally remove them; rinsing visible organic material with cold water, then washing in hot soapy water and rinsing to remove soap can clean most equipment and objects; it may be necessary to use a stiff brush to clean equipment with grooves and corners

Table 6-2 **Principles and Practices of Surgical Asepsis**	
Principles	**Practices**
All objects used in a sterile field must be sterile.	All articles are sterilized appropriately by dry or moist heat, chemicals, or radiation before use.
	Always check a package containing a sterile object for intactness, dryness, and expiration date. Sterile articles can be stored for only a prescribed time; after that, they are considered unsterile. Any package that appears already open, torn, punctured, or wet is considered unsterile.
	Storage areas should be clean, dry, off the floor, and away from sinks.
	Always check chemical indicators of sterilization before using a package. The indicator is often a tape used to fasten the package or contained inside the package. The indicator changes color during sterilization, indicating that the contents have undergone a sterilization procedure. If the color change is not evident, the package is considered unsterile. Commercially prepared sterile packages may not have indicators but are marked with the word *sterile*.
Sterile objects become unsterile when touched by unsterile objects.	Handle sterile objects that will touch open wounds or enter body cavities only with sterile forceps or sterile gloved hands.
	Discard or resterilize objects that come into contact with unsterile objects.
	Whenever the sterility of an object is questionable, assume the article is unsterile.
Sterile items that are out of vision or below the waist level of the nurse are considered unsterile.	Once left unattended, a sterile field is considered unsterile.
	Sterile objects are always kept in view. Nurses do not turn their backs on a sterile field.
	Only the front part of a sterile gown, from shoulder to waist (or table height, whichever is higher) and the cuff of the sleeves to 2 inches above the elbows are considered sterile.

(continued)

Table 6-2 **Principles and Practices of Surgical Asepsis (continued)**

Principles	Practices
	Always keep sterile gloved hands in sight and above waist level; touch only objects that are sterile.
	Sterile draped tables in the operating room or elsewhere are considered sterile only at surface level.
	Once a sterile field becomes unsterile, it must be set up again before proceeding.
Sterile objects can become unsterile by prolonged exposure to airborne microorganisms.	Keep doors closed and traffic to a minimum in areas where a sterile procedure is being performed, because moving air can carry dust and microorganisms.
	Keep areas in which sterile procedures are carried out as clean as possible by frequent damp cleaning with detergent germicides to minimize contaminants in the area.
	Keep hair clean and short or enclose it in a net to prevent hair from falling on sterile objects. Microorganisms on the hair can make a sterile field unsterile.
	Wear surgical caps in operating rooms, delivery rooms, and burn units.
	Refrain from sneezing or coughing over a sterile field. This can make it unsterile because droplets containing microorganisms from the respiratory tract can travel 1 m (3 ft). Some agencies recommend that masks covering the mouth and the nose should be worn by anyone working over a sterile field or an open wound.
	Nurses with mild upper respiratory tract infections refrain from carrying out sterile procedures or wear masks.
	When working over a sterile field, keep talking to a minimum. Avert the head from the field if talking is necessary.
	To prevent microorganisms from falling over a sterile field, refrain from reaching over a sterile field unless sterile gloves are worn and refrain from moving unsterile objects over a sterile field.
Fluids flow in the direction of gravity.	Unless gloves are worn, always hold wet forceps with the tips below the handles. When the tips are held higher than the handles, fluid can flow onto the handle and become contaminated by the hands. When the forceps are again pointed downward, the fluid flows back down and contaminates the tips.
	During a surgical hand wash, hold the hands higher than the elbows to prevent contaminants from the forearms from reaching the hands.
Moisture that passes through a sterile object draws microorganisms from unsterile surfaces above or below to the sterile surface by capillary action.	Sterile moisture proof barriers are used beneath sterile objects. Liquids (sterile saline or antiseptics) are frequently poured into containers on a sterile field. If they are spilled onto the sterile field, the barrier keeps the liquid from seeping beneath it.
	Keep the sterile covers on sterile equipment dry. Damp surfaces can attract microorganisms in the air.
	Replace sterile drapes that do not have a sterile barrier underneath when they become moist.
The edges of a sterile field are considered unsterile.	A 2.5 cm (1 in) margin at each edge of an opened drape is considered unsterile because the edges are in contact with unsterile surfaces.
	Place all sterile objects more than 2.5 cm (1 in) inside the edges of a sterile field.
	Any article that falls outside the edges of a sterile field is considered unsterile.
The skin cannot be sterilized and is unsterile.	Use sterile gloves or sterile forceps to handle sterile items.
	Prior to a surgical aseptic procedure, wash the hands to reduce the number of microorganisms on them.
Conscientiousness, alertness, and honesty are essential qualities in maintaining surgical asepsis.	When a sterile object becomes unsterile, it does not necessarily change in appearance.
	The person who sees a sterile object become contaminated must correct or report the situation.
	Do not set up a sterile field ahead of time for future use.

Source: Berman, Audrey J.; Snyder, Shirlee, *Kozier & Erb's Fundamentals of Nursing*, 9th Ed. © 2012. Reprinted and Electronically reproduced by permission of Pearson Education, Inc., Upper Saddle River, New Jersey.

III. OVERVIEW OF VITAL SIGNS

    A. Accurate measurement of vital signs (VS) is a basic nursing skill (taking temperature, pulse, respiration, and blood pressure)

        1. VS measurement provides objective data used to assess client's health conditions and the need for intervention

        2. Accuracy is essential because subtle changes in VS measurements may indicate a change in client condition

        3. Changes in one VS measurement often cause a change in another; for instance, one degree of body temperature elevation can cause an increase of 4–6 heartbeats per minute

        4. Most health care facilities have policies related to when VS are measured for a client; these policies set minimum standards for the health care facility

        5. When and how often to measure VS is mainly a nursing decision

        6. VS measurements need to be taken on admission, before and after any invasive procedure, and when a client's condition changes

        7. Nursing evaluation of VS measurements depends on client's baseline data, client VS trends, and cause-and-effect relationship between nursing intervention and client response

    B. Temperature

        1. Regulation: body core temperature remains within a constant range due to physiological balance between heat production and heat loss

            a. This process is regulated by a thermostatic arrangement in brain's hypothalamus

            b. The body's surface temperature is the skin temperature and is directly related to environment

            c. Heat production occurs through metabolism, muscle activity, thyroxine production, chemical thermogenesis (norepinephrine, epinephrine, and sympathetic stimulation), and fever

            d. Heat loss occurs through radiation, conduction, convection, and vaporization (evaporation)

        2. Normal ranges: normal range for oral temperature in an adult is 36.7°C (98°F) to 37°C (98.6°F); a client with a normal temperature is said to be **afebrile**

        3. Measuring: the type of measuring device and route determine procedure to follow when taking a client's temperature; common routes are oral, axillary, tympanic, and rectal; internal methods to evaluate core body temperature may be used in critical care areas

            a. Client age and condition will determine the route used; for instance, a client who has had oral surgery should not have temperature measured using oral method; a client with diarrhea should not have temperature evaluated using rectal method

            b. Current literature indicates rectal or tympanic (external) routes and bladder (internal) route are closest to body's core temperature, making them the optimal routes when a client has an elevated temperature (fever) unless contraindicated

            c. The axilla is the safest site to assess a newborn's temperature

        4. Alterations: body temperature can vary according to client's age, sex, activity, time of day, and emotions

            a. Newborn body temperature regulatory mechanisms are imperfect and as a result the temperature is influenced by environmental temperature

            b. Older adults have a slightly lower body temperature

            c. Women have a slightly higher temperature than men related to hormone activity

            d. Exercise and activity can increase body temperature because of an increase in muscle activity

            e. Variations in time of day temperature are related to client activity and metabolism of food; generally speaking, body temperature is lower when clients are sleeping; highest temperature is reached between 4:00 p.m. and 6:00 p.m.; lowest temperature occurs between 4:00 a.m. and 6:00 a.m.

    f. Heightened emotions increase body temperature by action of sympathetic nervous system

    g. Altered body temperature may also be associated with injury to hypothalamus (temperature regulatory centers) such as with head injury or tumors

    h. Pyrexia and hyperthermia are other similar terms used to describe a fever, and this state is often referred to as being **febrile**

        1) Hyperpyrexia is a body temperature above 41°C (105.8°F)

        2) A deviation from normal body temperature in this range indicates a disease process is occurring that has caused an increase in heat production and/or a decrease in heat loss

        3) Clinical signs and symptoms of elevated body temperature are associated with body's temperature regulatory mechanisms trying to maintain balance (see Table 6-3)

        4) Clinical signs of fever are associated with hypothalamic thermostatic changes from a normal level to a higher level in response to tissue destruction, pyrogenic substances, or dehydration

        5) Elevation of body temperature is considered a normal defense mechanism in response to pathogens; it interferes with pathogen's ability to replicate and grow

        6) An elevated body temperature should be treated with antipyretic medication and other nursing interventions when it interferes with body system functioning (see Table 6-3 again)

        7) The 4 commonly occurring types of fever are constant, remittent, intermittent, and relapsing

    i. Hypothermia describes a body temperature below normal; nursing measures for clients with hypothermia are associated with decreasing heat loss and promoting heat production, such as providing blankets, heat shields, and raising environmental temperature

Practice to Pass

Identify conditions that cause heat loss in a client and nursing interventions to prevent or control this problem.

Table 6-3 Signs of Fever and Nursing Interventions

Period	Clinical Symptoms	Nursing Interventions (any phase)
Onset (cold or chill phase)	Increased heart rate and respiratory rate; feeling cold with shivering; pale cold skin with "gooseflesh"; cessation of sweating	Monitor vital signs, intake and output, and skin color and temperature. Monitor white blood cell count, hematocrit, or other laboratory indicators of dehydration or infection. Remove excess blankets when client feels warm but provide warmth when chilled. Provide adequate nutrition and fluids (e.g., 2,500–3,000 mL daily) to meet increased metabolic demands and prevent dehydration.
Course (plateau phase)	Increased pulse and respiratory rate; absence of chills; skin feels warm; photosensitivity; aching muscles, malaise and weakness; increased thirst; lethargic, may be disoriented; may become dehydrated	Administer antipyretic medicine as prescribed. Limit physical activity to prevent heat production. Provide tepid bath to increase heat loss by conduction. Monitor for signs of dehydration. Provide safety measures if client disoriented from fever.
Defervescence (fever abatement/flush phase)	Skin warm and flushed; diaphoresis; decreased shivering; possible dehydration	Provide dry bedding and clothing. Provide oral care to keep mucous membranes moist.

Source: Berman, Audrey J.; Snyder, Shirlee, *Kozier & Erb's Fundamentals of Nursing*, 9th Ed. © 2012. Reprinted and Electronically reproduced by permission of Pearson Education, Inc., Upper Saddle River, New Jersey.

C. Pulse

1. Basic information about client's circulatory system can be obtained by assessing pulse

2. The **pulse** is caused by contraction of left ventricle of heart moving blood into arteries; this produces a pulse wave that can be palpated

3. In healthy people, pulse rate is the same as rate of ventricular contractions; in some types of heart disease, they differ

4. In a client with heart disease, it is important to measure both apical pulse rate and peripheral pulse rate for comparison (should be equal)

5. Pulse sites: peripheral pulse sites may be important to evaluate depending on client condition or age; the radial pulse is the most common site assessed due to accessibility (see Figure 6-2 and Table 6-4)

   a. Assess apical pulse whenever there is a variation from normal rate in a peripheral pulse, if client has cardiovascular disease or is taking a cardiac glycoside or beta-blocker medication, or for children under age 3 years

   b. To assess apical rate, place a clean stethoscope over apex of heart (left 5th intercostal space, midclavicular line, point of maximum impulse) and count heart beats for 1 minute

   c. A difference between radial pulse (peripheral) and apical pulse is referred to as a **pulse deficit**; an apical rate greater than the radial rate needs to be reported promptly, as it may indicate vascular disease or cardiac dysrhythmia

6. Rate: pulse rate can vary depending on the client's health status, age, sex, activity, medication, body build and position, stress and emotional factors, and pain

   a. A client experiencing stress or pain will have an elevated pulse whereas an athletic client's pulse may be lower; it is important to consider these factors when evaluating pulse rate, rhythm, and volume

Figure 6-2

Peripheral pulse sites.

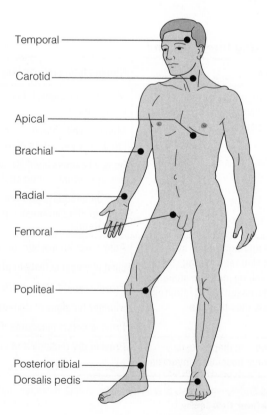

Temporal

Carotid

Apical

Brachial

Radial

Femoral

Popliteal

Posterior tibial
Dorsalis pedis

Table 6-4	Specific Pulse Sites and Nursing Implications	
Site	**Location**	**Nursing Implications**
Temporal	Above and lateral to the eye over the temporal bone	Easy accessibility especially for children
Carotid	Medial edge of the sternocleidomastoid muscle in the neck	Use when peripheral sites not palpable, such as with shock
Apical	Fourth to fifth intercostal space; left midclavicular line	Auscultate apical pulse routinely for children under 3
Brachial	Groove between biceps and triceps muscle at the antecubital fossa	Assess BP; measure during infant cardiac arrest
Radial	Thumb side of wrist	Evaluates hand circulation
Ulnar	Ulnar side of forearm at the wrist	Evaluates hand circulation
Femoral	Midway between symphysis pubis and anterior superior iliac spine	Used when peripheral sites not palpable, during CPR and with shock; for infants and children; to evaluate lower limb circulation
Popliteal	Behind the knee in the popliteal fossa	Evaluate lower leg circulation, when taking a thigh BP
Dorsalis pedis	Top of foot; between extension tendons of great and first toe	Evaluates circulation to foot

    b. Assess rate, rhythm, and volume by compressing an artery against an underlying bone with the pads of 3 fingers; using too much pressure may obliterate the pulse, while too little pressure may make it difficult to feel the pulse

    c. Specific terms are used to describe variation in rate

        1) A pulse that is below normal rate (60 in adults) is referred to as **bradycardia**

        2) A pulse that is higher than normal rate (greater than 100 in adults) is called **tachycardia**

  7. Rhythm: pulse should be regular with an equal time interval between beats; a variation in rhythm is labeled as irregular and could indicate a dysrhythmia

  8. Pulse volume or pulse amplitude: also called pulse force, refers to quality of pulsation felt from force of blood with each beat; it is the pulse strength; volume should remain constant with moderate pressure of fingers and is obliterated with greater pressure

    a. A scale of 0 to 3 is used to describe pulse volume; see Box 6-2

    b. Some health care facilities may use a different scale to measure pulse volume; be familiar with agency policy and use scale provided by agency

D. Respirations

  1. Respiratory rate (RR) is the number of breaths per minute and includes inspiration (breathing in) and exhalation (breathing out)

  2. Client factors that affect RR include age, activity, environmental temperature, body temperature, emotions, stress, body position, medication, and disease process

  3. Control of respiration occurs in several areas

    a. Respiratory centers in medulla oblongata

    b. Pons in brain

    c. Chemoreceptors located centrally in medulla and peripherally in carotid and aortic bodies that respond to oxygen, carbon dioxide, and hydrogen ion concentrations in arterial blood

Box 6-2	0: pulse is absent
	1: pulse is difficult to feel; thready or weak
Scale for Recording Pulse Volume	2: pulse has normal amplitude
	3: bounding pulse that is difficult to obliterate

4. Techniques for assessing RR include counting rate and evaluating depth and rhythm by watching movement of client's chest wall and/or placing a hand on client's chest wall
   a. Ensure that client is relaxed and unaware of assessment and in a position that supports maximum lung expansion, unless contraindicated by client's condition
   b. Count the rate for 30 seconds (then multiply by 2) unless it is irregular; then it should be counted for 1 full minute
   c. Consider findings in relation to client's normal breathing patterns, position, health problems, medications or therapies, and cardiovascular function
5. Quality: evaluate respirations for amount of effort and sound occurring with each cycle; normally there is no sound and respirations are effortless
   a. **Dyspnea** describes difficult and labored breathing
   b. Orthopnea describes ability to breathe only when head and chest are elevated; clients that have difficulty breathing in a prone or supine position may breathe better when sitting up
   c. Sounds are described such as stridor (harsh sound with inspiration), wheezing (high-pitched musical sound heard on expiration) and bubbling (gurgling sounds); these adventitious sounds may be present if airway is partially obstructed on inspiration
6. Rate, depth, and pattern: normally respirations are evenly spaced at an adult rate of 12 to 20 per minute (called **eupnea**)
   a. A respiratory rate that it below normal is referred to as **bradypnea**, while a rate above normal is called **tachypnea**
   b. Depth of respiration is described as normal, deep, or shallow
   c. Terms used to describe abnormal patterns are hyperventilation (increased amount of air in lungs characterized by prolonged deep breaths), hypoventilation (decreased in amount of air in lungs caused by shallow breathing), and Cheyne-Stokes breathing (gradual increase in depth of respirations followed by gradual decrease)
   d. Chest movements: abnormal movements include intercostal retractions, substernal retractions, and flail chest; these signs indicate a problem with air exchange due to an inflammatory response of bronchioles (asthma), fluid consolidation in lung fields, or a chest injury

E. Blood pressure (BP)
1. **Blood pressure** is a measure of force of blood as it flows through arteries
2. Assessment of BP provides information about circulatory system, specifically elasticity of arterial walls, efficiency of heart as a pump, and volume of circulating blood (cardiac output, peripheral vascular resistance, blood volume and viscosity)
3. The movement of blood in waves causes 2 pressure measurements; **systolic pressure** (resulting from contraction of heart's ventricles) and **diastolic pressure** (resulting from relaxation of heart ventricles)
4. The pulse pressure is the difference between systolic and diastolic BPs; is usually around 40 millimeters of mercury (mmHg); a consistently elevated pulse pressure occurs in arteriosclerosis; a low pulse pressure can occur in severe heart failure
5. American Heart Association recommends 2 blood pressure readings be taken; prior to assessing second reading, wait 1 minute; an average of 2 measurements is recorded
6. BP equipment: measures BP, which is recorded as a fraction, with systolic pressure written over diastolic pressure; equipment to measure BP may include:
   a. A sphygmomanometer with an attached BP cuff and a stethoscope; 2 types of sphygmomanometers are available
      1) An aneroid manometer which consists of a calibrated dial
      2) A calibrated cylinder filled with mercury (older, not often seen)
   b. An electronic sphygmomanometer is utilized without a stethoscope and does not require listening to sounds of client's BP

    c. A Doppler ultrasound stethoscope may also be used for assessment when sounds are difficult to hear, such as in infants and clients in shock; when a Doppler stethoscope is used, systolic BP is usually recorded with a large letter D (for Doppler) beside numeric value

    d. A BP cuff comes in a variety of sizes and cuff size is determined by size of client; the bladder of the cuff must have correct width and length for client's arm (bladder cuff encircles at least two-thirds of upper arm); if cuff is too wide, the resulting measurement may be low, and if it is too narrow the resulting measurement will be high

7. Measurement: adults and children

    a. BP can be measured directly (catheter placed in artery shows waves representing arterial pressure on a monitor) or indirectly (auscultated and palpated)

    b. The auscultatory (auscultated) method is most frequently used

        1) Apply BP cuff to client's left arm at heart level

        2) The right arm may be used if left arm is contraindicated because of a surgical procedure, cast, paralysis, mastectomy, or hemodialysis graft or fistula

        3) When establishing a client's baseline, measure BP in both arms

        4) Palpate over brachial pulse site and inflate cuff until it is 30 mmHg above where client's pulse disappeared

        5) Then place stethoscope over brachial artery and deflate cuff 2 to 3 mmHg/second while simultaneously watching manometer and listening to sounds heard through stethoscope; these sounds are called Korotkoff's sounds and consist of 5 phases

           a) Phase 1: first faint tapping or thumping sound heard; first tapping sound heard is systolic BP

           b) Phase 2: period during deflation when sounds have a muffled quality

           c) Phase 3: period when sound becomes crisper and again assumes a thumping sound

           d) Phase 4: the time when sound becomes muffled and has a soft blowing quality; American Heart Association recommends this sound be recorded as the diastolic blood pressure in children; in some instances, 3 numbers may be recorded, phase 1, 4, and 5

           e) Phase 5: last sound heard; this is the diastolic BP in adults

        6) If sounds cannot be heard, palpate the BP

        7) An elevated BP is referred to as **hypertension** (systolic BP 140 mmHg or diastolic BP 90 mmHg or higher); prehypertension occurs when systolic BP is 120–139 mmHg and diastolic BP is 80–89 mmHg; a BP that is below normal is referred to as **hypotension**

        8) **Orthostatic hypotension** refers to a significant drop in BP when client stands from a sitting position, or sits up from a recumbent position

        9) Factors affecting BP are age, exercise, stress, race, obesity, gender, medications, diurnal variations, and disease process

        10) The average BP in a healthy adult is 120/80 mmHg; it is important when providing care for clients to consider client's BP trends and client factors that affect BP

8. Causes for error: most errors in taking the BP are related to an improperly fitting BP cuff and improper procedure

    a. Elevating client's arm above heart can cause a low BP reading

    b. Deflating cuff too slowly will cause a high diastolic reading

    c. Deflating too fast will cause a low systolic with a high diastolic reading

    d. An improperly fitting cuff can provide erroneous results as previously outlined

    e. Health care workers responsible for BP assessment must ensure accuracy of results obtained; many clinical judgments are made based on BP readings

Practice to Pass

What assessment criteria will assist the nurse in determining if a newly admitted client's blood pressure is normal, although it is not consistent with established norms?

9. Interpreting abnormal findings: consider variations in client trends, such as if BP is elevated on more than 2 occasions, and whether there are client factors that could affect BP

F. **Special procedures/equipment**
   1. Cardiac monitor: provides information associated with cardiac function including rate, rhythm, and quality of heart contraction
   2. Doppler: an instrument that amplifies sound and is useful when assessing pulses that are difficult to palpate or a BP that is difficult to hear; this device has an ultrasound transducer and an audio unit that transmit sound of blood as it moves through blood vessels
   3. Pulse oximeter: a noninvasive device placed on a client digit or earlobe that provides information about oxygen saturation (SaO_2) (normal = 95–100%)
   4. Arterial line: provides information directly about a client's arterial BP; a catheter is inserted into an artery and the tip senses pressure and transmits this data to a machine that displays BP
   5. Hemodynamic monitoring: is used to assess a critically ill client's cardiovascular status; it is indicated when VS measurements are not adequate to evaluate a client's cardiac status; information received from this monitoring includes heart rate, arterial BP, central venous pressure, pulmonary pressures, and cardiac output (CO)

> **Practice to Pass**
>
> What variations in a client's pulse and respirations could be anticipated if the blood pressure was low because of bleeding?

IV. OVERVIEW OF BODY MECHANICS

A. **Scientific principles**
   1. **Body mechanics** are associated with the action and function of muscles that are used to maintain balance and posture of body during all activities involved in daily living
   2. In nursing practice, these principles are used to protect both nurse and client from injury to musculoskeletal and nervous systems
   3. These principles involve concepts of center of gravity, line of gravity, and base of support
      a. Body is more stable with a greater base of support
      b. Holding an object close to body requires less energy
      c. When a person moves, center of gravity shifts continuously in the direction of moving body parts
      d. Facing the direction of work and using pelvic tilt before an activity decreases risk for injury
      e. Balance depends on interrelationship between center of gravity, line of gravity, and base of support; if all body parts are balanced, less energy is used

B. **Correct body alignment**
   1. Bones and muscles of musculoskeletal system and central and peripheral nerves are responsible for body shape, form, and movement
   2. Related concepts
      a. Correct body alignment and posture require that body weight is centered and forces of gravity are balanced; when joints and muscles are not experiencing an extreme flexion or extension, or unusual stress, alignment is achieved and structures and internal organs are supported
      b. The usual line of gravity begins at top of head and bisects shoulders, trunk, and weight-bearing joints; the base of support is slightly anterior to sacrum
      c. Maintaining proper body alignment promotes functioning of respiratory, circulatory, renal, and gastrointestinal systems

C. Effective body movement

1. Balance and movement occur with coordinated muscle activity and neurologic integration; reticular formation integrates neural input that helps maintain body's balance
2. Equilibrium is a function of the vestibular apparatus of the ear
3. The cerebellum coordinates motor activities of movement, the cerebral cortex begins voluntary movement, and the basal ganglia maintain posture

D. Methods to protect the back

1. Nurses need to be mindful of proper body mechanics when providing care to clients
2. Measures to prevent back injury
   a. Maintain a wide base of support when assisting clients with position changes
   b. Avoid twisting movements of the spine
   c. Adjust height of work area when working
   d. Bend hips and knees to alter position of body
   e. When lifting, use large muscle groups of legs
   f. Hold objects close to body when lifting
   g. Employ mechanical devices when appropriate
   h. Use smooth and coordinated motions when working
3. Implement no-lift policies; 35 pounds is the maximum weight a nurse should attempt to lift
4. Utilize ceiling, mobile, and sit-to-stand lifts

V. OVERVIEW OF CARDIOPULMONARY RESUSCITATION

A. Cardiopulmonary resuscitation (CPR) is a basic emergency procedure for life support

1. The guidelines have changed from "Airway, Breathing, and Circulation" to "Circulation, Airway, Breathing"
2. It is used to establish circulation and ventilation to prevent irreversible brain damage resulting from anoxia
3. Guidelines were most recently revised in 2010
4. Do not look, listen, and feel for breathing as an early step

B. Basic life support (BLS)

1. BLS or CPR does not require use of any equipment, although mechanical devices may be used
2. It can be done with 1 or 2 people and involves 3 interrelated activities: restoring circulation, airway, and breathing
3. Most health care facilities require personnel to be trained in BLS
4. Three signs of cardiac arrest are **apnea** (absence of respirations), *asystole* (absence of carotid or femoral pulse), and dilated pupils

C. One- and two-person adult CPR for health care providers

1. Begin CPR after calling for help (if an automatic external defibrillator [AED] is available, obtain and use it once first if victim is unresponsive)
2. Turn client on his or her back and place on a board or hard surface
3. Begin chest compressions (push hard and push fast); 100 compressions per minute at a depth of 2 inches
4. Once compressions have been started, deliver one rescue breath; give significant tidal volume to produce a chest rise
5. Compression to ventilation ratio of 30 chest compressions to 2 ventilations; continue until an advance airway is placed
6. Minimize the frequency and duration of interruptions in compressions

7. Once an advanced airway (endotracheal tube, laryngeal mask airway [LMA], or esophageal-tracheal Combitube) is in place, provide 1 breath every 6–8 seconds (8–10 ventilations per minute); deliver 100 compressions per minute continuously ("push hard, push fast"), without pauses for ventilation

8. When there are 2 or more rescuers and client has an advanced airway, switch roles every 2 minutes to prevent fatigue; switch as quickly as possible (less than 5 seconds) to minimize interruptions in chest compressions

9. Performance errors and complications of CPR: complications associated with CPR include the following:
   a. Improper hand position during cardiac compressions can cause rib fracture
   b. Failure to adequately ventilate client due to improper head position can lead to hypoxia and gastric distention
   c. Poor oxygen profusion to vital organs may result in brain and tissue damage
   d. The body attempts to maintain homeostasis by shunting circulation to vital organs, resulting in less perfusion to periphery, which can result in distal tissue damage

D. **Infant and child resuscitation for health care providers**
   1. The compression depth is 1.5 inches for infants and 2 inches for children
   2. Do not assess a pulse in an unresponsive child who is not breathing; begin CPR; initiate CPR with chest compressions; 30 compressions with one rescuer or 15 compressions with 2 rescuers; depress the chest one-third to one-half the anterior–posterior diameter of chest
   3. Use a manual AED for infants
   4. Take care not to overextend infant's head when opening airway
   5. Rescuer may be required to place own mouth over mouth and nose of an infant to establish an airtight seal

E. **Termination of basic life support**
   1. CPR should be maintained until there is a return of respiration and a pulse or until directed by a physician to discontinue basic life support
   2. The only other acceptable reason for discontinuing CPR, once begun, is physical exhaustion of the rescuer

F. **Foreign body airway obstruction**
   1. Airway obstruction is a medical emergency that requires immediate attention
   2. Common causes
      a. A common cause of airway obstruction is the tongue falling back and blocking the airway; for this problem, the rescuer should position the unconscious, but breathing, client on either side to relieve the obstruction
      b. In other cases, food or other foreign objects can be aspirated into the airway resulting in obstruction; procedures to evacuate the foreign object are based on the client's age and body size
      c. Client education in the prevention of airway obstruction is an important nursing function
         1) Remind adults to chew food slowly and thoroughly before attempting to swallow
         2) When assisting older clients with eating, present foods with a consistency that facilitates swallowing and at an appropriate temperature
         3) Instruct parents to teach their children not to run and play while eating, and not to put foreign objects in their mouths
         4) Keep small objects away from children under the age of 3

        5) Avoid feeding peanuts, popcorn, and raisins (and other small nondissolving or hard items) to children under the age of 3; always cut a hot dog in half lengthwise, cutting it in round pieces creates pieces that are the size of the child's trachea

        6) Cut all other food products small enough for the child to easily swallow

3. Recognition

  a. When a client's airway is partially obstructed he or she may cough, have high-pitched sounds, and indicate there is trouble breathing by holding hands to the throat area

    1. As long as client is coughing strongly and VS are stable, no interventions are necessary

    2. It is important not to slap client on the back because this may move the foreign object further into client's airway

  b. If client is producing a high-pitched inspiratory stridor, the airway is almost obstructed; in this situation, client may only be able to produce a weak cough, as well as be unable to speak, appear cyanotic, and have irregular shallow breathing

  c. If client is not making any sound, the airway is totally obstructed and requires immediate action

4. Management for adults: performing the Heimlich maneuver should remove the foreign object

  a. If client is conscious and coughing, ask if he or she is choking; if client nods yes, ask if he or she wants help; intervene only if cough becomes silent, or respiratory difficulty is increased or is accompanied by stridor

  b. Stand behind client and wrap arms around client's waist; make a fist with one hand and place thumb side of fist against client's abdomen above navel and below xiphoid process, grasp fist with other hand and press fist into abdomen while thrusting upward; repeat this sequence rapidly until object is expelled or client becomes unconscious (then support client to ground, activate emergency medical system, and begin CPR)

  c. When discovering unconscious client on the ground, call for help and use tongue-jaw lift method to open mouth and inspect for presence of a foreign object causing obstruction; perform a finger sweep only if object is visualized; perform abdominal thrust to evacuate an object; straddle client's thighs and place heal of one hand on epigastric region below xiphoid process, then place second hand on top of the first quickly thrusting upward; repeat 6 to 10 times; if object is not removed try to ventilate client; if unsuccessful, repeat abdominal thrusts or try chest thrusts (see next)

  d. Clients who are obese or pregnant require chest thrusts instead of abdominal thrusts; make a fist and place thumb side against middle of client's sternum and grasp fist with other hand to deliver a quick backward thrust

5. Management for children: for children over the age of 1, the procedure is the same as for adults only performed more gently

6. Management for infants: to dislodge a foreign object from an infant's airway; do the following:

  a. Hold infant over arm with head lower than trunk supporting the head by holding jaw firmly in the hand, then rest infant's body on forearm

  b. Deliver 5 back blows with heel of hand between infant's scapula

  c. If object is not evacuated, turn infant to a supine position and place 2 fingers over sternum (position for chest compressions) and deliver 5 chest thrusts

  d. Continue to alternate between back blows and chest thrusts until object is expelled

  e. If infant becomes unconscious from lack of oxygen, add attempts to ventilate to the sequence; do not perform blind finger sweeps

Case Study

A 35-year-old client with type 1 diabetes mellitus was admitted to the medical unit with an ulcer on the bottom of the foot that is not healing. The client injured the foot 2 weeks prior to admission by stepping on a stick while gardening. The client's vital signs are oral temperature 39°C (102.2°F), pulse 110, respirations 24, and blood pressure 130/90. There is a large amount of purulent drainage from the circular wound on the bottom of the right foot measuring approximately 7 cm. The affected foot is swollen, red, and warm to touch. The client states it is very painful.

1. What diagnostic tests are likely to be ordered for this client?

2. Based on the information given, describe the body's defense mechanism initiated in response to injury.

3. Identify possible nursing diagnoses that may be applicable for this client and the criteria to support the diagnoses.

4. Identify expected outcome criteria based on the nursing diagnoses identified.

5. Describe nursing interventions related to the prevention of the spread of microorganisms.

For suggested responses, see page 307.

POSTTEST

1 A client had oral surgery following a motor vehicle crash, and the nurse assessing the client finds the skin flushed, warm, and diaphoretic. Which of the following would be the best method to assess the client's body temperature?

1. Oral
2. Axillary
3. Forehead temperature strip
4. Rectal

2 The nurse is preparing to change a client's sterile dressing. Which of the following nursing actions will increase the client's risk of developing an infection?

1. Verbally describing to the client and family each phase of the dressing change process while performing it
2. Checking that sterile dressing packages are intact before opening
3. Opening gauze pads packages before putting on sterile gloves
4. Ensuring that the table that will hold the sterile field is dry

3 Which action would the nurse take to use a wide base of support when assisting a client to get up from a chair?

1. Bend at the waist, place arms under the client's arms, and lift.
2. Face the client, bend knees, place hands on client's forearms, and lift.
3. Spread the feet apart before touching the client.
4. Tighten the pelvic muscles before assisting the client.

4 A nurse is giving a client a bed bath. Which of the following nursing actions will assist the nurse in preventing a back injury?

1. Narrow the base of support.
2. Raise the bed to a comfortable position.
3. Move the client to the opposite side of the bed.
4. Position self near the client's head.

5 When providing care to a client, which of the following will place the nurse at risk for contamination from the client's body fluids?

1. Providing a back massage
2. Feeding a client
3. Providing hair care
4. Providing oral hygiene

6 A nurse finds a client unresponsive in bed and is preparing to open the client's airway. Which of the following methods to open the airway would be most appropriate to use?

1. The jaw-thrust maneuver
2. The head tilt–chin lift procedure
3. The chest thrust maneuver
4. The chin to sternum method

7 After correctly positioning a client for a urinary catheterization procedure, the nurse sets up a sterile field and places the kit supplies on the area. The nurse hears a page to respond to another client who has fallen in the hallway. Which of the following would be the most appropriate nursing action?

1. Ensure the client's safety, cover the field with a sterile towel, and respond to the other client.
2. Continue quickly with the procedure, and then assist the other client, checking back with the first client as soon as possible.
3. Ensure the client's safety, discard the sterile equipment, and respond to the other client.
4. Explain the situation to the client needing catheterization, leave the sterile supplies in place, and attend to the other client.

8 The nurse is unable to palpate a client's pedal pulse in an edematous right lower extremity. Which of the following would be the best nursing action at this time?

1. Notify the provider of the inability to detect pedal pulses.
2. Check the temperature of the lower extremities.
3. Use a Doppler to check for the pedal pulse.
4. Measure the right lower extremity and compare it to the left.

9 Several clients are being admitted to the hospital unit at one time. There is only one private room available. Which client has the highest priority for being admitted to this private room?

1. A client admitted for elective surgery who requested a private room prior to admission.
2. A client who has a large infected abdominal wound.
3. A client who has a communicable respiratory infection.
4. A client who is under the age of 12.

10 A nurse is preparing a teaching plan for a family member who will be caring for a client with an abdominal incision. Which of the following concepts would have the first priority in the teaching plan?

1. Surgical asepsis
2. Demonstration in sterile gloving technique
3. Hand washing
4. Signs of healing

➤ *See pages 147–148 for Answers and Rationales.*

ANSWERS & RATIONALES

Pretest

1 **Answer: 3** **Rationale:** For infections spread by direct contact or by contact with infected items, the nursing staff would implement contact precautions. All other precautions listed are not necessary. Standard precautions, which are not listed as an option, would also be used. **Cognitive Level:** Applying **Client Need:** Safety and Infection Control **Integrated Process:** Nursing Process: Implementation **Content Area:** Fundamentals **Strategy:** The critical phrase is *spread through close physical contact.* Use knowledge of Centers for Disease Control (CDC) guidelines to assist in selecting appropriate infection control measures. **Reference:** Berman, A., & Snyder, S. J. (2012). *Kozier & Erb's fundamentals of nursing: Concepts, process, and practice* (9th ed.). Upper Saddle River, NJ: Pearson Education, pp. 692–693.

2 **Answer: 3** **Rationale:** Using the principle of medical asepsis, the client who should be assessed first is the client most at risk for infection. A client who is severely neutropenic has lost normal body defense mechanisms for resisting infection. The nurse needs to consider the client's ability to resist organisms, as well as risks for infecting others, when planning care. **Cognitive Level:** Applying **Client Need:** Safety and Infection Control **Integrated Process:** Nursing Process: Planning **Content Area:** Fundamentals **Strategy:** The core issue of the question is knowledge of medical asepsis. Recall that knowledge of medical asepsis is essential to safe nursing practice. **Reference:** Kozier, B., Erb, G., Berman, A., & Snyder, S. J. (2012). *Kozier & Erb's fundamentals of nursing: Concepts, process, and practice* (8th ed.). Upper Saddle River, NJ: Pearson Education, p. 677.

3 **Answer: 2** **Rationale:** An endogenous infection is one in which the source is the client. An exogenous source would be from the hospital or hospital personnel, other clients, or contaminated IV fluids. **Cognitive Level:** Applying **Client Need:** Safety and Infection Control **Integrated Process:** Nursing Process: Assessment **Content Area:** Fundamentals **Strategy:** The critical word in the question is *endogenous*. Recall potential sources of infection and use the process of elimination in making a selection about this type of infection. **Reference:** Berman, A., & Snyder, S. J. (2012). *Kozier & Erb's fundamentals of nursing: Concepts, process, and practice* (9th ed.). Upper Saddle River, NJ: Pearson Education, p. 672.

4 **Answers: 1, 2, 4** **Rationale:** Goggles are worn only when there is danger of splashing of body fluids. Head covers are commonly used in surgery. All of the other equipment would be appropriate for the nurse to wear in this situation to prevent the spread of the organism. **Cognitive Level:** Applying **Client Need:** Safety and Infection Control **Integrated Process:** Nursing Process: Implementation **Content Area:** Fundamentals **Strategy:** The critical phrases are *infection spread by droplets* and *hands were scratched*. Use knowledge of medical asepsis and Centers for Disease Control (CDC) precaution guidelines to select appropriate protection when caring for clients. Remember that droplet precautions recommend use of a mask when within 3 feet of a client. **Reference:** Berman, A., & Snyder, S. J. (2012). *Kozier & Erb's fundamentals of nursing: Concepts, process, and practice* (9th ed.). Upper Saddle River, NJ: Pearson Education, pp. 695–699.

5 **Answer: 1** **Rationale:** The oral temperature would be the most appropriate method for this client. Although the rectal method is the most accurate way to assess a client's temperature, this client has diarrhea, and insertion of a thermometer may further stimulate the bowel. The axillary method and using heat-sensitive tape may not provide as precise a measurement as the oral route. **Cognitive Level:** Applying **Client Need:** Safety and Infection Control **Integrated Process:** Nursing Process: Assessment **Content Area:** Fundamentals **Strategy:** The critical phrase is *vomiting and diarrhea*. To make a selection, recall the indications for use of the various routes and their accuracy. **Reference:** Berman, A., & Snyder, S. J. (2012). *Kozier & Erb's fundamentals of nursing: Concepts, process, and practice* (9th ed.). Upper Saddle River, NJ: Pearson Education, pp. 540–541.

6 **Answer: 2** **Rationale:** The nurse should recognize that a pulse volume of 1 indicates the client's pulse is difficult to feel and thready, and that the client's circulatory status is altered. The first action is to check the client's condition and circulatory status. If the nurse notified the provider first, the nurse would be reporting on another nurse's assessment, which is not an appropriate nursing practice. The other options are not applicable to this situation. **Cognitive Level:** Applying **Client Need:** Reduction of Risk Potential **Integrated Process:** Nursing Process: Assessment **Content Area:** Fundamentals **Strategy:** The critical phrase is *pulse volume is described as 1*. To choose correctly, recall that a pulse with a volume of 1 is thready, 2 is weak, 3 is normal, and 4 is bounding. **Reference:** Berman, A., & Snyder, S. J. (2012). *Kozier & Erb's fundamentals of nursing: Concepts, process, and practice* (9th ed.). Upper Saddle River, NJ: Pearson Education, p. 548.

7 **Answer: 2** **Rationale:** Removing blankets from the client will assist in heat loss through the skin. Offering fluids will prevent dehydration. Placing ice bags on the client is likely to cause shivering, which would increase heat production and reduce local circulation. Restricting fluid intake is not an appropriate nursing intervention for treating a fever. **Cognitive Level:** Applying **Client Need:** Reduction of Risk Potential **Integrated Process:** Nursing Process: Implementation **Content Area:** Fundamentals **Strategy:** The core issue of the question is the most effective method of treating an elevated temperature. Use knowledge of appropriate nursing interventions for clients with alterations in body temperature to select the correct action to take with febrile clients. **Reference:** Berman, A., & Snyder, S. J. (2012). *Kozier & Erb's fundamentals of nursing: Concepts, process, and practice* (9th ed.). Upper Saddle River, NJ: Pearson Education, p. 537.

8 **Answer: 4** **Rationale:** A pulse deficit of 16 beats less in the peripheral pulses is indicative of the heart firing ectopic beats and is of greatest concern. This symptom warrants notifying the primary health care provider. Mild tachycardia is commonly noted in clients who are febrile. The increased temperature results in an increase in the heart rate. When a client is asleep, the heart rate decreases. An 18-month-old infant will normally have a heart rate of 120 beats/minute. **Cognitive Level:** Applying **Client Need:** Reduction of Risk Potential **Integrated Process:** Nursing Process: Assessment **Content Area:** Fundamentals **Strategy:** The critical words in the question are *greatest concern*. Recall the significance of common variations in pulse rates and volumes to enable you to recognize significant changes and take appropriate action. **Reference:** Berman, A., & Snyder, S. J. (2012). *Kozier & Erb's fundamentals* *of nursing: Concepts, process, and practice* (9th ed.). Upper Saddle River, NJ: Pearson Education, p. 553.

9 **Answer: 3** **Rationale:** If the client is able to cough, the nurse should stand and observe the client to determine if he is able to dislodge the food. The nurse should intervene only if the client cannot cough. The attempt to dislodge the food should occur only if the client is unable to cough and talk. Laying the client on the floor to dislodge the food is only done if the client has become unconscious. Slapping the choking individual on the back is not necessary. The client should cough to try to dislodge the food. **Cognitive Level:** Applying **Client Need:** Physiological Adaptation **Integrated Process:** Nursing Process: Planning **Content Area:** Fundamentals **Strategy:** The critical words are *coughing loudly.* To make a selection, recall the steps in recognition and management of foreign body airway obstruction. Remember not to interfere with the cough efforts of a client when the cough is strong. **Reference:** Berman, A., & Snyder, S. J. (2012). *Kozier & Erb's fundamentals of nursing: Concepts, process, and practice* (9th ed.). Upper Saddle River, NJ: Pearson Education, p. 735.

10 **Answer: 2** **Rationale:** The depth of chest compressions for an adult is 2 inches. Thus the correct answer is 2, which is the minimum depth of compressions in the adult client according to the 2010 American Heart Association Guidelines. **Cognitive Level:** Applying **Client Need:** Physiological Adaptation **Integrated Process:** Teaching and Learning **Content Area:** Fundamentals **Strategy:** The critical words in the question are *depth* and *adult.* Use knowledge of CPR to arrive at the correct answer. **Reference:** American Heart Association. (2010). *American Heart Association guidelines for CPR and ECC.* Retrieved January 27, 2012, from www.heart.org/cpr

Posttest

1 **Answer: 4** **Rationale:** A client who has undergone oral surgery should not have the temperature taken by the oral method. The client is exhibiting signs and symptoms of elevated body temperature, and the rectal method is the best choice. A forehead temperature strip and the axillary method does not give as precise measurements as the rectal route in a client at risk for infection or other causes of hyperthermia. **Cognitive Level:** Applying **Client Need:** Basic Care and Comfort **Integrated Process:** Nursing Process: Assessment **Content Area:** Fundamentals **Strategy:** The critical words are *oral surgery* and *best method.* Recall accurate measurement of vital signs as a basic nursing skill to make a selection. **Reference:** Berman, A., & Snyder, S. J. (2012). *Kozier & Erb's fundamentals of nursing: Concepts, process, and practice* (9th ed.). Upper Saddle River, NJ: Pearson Education, pp. 539–540.

2 **Answer: 1** **Rationale:** While working over a sterile field, talking should be kept to a minimum and the head should be averted from the field if talking is necessary.

The other options represent correct actions when using sterile or surgical aseptic technique. **Cognitive Level:** Analyzing **Client Need:** Safety and Infection Control **Integrated Process:** Teaching and Learning **Content Area:** Fundamentals **Strategy:** The critical words are *surgical aseptic technique.* Recall the principles and practices of surgical asepsis to enable you to provide safe care and appropriate family education. **Reference:** Berman, A., & Snyder, S. J. (2012). *Kozier & Erb's fundamentals of nursing: Concepts, process, and practice* (9th ed.). Upper Saddle River, NJ: Pearson Education, p. 700.

3 **Answer: 3** **Rationale:** A wide base of support is achieved by spreading the feet apart to lower the center of gravity. **Cognitive Level:** Applying **Client Need:** Safety and Infection Control **Integrated Process:** Nursing Process: Implementation **Content Area:** Fundamentals **Strategy:** The critical term is *wide base of support.* Recall knowledge of scientific principles of body mechanics to enable you to select effective measures to protect the back and prevent injury. **Reference:** Berman, A., & Snyder, S. J. (2012). *Kozier & Erb's fundamentals of nursing: Concepts, process, and practice* (9th ed.). Upper Saddle River, NJ: Pearson Education, p. 1148.

4 **Answer: 2** **Rationale:** To prevent back strain for the nurse, the bed should be raised to a comfortable position. A nurse should stand with a wide base of support, work as closely as possible to an object, and avoid twisting motions. **Cognitive Level:** Applying **Client Need:** Safety and Infection Control **Integrated Process:** Nursing Process: Implementation **Content Area:** Fundamentals **Strategy:** The core issue of the question is how to prevent back injury while leaning over. Recall scientific principles of body mechanics to select effective measures to protect the back and prevent injury. **Reference:** Berman, A., & Snyder, S. J. (2012). *Kozier & Erb's fundamentals of nursing: Concepts, process, and practice* (9th ed.). Upper Saddle River, NJ: Pearson Education, p. 1148.

5 **Answer: 4** **Rationale:** Providing oral hygiene is a procedure that exposes the nurse to a client's body fluids. The other responses do not require the use of gloves because contact with body fluids is not a concern. **Cognitive Level:** Applying **Client Need:** Safety and Infection Control **Integrated Process:** Nursing Process: Implementation **Content Area:** Fundamentals **Strategy:** The core issue of the question is basic knowledge of standard precautions. Understanding of Centers for Disease Control (CDC) guidelines for precautions will assist you in selecting appropriate infection control measures. **Reference:** Berman, A., & Snyder, S. J. (2012). *Kozier & Erb's fundamentals of nursing: Concepts, process, and practice* (9th ed.). Upper Saddle River, NJ: Pearson Education, p. 693.

6 **Answer: 2** **Rationale:** The method of choice for opening the airway is the head tilt–chin lift procedure. The jaw-thrust maneuver should be used when neck injury is possible. The chest thrust maneuver is implemented to clear an airway of a foreign body. Moving the chin down onto the sternum will not open the airway. **Cognitive Level:** Applying **Client Need:** Physiological Adaptation **Integrated Process:** Nursing Process: Implementation **Content Area:** Fundamentals **Strategy:** The critical words are *unresponsive* and *open the client's airway*. Recall the correct techniques for cardiopulmonary resuscitation to enable you to correctly manage common airway emergencies. **Reference:** American Heart Association. (2010). *American Heart Association guidelines for CPR and ECC.* Retrieved January 29, 2012, from www.heart.org/cpr

7 **Answer: 3** **Rationale:** A client fall is a potential medical emergency; however, the nurse's first responsibility is ensuring the safety of the client being attended to. Sterile equipment is considered contaminated if left unattended and therefore must be thrown away. The nurse needs to prioritize care appropriately; thus, the nurse needs to respond to the client who fell rather than continue with the catheterization. **Cognitive Level:** Applying **Client Need:** Safety and Infection Control **Integrated Process:** Nursing Process: Implementation **Content Area:** Fundamentals **Strategy:** The critical phrase is *most appropriate nursing action.* This tells you that there may be more than one way to proceed but that one has a better rationale than the others. Understanding rules of surgical asepsis would enable you to know that sterile supplies cannot be unattended, and critical thinking skills would direct you to correctly prioritize care for the 2 clients. **Reference:** Berman, A., & Snyder, S. J. (2012). *Kozier & Erb's fundamentals of nursing: Concepts, process, and practice* (9th ed.). Upper Saddle River, NJ: Pearson Education, pp. 702–705.

8 **Answer: 3** **Rationale:** To ensure that lower extremity circulation is intact, the nurse should verify the presence of the pedal pulse. Although checking the lower extremity temperature and measuring circumference will provide data on circulation, it does not ensure a pedal pulse is present. It is inappropriate to notify the provider without first gathering all appropriate data.

Cognitive Level: Applying **Client Need:** Reduction of Risk Potential **Integrated Process:** Nursing Process: Assessment **Content Area:** Fundamentals **Strategy:** The critical words are *best nursing action.* Recall that the use of a Doppler to assess peripheral pulses is an essential skill related to physical assessment. **Reference:** Berman, A., & Snyder, S. J. (2012). *Kozier & Erb's fundamentals of nursing: Concepts, process, and practice* (9th ed.). Upper Saddle River, NJ: Pearson Education, pp. 549–550.

9 **Answer: 3** **Rationale:** The client with the airborne infection can spread this infection simply by breathing and requires isolation in a private room. The client with the abdominal wound would not be as likely to spread this organism when the wound is dressed. The clients in the other options have no medical need for a private room. **Cognitive Level:** Applying **Client Need:** Safety and Infection Control **Integrated Process:** Nursing Process: Implementation **Content Area:** Fundamentals **Strategy:** The critical term is *highest priority.* Recall Centers for Disease Control (CDC) precaution guidelines to enable you to make safe room assignments. **Reference:** Berman, A., & Snyder, S. J. (2012). *Kozier & Erb's fundamentals of nursing: Concepts, process, and practice* (9th ed.). Upper Saddle River, NJ: Pearson Education, p. 684.

10 **Answer: 3** **Rationale:** Hand-washing technique is the single most important procedure in reducing the spread of microorganisms. The other options may also be part of the teaching plan but have a lesser priority if they are used compared to basic hand washing. **Cognitive Level:** Applying **Client Need:** Safety and Infection Control **Integrated Process:** Teaching and Learning **Content Area:** Fundamentals **Strategy:** The critical term is *first priority.* Recall basic principles of infection control to direct you to set hand washing as the priority for client and family education. **Reference:** Berman, A., & Snyder, S. J. (2012). *Kozier & Erb's fundamentals of nursing: Concepts, process, and practice* (9th ed.). Upper Saddle River, NJ: Pearson Education, pp. 685–686.

References

American Heart Association. (2010). *American Heart Association guidelines for CPR and ECC.* Retrieved January 27, 2012, from www.heart.org/cpr

Berg, R. A., Hemphill, R., Abella, B. S., Aufderheide, T. P., Cave, D. M., Hazinski, M. F., et al. (2010). Part 5: Adult basic life support: 2010 American Heart Association guidelines for cardiopulmonary resuscitation and emergency cardiovascular care. *Circulation.* 2010; 122 (suppl 3): S685–S705.

Ball, J., & Bindler, R. (2010). *Child health nursing: Partnering with children and families.* (2nd ed.) Upper Saddle River, NJ: Pearson Education.

Berman, A., & Snyder, S. J. (2012). *Kozier & Erb's fundamentals of nursing: Concepts, process, and practice* (9th ed.). Upper Saddle River, NJ: Pearson Education.

D'Amico, D. & Barbarito, C. (2012). *Health and physical assessment in nursing* (2nd ed.). Upper Saddle River, NJ: Pearson Education.

Smith, L. (2005). Practice guidelines: New AHA recommendations for blood pressure measurement. *American Family Physician.* 72(7): 1391–1398.

Waters, T. R., Nelson, A., Hughes, N., & Menzel, N. (2009). *Safe patient handling training for schools of nursing.* Retrieved January 27, 2012, from http://www.cdc.gov/niosh/docs/2009-127/

ANSWERS & RATIONALES

Meeting Basic Human Needs

7

Chapter Outline

Safety: Risks According to Developmental Level

Using Restraints to Promote Safety

Maintaining Hygiene

Meeting Oxygenation Needs

Meeting the Client's Need for Sleep

Meeting Nutritional Needs

Meeting Urinary Elimination Needs

Meeting Bowel Elimination Needs

Objectives

➤ Identify principles of safety promotion based on an individual's developmental level.

➤ Describe the different types of restraints and their appropriate use.

➤ Review basic fire safety prevention measures for use in both the home and hospital setting.

➤ Describe the importance of and methods for promoting hygiene.

➤ Identify factors that affect oxygenation, alterations in oxygenation, and nursing interventions that promote adequate air exchange.

➤ Describe sleep alterations and associated health promotion activities.

➤ Describe basic nutritional requirements, therapeutic diets, and clinical signs of altered nutrition.

➤ Specify the common problems, diagnostic tests, and health promotion activities for urinary elimination.

➤ Specify the common problems, diagnostic tests, and health promotion activities for bowel elimination.

NCLEX-RN® Test Prep

Use the accompanying online resource, NursingReviewsandRationales, to test yourself with hundreds of NCLEX®-style practice questions.

Review at a Glance

aerobic capacity ability of body to take in oxygen and transport it to various organs of body

anemia a condition in which blood is deficient in red blood cells and causes a reduced capacity to carry oxygen

atherosclerosis buildup of fatty plaques along walls of arteries

cardiac output amount of blood pumped by heart each minute (usually 4–8 liters in an adult)

catalyze accelerate a chemical reaction

cerumen wax-like substance secreted by glands of external ear

circadian synchronization status of being awake when physiological and psychological rhythms are most active and asleep when they are most inactive

clubbing a condition in which base of nails become swollen, angle between nail and base is 180 degrees or greater, and ends of fingers and toes increase in size

diffusion movement of gases or other particles from an area of greater pressure or concentration to an area of lower concentration or pressure

dyspnea labored or difficult breathing

epidermis outer epithelial layer of skin

hyperventilation increased respirations accompanied by decreased carbon dioxide levels associated with pathologies including asthma, pulmonary embolism, or edema

hypoventilation reduced rate and depth of respirations that causes an increase in carbon dioxide

intercostal retraction indrawing chest movement of muscles between the ribs

Kegel exercises pelvic floor muscle exercises that can reduce episodes of incontinence

Kussmaul's breathing a particular type of breathing that includes deep, pauseless respirations associated with diabetic acidosis

orthopnea positional breathing discomfort associated with lying down

oxyhemoglobin compound of oxygen and hemoglobin

paronychia infection of tissue surrounding a nail

petechiae pinpoint red areas or bleeding in skin, associated with platelet deficiencies

polysaccharides branched chains of glucose molecules (e.g., starches)

pressure ulcer erosion of skin occurring over a bony prominence

pruritus itching

sedentary physical state characterized by little exercise or exertion

substernal retraction indrawing chest movement of muscles beneath the sternum

PRETEST

1 Parents of a group of toddlers are participating in a safety education class to prevent injuries. Which topic should the nurse include in the safety teaching session regarding toddlers?

1. Physical capacities and curiosity
2. Slow reflexes
3. Difficulty in reading
4. Social and personality development

2 A nurse on the unit observes that the night shift nurse has placed restraints on multiple clients. In which situations would the nurse conclude that the use of restraints is appropriate? Select all that apply.

1. Child who is hyperactive
2. Infant with a recent cleft palate repair who is trying to suck his thumb
3. Client with a developmental disability who is alert but still weak
4. Adult client who is severely anxious about test results
5. Cognitively impaired young adult client who fell 3 times even with bed alarm on

3 An older adult client on bed rest for a few days has been incontinent. The client now reports pruritis and excessively dry skin, particularly in the area of the lower back. To what skin problem would the nurse recognize that the client is most susceptible?

1. Erythema
2. Ammonia dermatitis
3. Contact dermatitis
4. Petechiae

4 The nurse instructs a client on the use of an incentive spirometer. The nurse evaluates that the client understood the instructions if the client performs which action?

1. Maintains a supine position while using the spirometer and inhales slowly with lips pursed around mouthpiece
2. Inhales rapidly, exhales into spirometer to reach the indicator mark, and waits 10 seconds before repeating the process
3. Exhales completely, places mouth around mouthpiece before inhaling slowly to reach the indicator mark, removes mouthpiece, holds breath, and exhales slowly
4. Purses lips tightly around mouthpiece, inhales slowly and deeply, and exhales slowly into the device until spirometer reaches indicator mark

5 A client reports having difficulty sleeping since admission to the hospital. Which nursing interventions would the nurse use for this client? Select all that apply.

1. Provide client with a warm beverage such as coffee or tea before bedtime.
2. Promote a bedtime routine as similar to client's home routine as possible.
3. Dim lighting in the client's room and close the door to the hallway at bedtime.
4. Change client's gown, offer a back rub, and straighten the bed linens prior to bedtime.
5. Encourage a long, brisk walk in the hallway before bedtime.

6 A client is being discharged with oxygen therapy via a nasal cannula. Which instruction should the nurse give to the client and family?

1. Use battery-operated equipment instead of electrical equipment.
2. Use petroleum jelly for the nares to prevent chafing.
3. Wear cotton clothing to avoid static electricity.
4. Use baby oil to protect the facial skin.

7 A client shares with the nurse an inability to sleep through the night since admission 3 days ago to the hospital. Which factor is most likely to have a negative effect on the client's sleep pattern?

1. Presence of pain
2. Absence of unfamiliar stimuli
3. Ability to talk about day's events
4. Moderate fatigue

8 An older adult client who is bedridden states being constipated. What instruction should the nurse provide to assist this client?

1. Decrease fluid intake before bedtime.
2. Encourage bland and low-residue foods.
3. Avoid beverages with caffeine.
4. Drink hot liquids and increase intake of water and fruit juices.

9 A client is experiencing occasional urinary urgency and incontinence, and the nurse is working with the client on bladder training. Which accomplishment would indicate to the nurse that the client has achieved the expected outcome?

1. Voids every time there is an urge
2. Practices deep, slow breathing until the urge to void diminishes
3. Uses adult disposable briefs continuously
4. Uses protector pads only when going out

10 A client is on a full liquid diet following gastric surgery. Which food brought to the client by a family member indicates to the nurse that dietary teaching is effective?

1. Homemade clam chowder with potatoes
2. Custard
3. Soft cake
4. Chopped vegetables

➤ *See pages 183–184 for Answers and Rationales.*

I. SAFETY: RISKS ACCORDING TO DEVELOPMENTAL LEVEL

A. Infant, toddler, and preschooler

1. Home accidents
   a. In infants, common accidents are suffocation, falls, choking, drowning, and burns; infants are completely dependent on caregivers and are unaware of dangers in environment
   b. Among toddlers and preschoolers, common accidents include poisoning, falls, burns, playground and street-related injuries; because of their increased activity, curiosity, and immaturity, they are more susceptible to injury
2. Health education for parents is a high priority and should include several elements
   a. Knowledge of child's developmental abilities (e.g., infant's dependency, toddler's mobility and curiosity, preschooler's increased activity, and clumsiness)
   b. Control of environment (i.e. safe use of infant care equipment; cover electric outlets; coil electrical cords out of reach; keep cleaning supplies and medicines locked)
   c. Supervision (swimming, playgrounds)
   d. First aid measures
3. Safety education for child should include playing in safe areas, dangers of playing with matches, avoiding strangers, and obeying traffic signals

B. School-age child
1. Transportation- or recreation-related injuries: not wearing seatbelts, helmets or life-preservers; school-age children are active and may not pay attention to directions
2. Sports-related injuries: drowning, accidents while biking, skateboarding, or playing ball—usually related to intense competition and not obeying rules
3. Environmental-related injuries: may play or experiment with fire or firearms

C. Adolescent
1. Substance abuse: experimentation with drugs and risk-taking, often because of peer pressure
2. Volatile behavior and sometimes violence
3. Recklessness in driving, sports, and lifestyle choices such as unprotected sex, which are often influenced by the following:
   a. Feelings of immortality
   b. A distortion in adolescent egocentric thinking
   c. A notion they are invulnerable to risks that affect others
4. Safety education includes importance of seatbelts, avoiding use of drugs and drinking and driving, and solving problems without violence

D. Adult
1. Lifestyle habits: exposure to the sun, not wearing a seatbelt, or driving while intoxicated
2. Stress-related illnesses: inability to cope with stress can precipitate suicide, road rage, and accident proneness
3. Safety education includes health screenings, exercise, preventive care, and diet

E. Older adult
1. Accidents from falls, driving, and thermal injuries
   a. Visual difficulties, decreased hearing, slower reflexes, poor balance and coordination, impaired mobility, and changes in depth perception contribute to falls and driving incidents
   b. Neurologic disorders such as Parkinson's disease or stroke lead to difficulty with movement and weakness, predisposing the person to falls
   c. Diseases of the spinal cord, nerves, or nervous system interfere with ability to feel discomfort and can lead to thermal injuries
   d. Safety education includes home safety (no throw rugs, adequate lighting, no clutter), proper temperature control on hot water heater, assessment of ability to drive, and importance of diet and exercise to maintain health and strength
2. Change in mental status related to multiple medications
   a. Older clients taking antihypertensives or diuretics may have postural hypotension; narcotics, hypnotics, sedatives, and tranquilizers cause drowsiness and impaired awareness of the surroundings
   b. Older adult clients are more at risk for polypharmacy—mixing of multiple medications, leading of any of the following:
      1) Additive effects (similar effects being enhanced)
      2) Potentiating effects (effects of 2 drugs taken together are greater than the singular effect of each drug)
      3) Paradoxical effects (effects opposite those that are expected)
   c. Safety education includes importance of using one pharmacy and telling all health care providers about all prescription, over-the-counter, and herbal products used

F. Potential risks across the lifespan
1. Falls account for the majority of injuries, especially to clients in a health care agency who have disease processes that cause weakness, mobility difficulties, or who take multiple medications; clients in unfamiliar environments need frequent safety information

      2. Client-caused accidents: self-inflicted cuts and injuries, setting fires, burns; these can be related to psychological dysfunction, risk-taking behaviors, cognitive deficits, and developmental disabilities

      3. Ingestion of foreign substance or poisoning: can be related to improper disposal or storage of substances or lack of precautionary measures

  G. **Safety risks specific to health care settings**

      1. Equipment: caused by malfunction, disrepair, misuse; accidents can result from electrical equipment not properly grounded or with frayed cords, wheelchairs or beds not properly maintained, and improper use of lifting devices; follow agency protocols and procedures to minimize these risks

      2. Errors in medication administration: take safeguards in administering medications, including no distractions during medication preparation and positive patient identification (PPID) using 2 unique client identifiers (such as name and date of birth or medical record number) before medication administration

      3. Failure of staff to follow safety guidelines and protocols; take care to follow agency protocols, and alert management regarding threats to safety that are unit-based or system-based in health care agency

  H. **Fire safety**

      1. Preventive measures for home

         a. Focus on teaching: emergency phone numbers, maintenance of smoke alarms and fire extinguishers, importance of family "fire drills"; careful disposal of burning cigarettes or use of matches; grease fire prevention; smoking in restricted places such as when oxygen is in use leads to fires

         b. If there is a fire, teach precautions such as: close windows and doors to contain fire, cover nose and mouth with damp cloth when leaving a smoke-filled area, and stay as close to the ground as possible

      2. Preventive measures for hospital or agency

         a. Be aware of safety precautions and fire prevention practices; know categories of fire and the correct type of extinguisher to use for each; participate in practice fire drills and evacuation procedures

         b. Use the acronym RACE to recall what to do in an actual fire

            1) Remove clients from danger

            2) Activate the fire alarm

            3) Contain the fire

            4) Evacuate the area (horizontal evacuation should be done if possible before vertical evacuation)

II. USING RESTRAINTS TO PROMOTE SAFETY

  A. **Overall objectives**

      1. Reduce risk of client injury from falls: for example, a postoperative client being transported on a stretcher or a client who is confused, agitated, and climbing out of bed might need restraints if alternatives to restraints have been exhausted

      2. Prevent interruption of therapy such as traction, IV infusions, or drainage tubes; e.g., a child who pulls at sterile dressings may need to have a restraint

      3. Prevent a confused or agitated client from removing therapeutic devices, e.g., a client who keeps taking off an oxygen mask or pulling out a gastric feeding tube

      4. Reduce risk of injury to others by client; e.g., ingestion of illicit substances causes a client to become combative when hallucinating

  B. **Guidelines for using restraints**

      1. Follow regulations; use restraints as a last resort and apply only under a health care provider's written prescription; always check prescriptions; document necessity of restraints, observations, and care given; reevaluate use according to policy

2. For all restraints, maintain a snug fit by making sure there are 1 to 2 finger-widths between client's body parts and the restraint; check adequacy of circulation and skin condition at least every hour; ensure call bell is within reach

3. Remove restraints every 2 hours to allow for exercise, toileting, and to check skin condition and circulation; attach restraints to bed frame but never to a movable part of bed; do not use restraints in place of nursing supervision; use least restrictive type of restraint

4. Use caution when removing restraints from an agitated client to prevent injury to client or staff

C. **Types of restraints**

1. Chemical restraints: consist of medication (such as sedatives, anxiolytics, neuroleptics) to control socially disruptive behavior; the primary goal is to prevent client from injuring self or others

2. Side rails: used to confine clients in bed

   a. Ensure that there is a written prescription before using in health care facilities

   b. Explain to client and family the purpose of side rails; do not use them as a punishment

   c. Half or three-quarter rails may be better than full-length rails for confused or agitated clients who might be injured climbing over rails or falling at end of bed; keep bed in lowest position

3. Bed enclosure

   a. Requires an order

   b. Has a top and zippered sides to keep client in bed while allowing full movement in bed

4. Jacket: vest or chest restraint

   a. Select correct size; explain purpose to client and family; place restraint over client's gown and follow manufacturer's recommendations

   b. Tie straps to nonmovable parts of bed or wheelchair; do not tie vest to head of bed or side rails

   c. Ensure safe positioning of client to promote proper breathing

5. Belt or waist restraint

   a. Check that belt is in good condition; attach belt around waist; if belt has a buckle, place it so it does not interfere with client's comfort

   b. Tie strap to nonmovable part of bed or chair; use belts when transporting clients in stretchers or wheelchairs

6. Extremity: may be a mitt or hand, wrist, ankle, or elbow restraint; always follow manufacturer's recommendations for application

   a. Mitt: used to interfere with manual dexterity; ensure client can flex fingers slightly and circulation is maintained; secure wrist ties and attach to bed frame or chair

   b. Wrist or ankle: used to restrict arm or leg movement; follow recommendations and pad bony prominences when using commercial restraints

   c. Elbow: used to prevent lower arm flexion; check that tongue blades in pockets are intact and ends are covered or padded; wrap restraint snugly around arm and secure properly; for small infants or children, pin restraints to shirt

D. **Alternatives to restraints**

1. Orient client and families to surroundings; prior to administering care, explain all procedures and treatments

2. Encourage family and friends to stay, or utilize constant companions for clients who need supervision; familiarity with caregivers may reduce agitation

3. Assign confused or disoriented clients to rooms near nurse's station; observe frequently and identify factors that precipitate client's confusion or agitation

4. Provide appropriate and meaningful visual and auditory stimuli; avoid overstimulating client; offer diversionary activities such as preschool sewing cards, picture books, or ask client to fold face cloths or small towels as a simple repetitive task

5. Eliminate bothersome therapies and treatments as soon as possible, for example, catheters and drains
6. Use relaxation techniques; approach client in a calm, nonthreatening manner
7. Institute exercise and ambulation schedules as condition allows
8. Maintain toileting routines to decrease falls related to elimination needs
9. Consult with physical and occupational therapists to enhance client's ability to carry out activities of daily living (ADLs), which help increase client's sense of accomplishment and reduce dependency
10. Evaluate all client medications to determine if each is having desired effect; check for adverse effects such as restlessness, confusion, perceptual difficulties, and dizziness
11. Conduct ongoing assessment and evaluation of client's care and ongoing response to care; factors such as client's environment and presence of familiar faces may promote relaxation or precipitate agitation; try to determine causes of sundowner's syndrome (nocturnal wandering and disorientation when darkness falls, associated with dementia), such as poor eyesight, hearing, and pain

III. MAINTAINING HYGIENE

A. Functions of the skin

1. Protection: skin is body's first line of defense because it covers underlying tissues and acts as a barrier to microorganisms
2. Sensation: pain, temperature, and pressure are transmitted as sensations through nerve receptors
3. Temperature regulation: when body temperature drops and heat must be conserved, superficial skin blood vessels constrict; cooling of body occurs through evaporation and when blood vessels dilate, heat is radiated and conducted away from body
4. Excretion and secretion: sweat (composed of water, chloride, potassium, glucose, and urea) is excreted through skin; sebum, an oily substance secreted by skin, contains chemicals that are toxic to bacteria; acid pH of skin secretions inhibits bacterial growth

B. Skin care

1. Developmental changes: age and ability influence one's skin care practices
   a. A newborn requires only sponge baths, not tub baths; newborn should be dried immediately and wrapped to prevent heat loss, especially since shivering starts at a lower body temperature and there is greater body surface area for heat loss compared to adults
   b. A toddler depends on caregiver to provide care; however, a toddler may want to try doing things independently (such as brushing teeth)
   c. An older adult who is frail may be dependent but may still be able to identify skin care preferences; excessive bathing can contribute to dry skin
2. Cultural considerations
   a. Hygiene practices vary considerably among different cultures; in some cultures, daily bathing is a ritual, while in others, a weekly routine is acceptable
   b. Other examples of differences are use of deodorants and preference for tub bath or shower
   c. Some cultures worry about hot and cold imbalances as a cause of illness
   d. Bathing may be avoided with some body conditions; for instance, some cultures avoid bathing during menstruation and childbirth
 3. Common skin problems: presence of these problems alerts nurse to type of skin assessment and care needed
   a. Excessive dryness: flaky and rough skin may crack, disrupting integrity of skin; may be accompanied by **pruritus** (itching)

   b. Abrasions: **epidermis** (superficial layer of skin) is rubbed or scraped off

   c. Ammonia dermatitis (diaper rash): reddened skin that may be excoriated, caused by skin bacteria reacting to urea in urine

   d. Contact dermatitis: reddened skin, accompanied by pruritus that may result in infection if scratched

   e. Erythema: redness of skin associated with rashes, infections, and allergic responses

   f. **Pressure ulcer**: a skin lesion, often over bony prominences caused by decreased circulation

C. Providing specific hygiene interventions

   1. Partial bed bath: client may do certain portions of bed bath as desired or as condition permits; includes only parts that may cause discomfort or odor if not washed, e.g., face, hands, axilla, perineum

     a. Prepare client by explaining procedure; provide privacy and have necessary equipment; position client for safety and easy access

     b. Wash face, rinse, and pat dry gently

     c. Assist client to immerse hands (may be one hand at a time) in wash basin to clean them; remove from basin and dry hands

     d. Wash client's chest and axilla, rinse, and pat dry; assist female clients to wash under breasts if needed; apply deodorant as desired

     e. Assist client to turn to side or prone if able; wash, rinse, and dry back, buttocks, and gluteal folds

     f. Assist client back to supine position; determine if client is able to do perineal care; assist as necessary; follow procedure for perineal care

     g. Assist client to put on clean gown and return client to comfortable position

     h. Document observations

   2. Complete bed bath: nurse washes client's entire body; may use a commercial product such as bath-in-a-bag; also provides opportunity for additional client assessment or teaching

     a. Explain procedure to client; if desired, a family member may assist with bath; prepare environment: close curtains and windows, elevate bed to a safe position; if appropriate, have client in a semi-sitting position

     b. Offer bedpan or urinal to client

     c. Prepare equipment

     d. Place bath blanket over client and remove bed linens; remove client's gown

     e. Wash client's eyes with water only, wiping from inner canthus to outer; use a separate corner of washcloth for each eye; dry eyes well; wash face and use soap only as directed by client; rinse and pat gently; wash, rinse, and dry ears and neck

     f. Place bath towel lengthwise under arm; wash using long firm strokes starting from wrists, rinse and dry arms, and then axilla; repeat with other arm

     g. Place towel on bed and put basin on top; immerse and wash client's hand in basin; pay attention to spaces between fingers; dry gently

     h. Fold bath blanket down to client's pubic area and replace it with a bath towel; wash, rinse, and dry chest and abdomen; for female clients, pay particular attention to area under breasts; avoid undue exposure; replace bath blanket

     i. Fold bath blanket over one leg; place bath towel under other leg; wash using long strokes starting from ankle to knee to thigh; rinse and dry; repeat with other leg

     j. Wash feet by placing each foot in basin, rinse, dry, and repeat with other foot; clean and dry well between toes

     k. Assist client to a side-lying position; place a towel alongside back and buttocks; cover client with bath blanket; wash, rinse, and dry back, buttocks, gluteal folds, and back of upper thighs

    l. Pay particular attention to skin over bony prominences and check for beginning skin problems such as pressure ulcer or ammonia dermatitis

    m. Change water and perform perineal care (see perineal care procedure)

    n. Assist client with other hygiene practices: use of deodorant, lotions, powder as appropriate; assist with mouth care or shaving

    o. Help client put on a clean gown; remove and replace bed linens; store equipment; clean up environment

    p. Document activity tolerance and observations such as reddened areas over bony prominences, irritation, or inflammation

3. Perineal care

    a. Explain procedure to client; ensure privacy; prepare equipment

    b. Assist client to a back-lying position with knees flexed and spread apart; drape and keep client warm

    c. Don gloves and inspect perineal area

    d. For females

        1) Using washcloth, clean labia majora, then spread labia to clean folds between labia majora and labia minora

        2) Use separate quarters of washcloth per stroke, wiping from pubis down to rectum (front to back)

        3) Rinse area well by pouring warm water over area or use a clean washcloth; dry area gently and well

    e. For males

        1) Wash and dry penis with firm strokes

        2) If uncircumcised, retract foreskin or prepuce and cleanse glans penis (tip); replace foreskin after cleaning

        3) Wash and dry scrotum

    f. Assist client to turn away; clean anal area with toilet paper or disposable wipes before washing as necessary; rinse and dry; apply perineal pad or diaper as needed

    g. In some settings, a special peri-wash solution may be used to perform perineal care

    h. Document any observations such as inflammation or discharge

4. Nail and foot care

    a. Nail care: prepare equipment; do one hand at a time; soak in warm water if nails are hard; cut or file straight across to prevent ingrown nails (never cut nails of a client with diabetes mellitus [DM]); file to round corners and push cuticles back gently; wash and dry; document observations such as **paronychia** (infection of tissue surrounding nail) or abnormal discolorations; refer client with DM to a podiatrist as needed

    b. Foot care: wash each foot in washbasin and cleanse between toes (see total bed bath); rub callused areas with washcloth; clean nails using a wooden stick; if agency permits, trim nails; rinse and dry gently; repeat procedure for other foot; apply lotion or powder as necessary; document observations such as breaks in skin and pressure areas

5. Oral care

    a. For a client who can do oral care independently: prepare equipment; assist client to a Fowler's position and place towel on chest; assist as needed

    b. For a client who needs assistance

        1) Brushing teeth: place moist toothbrush bristles at a 45-degree angle against teeth; move bristles back and forth; repeat for all tooth surfaces; gently brush tongue if coated; hand water cup to client for rinsing and ask to spit into emesis basin

        2) Flossing teeth: use disposable gloves; stretch floss and move it up and down between all teeth from top of crown to gum line; have client rinse mouth;

dispose of equipment, and document any abnormalities noted such as excessive bleeding or inflammation of gums

   3) Cleaning artificial dentures: prepare equipment and obtain a denture container and washcloth; place client in semi-Fowler's position; put on gloves; remove top dentures (move plate up and down gently to break suction then place it in container) and lower dentures (lift one side gently and then the other); clean and rinse dentures in sink carefully; dispose of equipment; document abnormalities such as irritated mucous membranes and ill-fitting dentures

c. For a client requiring total care

   1) Assemble equipment; place client in side-lying position so fluid can easily flow out or pool in side of mouth for suctioning; place a towel under client's chin and a curved basin against chin; use gloves

   2) Clean client's teeth as per procedure above; brush gently; flush client's mouth with water and let fluid drain from mouth; ensure all fluid drains out, otherwise use gentle suction or another syringe to remove it; some agencies use mouth care products with suction attached

   3) Inspect and clean the oral tissues; use an applicator or a tongue blade wrapped with gauze (moistened with mouthwash) to cleanse inside of cheeks, roof, and base of mouth and tongue; rinse client's mouth

   4) Discard gloves and other equipment; reposition client and ensure comfort

   5) Lubricate client's lips with petroleum jelly

   6) Record special mouth care including any solution used; document observations such as dryness or inflammation

6. Hair and scalp care

   a. Brushing hair: use a hairbrush with soft bristles; remove tangles gently, working from ends of hair, then middle to ends, then scalp to ends; use a wide pick comb for very curly hair, such as hair of some African Americans

   b. Shampooing hair

   1) Assist client as necessary; check whether order is necessary; if shampooing a client who is on bedrest, assemble equipment

   2) Ensure that client is warm; use a bath blanket; check water temperature

   3) Put waterproof sheet and towel on bed; place shampoo basin or tray and pad area where client's neck will rest; position client's head in basin or tray; position the receiving receptacle to collect draining water

   4) Cover client's eyes with a washcloth

   5) Shampoo hair and massage all areas of scalp working from hairline to neckline with pads of fingertips; rinse well and squeeze out as much water as possible

   6) If hair is matted or tangled with blood, consider using dry shampoo or hydrogen peroxide mixture for cleaning; note that hydrogen peroxide can change hair color

   7) Rub hair thoroughly with a towel; remove shampoo basin and wrap hair with dry towel; if desired, use hairdryer and ensure client comfort

   8) In general, shampooing should be done at least once per week

7. Care of eyes, ears, and nose

   a. Eye care: soften dried secretions with a moistened washcloth; wipe loosened secretions from inner to the outer canthus

   b. Ear care: wash auricles during bed bath; if **cerumen** visible, loosen it by retracting auricles downward then remove with a damp washcloth

   1) Unconscious client: if corneal reflex impaired, apply moist compresses over eye every 2 to 4 hours; clean each eye with a moistened washcloth; instill ordered ophthalmic ointment or artificial tears

2) Removable prosthetic (artificial) eye: use gloves; exert slight pressure below eyelid to overcome suction and remove artificial eye; clean socket and tissues around eye with moistened washcloth; clean artificial eye with warm normal saline and rinse; to reinsert prosthetic eye, retract eyelids and exert pressure on supraorbital and infraorbital bones; hold prosthetic eye with index finger and thumb of other hand and slip it gently into socket

   c. Nasal care: ask if client wishes to blow nose using tissue; nares or nostrils can be cleaned with damp washcloth

D. Care of the client's room environment

  1. Making an occupied bed

    a. Explain procedure and enlist client's cooperation; gather clean linen; have a linen hamper in room; draw curtains and place bed at a comfortable working height

    b. Remove call bell or other devices attached to bed linens; lower rail on nearest side of bed after determining that opposite side rail is up and locked

    c. Loosen all top linen at foot of bed; replace top sheet with bath blanket; fold spread or blanket and place on chair

    d. Put head of bed as flat as client can tolerate; move mattress up on bed; ask client to turn to distant side and adjust pillow under head; loosen old linen and fold draw sheet and bottom sheet toward center of bed; place new bottom sheet and draw sheet on bed and fan-fold the half to be used for other side of bed; tuck sheets and miter corners if using flat sheet

    e. Raise near side rail; assist client to roll over fan-folded sheets toward nurse; move pillow towards clean side; move to other side and lower side rail; remove used linens and place in linen hamper; unfold fan-folded clean linen; pull sheets to prevent wrinkles and tuck under mattress or make mitered corners

    f. Reposition client at center of bed; remove and replace pillowcase, then reposition for client's comfort

    g. Replace bath blanket with top sheet; place blanket and then bedspread on top; tuck in sheet, blanket, and spread at foot of bed, making room for movement of client's feet, and miter corners; fan-fold top covers to client's upper chest or waist-line as desired

    h. Place bed in lowest position; restore side rails to original position; replace call bell within client's reach; and put client items within safe reaching distance

  2. Making an unoccupied bed

    a. Gather equipment; assist client out of bed if necessary; assess client and ensure safety and comfort

    b. Remove call bell or drainage equipment attached to bed linens

    c. Loosen bed linens systematically starting from top of bed on one side and finishing at head of bed on other side; remove pillowcases, place in linen hamper and place pillows on bedside chair

    d. Fold reusable linens on bed into fourths; roll all soiled linen and dispose directly into linen hamper

    e. Move mattress up in the bed if needed; place folded bottom sheet on top of bed with hem side down; unfold and tuck fitted or contoured sheet on one side

    f. If needed, place a plastic or waterproof pad on top of bed extending from approximately client's middle back to mid-thigh; cover with a cloth draw sheet and tuck one side

    g. Place top sheet hem-side up on top of bed, then blanket or bedspread, unfold and tuck them in at foot of bed and miter corner on this side

    h. Move to other side of bed; repeat procedure for securing bottom sheet

    i. Spread remainder of linens; make a vertical or horizontal toe pleat in top linens for added foot room; tuck top linens under foot of mattress; miter bottom corners;

fold top of top sheet over blanket and bedspread providing a cuff; if client is getting back to bed, fan-fold top linens to center; place bed in a low position

   j. Replace pillowcases; attach call bell; place bedside table and over-bed table where client can reach them; tidy the room

 3. Keep area clutter-free: arrange furniture to avoid accidents, for example, no furniture in middle of room; remove unnecessary objects; keep obstacles out of the way

4. Keep objects needed by client nearby; put items for activities of daily living within reach, e.g., client's eyeglasses, cane, fluids, and call bell

5. Control odors: provide good ventilation; remove and dispose of offensive waste products appropriately; use room deodorizers as necessary

IV. MEETING OXYGENATION NEEDS

A. Overview of anatomy and physiology of cardiovascular and respiratory systems

Practice to Pass

The nurse is admitting a young child with burns to the unit. What safety precautions should the nurse implement?

1. Cardiovascular
   a. Structure
      1) Heart
         a) A hollow, cone-shaped organ within mediastinum, bordered laterally by lungs, posteriorly by spine, and anteriorly by sternum; it is covered by pericardium and has 3 layers: epicardium, myocardium, and endocardium
         b) Four chambers: upper chambers (atria) and lower chambers (ventricles) are separated by tricuspid (right) and bicuspid ormitral (left) valves; interventricular septum separates the 2 sides; semilunar valves (pulmonic on right and aortic on left) separate ventricles from great vessels
      2) Blood vessels
         a) Arteries: elastic vessels that carry blood away from heart
         b) Veins: carry blood back to heart
         c) Capillaries: smallest vessels, form connection between arterioles and venules
   b. Function: heart serves as a system pump, moving oxygenated blood and nutrients through arteries to tissues, and deoxygenated blood and wastes from tissues through veins

2. Conduction system: controls electrical activity and contraction of heart
   a. Sinoatrial (SA) node: primary pacemaker located where superior vena cava enters right atrium; initiates impulses conducted throughout heart resulting in ventricular contraction
   b. Atrioventricular (AV) node: specialized muscle tissue located in floor of right atrium near interatrial septum
   c. AV bundle or bundle of His and Purkinje fibers: ventricular conduction fibers

3. Respiratory system
   a. Structure
      1) Upper respiratory tract: mouth, nose, pharynx, larynx
      2) Lower respiratory tract: trachea, lungs (bronchi, bronchioles, and alveoli), pulmonary capillary network, and pleura (visceral and parietal)
   b. Function
      1) Pulmonary ventilation or breathing: inspiration (inhalation)—air flows into lungs and expiration (exhalation)—air moves out of lungs
      2) Alveolar gas exchange: after alveoli are ventilated, **diffusion** (movement) of oxygen occurs from alveoli into pulmonary blood vessels
      3) Transport of oxygen (O_2) and carbon dioxide (CO_2): O_2 is transported from lungs to tissues and CO_2 is transported from tissues back to lungs; O_2 combines with hemoglobin in red blood cells and is then carried to tissues as **oxyhemoglobin** (a compound of O_2 and hemoglobin)

B. Factors affecting oxygenation

1. Environment
   a. Altitude: higher altitude increases respiratory and cardiac rate and respiratory depth due to decreased O_2 levels
   b. Heat: causes peripheral vessel dilation, increased blood flow to skin and decreased resistance to blood flow; this increases cardiac output to raise blood pressure (BP); rate and depth of breathing also increase
   c. Cold: vasoconstriction occurs and BP elevates; this decreases cardiac action because of reduced need for O_2
   d. Air pollution: leads to symptoms such as coughing, choking, and difficulty breathing

2. Developmental factors affecting oxygenation
   a. Premature infants: inadequate respiratory function is caused by immature lungs; stimulation of respiratory center of brain is immature; gag and cough reflexes are weak
   b. Infants and toddlers: have smaller airway passages, which contributes to obstruction by foreign objects such as peanuts, coins, and small toys; diseases such as cystic fibrosis and asthma lead to difficulty breathing and adversely affect oxygenation
   c. School-age children: because of exposure to infectious agents at school and play, there is a tendency to develop upper respiratory problems
   d. Adolescents: at puberty, heart and lungs increase considerably in size and heart rate drops
   e. Young and middle-aged adults: **aerobic capacity** (ability of individual to provide O_2 to body's organs) and **cardiac output** (CO) (amount of blood pumped by heart each minute [4–8L]) show age-related changes during work or exercise starting at age 35 to 40; loss of blood vessel elasticity may contribute to hypertension, which affects oxygenation; **atherosclerosis** (plaque build-up in arterial walls) is a factor that decreases blood flow, particularly to heart muscle
   f. Older adults: chest wall becomes more rigid and lungs are less elastic, so more air is retained in lungs at expiration; cough effectiveness decreases; protective cilia become less effective increasing susceptibility to upper respiratory infections; decreased respiratory reserve increases risk for exercise intolerance; blood flow may be impaired because of hypertension, atherosclerosis and obstructive lung disease

3. Lifestyle factors affecting oxygenation
   a. Nutrition: high fat and salt intake may increase risk for heart disease and inadequate diet can lead to **anemia** (insufficient red blood cells)
   b. Physical exercise: increases rate and depth of respirations and cardiac rate, thus increasing supply of O_2 in body
   c. Smoking: nicotine increases heart rate, BP, and peripheral resistance; vasoconstriction occurs and decreases oxygenation to tissues
   d. Substance abuse: alcohol is a respiratory depressant and slows respirations; long-term use increases BP and tendency for malnutrition and anemia; narcotics (opioids) such as morphine decrease respiratory rate and depth
   e. Anxiety: in moderate and severe anxiety, hyperventilation occurs, arterial pressure of O_2 rises and pressure of CO_2 falls; client often experiences light-headedness, numbness of fingers and toes; epinephrine and norepinephrine released under stress increase BP and heart rate
   f. Overall health status: cardiovascular disease causes compromise in O_2 transport; respiratory disease affects oxygenation of blood

C. Alterations in respiratory functioning

1. **Hyperventilation**: increased movement of air into and out of lungs
    a. Causes: stress, metabolic acidosis may cause **Kussmaul's breathing**, a type of hyperventilation
    b. Signs and symptoms: increased rate and depth of respiration, more CO_2 is eliminated than normal
2. **Hypoventilation**: inadequate alveolar ventilation
    a. Causes: alveolar collapse, airway obstruction, or side effect of some drugs
    b. Signs and symptoms: inadequate alveolar ventilation; CO_2 retained in bloodstream; can lead to hypoxia; confusion, lethargy, or somnolence may be noted
3. Hypoxia: inadequate amount of O_2 transported to the tissues
    a. Causes: diseases such as anemia, pulmonary edema, heart failure; drugs such as anesthetics
    b. Signs and symptoms: rapid pulse; rapid shallow respirations, **dyspnea** (labored or difficult breathing); flaring of the nostrils, restlessness; **substernal** or **intercostal retractions** (retractions under and between ribs occurring with respirations), and cyanosis; in chronic hypoxia, client may experience fatigue, lethargy, and have **clubbing** (changes in appearance of ends of fingers and toes with angle of nail bed to digit 180 degrees or greater; associated with hypoxia)
4. Cyanosis
    a. Causes: severe anemia, respiratory tract obstruction, heart disease, cold environment; a very late indicator of hypoxia
    b. Signs and symptoms: bluish discoloration of skin, nail beds, and mucous membranes
5. Pain: chest pain can impair breathing patterns and respiratory functioning
    a. Causes: respiratory diseases such as pneumonia, pulmonary embolism, advanced bronchogenic carcinoma, and heart conditions, such as coronary artery disease, and angina
    b. Signs and symptoms: reports of pain that may be dull, aching, persistent or localized/radiating; discomfort accompanied by pallor, rapid or slowed breathing; anxiety; rapid heart rate; may be enhanced by either inhalation or expiration
6. **Orthopnea**: (positional breathing discomfort associated with lying down)
    a. Causes: respiratory and cardiac diseases, airway obstruction
    b. Signs and symptoms: difficulty breathing except when in a sitting or upright position
7. Wheezing
    a. Causes: severely narrowed bronchus
    b. Signs and symptoms: high-pitched, continuous musical, rasping, or whistling sounds heard during inspiration or expiration; does not clear with coughing
8. Cough: natural lung clearance mechanism to remove secretions
    a. Causes: excessive sputum production; allergies; pulmonary diseases
    b. Signs and symptoms: forced exhalation and clearing of airway passages
9. Hemoptysis
    a. Causes: pulmonary infection, lung carcinoma (cancer), abnormalities of heart or blood vessels
    b. Signs and symptoms: bright red frothy blood from lungs mixed with sputum; initial symptoms include tickling in throat, salty taste, a burning or bubbling sensation in chest

D. Nursing interventions to promote oxygenation

1. Positioning: Fowler's position (elevated head of bed) allows maximum chest expansion that eases respirations in clients with dyspnea; turn clients from side to side every 1 to 2 hours to allow alternate sides of chest to expand
2. Decrease anxiety: promote relaxation techniques, alleviate pain by using distraction or guided imagery as adjuncts to analgesics

3. Deep-breathing and coughing: teach clients breathing techniques to assist in clearing fluid from lungs and to promote oxygenation
   a. Assume a comfortable position: sitting or supine position with knees flexed
   b. Place one hand on abdomen just below ribs
   c. With mouth closed, breathe in deeply through nose to a count of 3; concentrate on feeling abdomen rise
   d. Purse lips and breathe out slowly and gently; concentrate on feeling abdomen fall and tighten abdominal muscles; count to 7 during exhalation
   e. Repeat several times (about 10 times initially) and gradually increase to 5 to 10 minutes four times a day
   f. For coughing: inhale deeply and hold breath for a few seconds, lean forward and cough rapidly, using abdominal, thigh and buttock muscles (coughing is contraindicated in postoperative eye, ear, neck, or brain surgery, or in other clients who have risk of increased intracranial pressure)

4. Suctioning: oro/nasopharyngeal, tracheal
   a. See Box 7-1 for procedure
   b. Limit suctioning to 10 seconds (some texts say 15) because no O_2 exchange occurs during this part of procedure; allow rest periods between suctioning to allow client to inhale O_2
   c. Assess for dysrhythmias or cyanosis as grave indicators of inadequate oxygenation; hyperoxygenate before suctioning, between attempts, and when suctioning is complete

---

| **Box 7-1**

Suctioning Technique | • Prepare equipment: portable or wall suction with tubing and collection container; sterile normal saline or water with a sterile disposable container for fluids; sterile gloves; water soluble lubricant; Y-connector; sterile gauzes; disposal bag; and goggles or face shield if appropriate.
• Select appropriate sterile suction catheters usually #12 to #18 for adults; #8 to #10 for children; and #5 to #8 for infants.
• Set pressure on suction gauge; use lowest amount of suction on wall unit to clear secretions: adults: 80–120 mmHg; children: 80–100 mmHg; premature infants: 40–80 mmHg; neonates: 60–80 mmHg.
• Explain procedure to client. Position a conscious client in a semi-Fowler's or an unconscious client in a lateral position with head turned towards nurse.
• Put on sterile gloves, maintain sterility of dominant hand and connect sterile catheter to suction.
• Measure distance between client's nose and earlobe (approximately 13 cm or 5 in. in adults) and mark position with fingers of sterile gloved hand. Test pressure and patency by placing nondominant thumb or finger on port or open branch of the Y-connector.
• Hyperoxygenate client with deep breaths or bag-valve-mask device (Ambu bag).
• Lubricate catheter tip with sterile water or saline (or for nasopharyngeal suctioning may use the lubricant).
• Insert catheter:
  • For oropharyngeal suctioning: pull tongue forward with gauze; introduce and advance catheter along one side of mouth into oropharynx.
  • For nasopharyngeal suctioning: introduce catheter through nostril or naris and advance to recommended distance.
  • For tracheal suctioning, insert during inhalation because epiglottis is open; continue to advance catheter to approximately 20 cm or until resistance is met; pull back slightly (expect client to cough during insertion).
• Do not apply suction while inserting catheter.
• Apply nondominant gloved thumb or finger to port to start suction and gently rotate catheter between thumb and forefinger. Apply and release suction |

intermittently during the withdrawing movement of catheter; allow 20- to 30-second intervals between each suction and limit each suctioning to 10 seconds maximum (some sources say 15).

- Hyperoxygenate client between suction attempts and at completion of procedure.
- For oropharyngeal suctioning, it may be necessary to suction secretions that collect in buccal cavity.
- Clean catheter by wiping off secretions with sterile gauze; flush catheter with sterile water; relubricate and repeat suctioning until air passage is clear. Alternate nares for repeat suctioning. Encourage client to breathe deeply and cough between suctions.
- Provide nasal or oral hygiene. Dispose of equipment.
- Assess effectiveness of suctioning: observe respiratory rate, skin color, dyspnea, and level of anxiety. Document relevant information.

5. Chest physiotherapy: percussion, vibration, postural drainage (often done by respiratory therapist unless nurse is authorized and competent to perform)
   a. Percussion or clapping: explain procedure and encourage client to breathe slowly and deeply; place client in a comfortable sitting or side-lying position; cover area with a gown or towel; cup hands, alternately flex and extend wrists rapidly to percuss affected lung segments for 1 to 2 minutes
   b. Vibration: vigorous or high-frequency quivering on chest wall, used alternately with or after percussion; explain procedure to client and position according to lung segment to be treated; encourage client to breathe slowly and deeply; place hands one on top of other with palms down; during exhalation, tense hand and arm and using mostly the heel of one hand, vibrate or shake hands against client's chest; stop vibrating when client inhales; after each vibration, encourage client to cough and expectorate; vibrate 5 times over each lung segment
   c. Postural drainage: use of gravity to drain secretions from respiratory tract; explain procedure and position client so head is lower than chest; place sputum container and wipes within client's reach; do percussion and vibration for 5 minutes and allow 5 minutes for drainage; encourage client to cough and expectorate; instruct client to turn to other side then to supine position, and repeat procedure; assist client to a sitting position and offer mouth care; document observations
6. Care of client with chest tubes: needed when air (pneumothorax), blood (hemothorax), or excessive fluid (pleural effusion) collects in pleural space
   a. Maintain water seal and patency of drainage system: tape connector sites; provide a straight line of tubing from bed to collection system, no kinks in tubing; do not use pins or restrain tubing
   b. Assess client's vital signs, respiratory and cardiovascular status regularly
   c. Maintain integrity of drainage system: disposable system or suction bottles below level of bed; maintain suction control to create gentle bubbling in suction control chamber (if fluid filled) or set dial on suction control chamber if using a "dry" system
   d. Do not strip chest tubes unless there is a prescription for this and if agency policy permits (most do not) because excessive negative pressure can damage lung tissue; if ordered, stripping is done by pinching tube close to client's chest with one hand, lubricating thumb and forefinger to compress and sliding down toward receptacle
   e. Keep sterile water, rubber-tipped clamps (if agency policy allows), and sterile dressing materials (dry gauze, petrolatum gauze, and tape) near client; if disconnection

occurs, reattach after wiping ends quickly with alcohol or place chest tube distal end in sterile water to restore underwater seal; clamp chest tube only if agency policy dictates (could cause tension pneumothorax); if chest tube is pulled out inadvertently, apply a sterile dressing to wound immediately; if air can be heard leaking from site, dressing should not be occlusive (if air cannot escape, it can lead to a tension pneumothorax)

   f. Mark drainage on receptacle every shift and read at eye level; report if drainage exceeds 100 mL/hr

   g. Monitor for subcutaneous emphysema; palpate around dressing for crackling sensation or sound, which indicates air in subcutaneous tissues caused by a poor seal at chest tube insertion site

   h. Document amount and color of drainage on intake and output record and progress notes, respectively

7. Oxygen therapy: when O_2 therapy is used, follow certain safety precautions (see Box 7-2)

   a. Check health care provider prescription and assess client's respiratory and cardiovascular status

   b. Explain procedure to client and place client in a semi-sitting position

   c. Set up O_2 equipment: attach flow meter to wall outlet or portable O_2 cylinder; fill humidifier with water and attach to base of flow meter; attach delivery system (cannula or face mask) and tubing to flow meter; turn on O_2 at prescribed rate

   d. Cannula: put cannula over client's face with outlet prongs fitting the nares and elastic band around head; pad bands over ears and under cheekbones as necessary

   e. Face mask: guide mask toward client's face and apply it from nose downward; mold mask to face; secure elastic band around client's head and pad band over ears as needed

   f. Assess the client's respiratory and cardiovascular status regularly; check client's nares for irritation if cannula is used, facial skin if with a face mask; document observations

   g. Check flow of O_2 and level of water in humidifier regularly

   h. Document O_2 saturation level obtained by pulse oximetry every 8 hours; also document amount of O_2 on flowsheet and client response to O_2 therapy in progress notes

Practice to Pass

A client with chest tubes is admitted to the nursing unit. How would the nurse care for this client?

Box 7-2	
Safety Precautions During Oxygen Therapy	• No smoking is allowed at any time when oxygen is in use; place cautionary signs on appropriate doors, in client's room, and on oxygen equipment. • Instruct client and visitors not to smoke and discuss possible consequences of smoking when oxygen is in use. If necessary, remove matches, lighters, and ashtrays. • If O_2 therapy is used at home, instruct family members or caregivers to smoke only outside. • Avoid materials that generate static electricity such as woolen blankets and synthetic fabrics; instead use cotton fabrics for linens and clothing of clients and caregivers. • Avoid use of volatile, flammable substances such as acetone in nail polish removers, alcohol, ether, and oils near clients using O_2. • Make sure electric devices such as radios, razors, hearing aids, heating pads, and televisions are in good working order to prevent short-circuit sparks. • Ensure that electric monitoring equipment, diagnostic equipment, and suction machines are properly grounded. Disconnect any ungrounded equipment. • Personnel need to be aware of location of fire extinguishers and be able to use them properly.

8. Incentive spirometer (IS)
   a. Check health care provider prescription; assist client to a sitting or Fowler's position and explain procedure
   b. Assemble equipment; set marker at recommended volume goal
   c. Instruct client to place mouth tightly around mouthpiece
   d. Instruct client to inhale slowly and maintain a steady flow as if pulling through a straw; encourage client to raise and maintain flow rate indicator
   e. Instruct client to remove mouthpiece but hold breath for 2 to 3 seconds and then exhale slowly through pursed lips
   f. Have client repeat the procedure a few times and then cough; encourage to use 5 to 10 times hourly; keep IS within reach of client; document IS use in client record
9. Frequent reassessment: monitor respiratory rate, O_2 saturation, lung sounds, and other respiratory data at least once per 8 hours and more frequently as needed to detect subtle changes; monitor trends and report accordingly

V. MEETING THE CLIENT'S NEED FOR SLEEP

A. Physiology of sleep

1. Circadian rhythm: rhythmic repetition of patterns each 24 hours; sleep is a complex biologic rhythm; a person whose biologic clock coincides with sleep–wake patterns is in **circadian synchronization**
2. Sleep regulation: centers in lower portion of brain actively inhibit wakefulness, causing sleep
3. Types and stages of sleep: 2 types of sleep are NREM (non–rapid eye movement) and REM (rapid eye movement); see Box 7-3 Types of Sleep
4. Nocturnal erections: both erections and emissions start around adolescence and occur during REM sleep

B. Normal sleep requirements and patterns

1. Neonates: newborns sleep an average of 16 to 18 hours per day, divided into about 7 sleep periods; most non-REM sleep is spent in Stages III and IV and nearly 50% is in REM sleep
2. Infants: range of sleep is from 12 to 22 hours; periods of wakefulness increase with age; by 4 months, infants sleep through night and nap during day; at end of first year,

---

Box 7-3
 	
Types of Sleep
	• NREM: deep and restful sleep characterized by decrease in physiologic functions: BP and pulse decreases, skeletal muscles relax, basal metabolic rate decreases, brain waves become slower; characterized by 4 stages
	  • Stage I: very light sleep, relaxed and drowsy, floating sensation, eyes roll from side to side, lasts only a few minutes
	  • Stage II: light sleep, easily roused, slight decrease of pulse and respirations, lasts 10 to 15 minutes
	  • Stage III: medium-depth sleep, less easily aroused, pulse and respirations and other physiologic functions such as BP and temperature continue to fall; skeletal muscles are relaxed, reflexes diminished, and snoring may occur
	  • Stage IV: called delta sleep; deepest sleep stage, difficult to arouse, rarely moves and muscles completely relaxed; dreaming may occur; may last about 30 minutes
	• REM sleep: usually occurs every 90 minutes and lasts 5 to 30 minutes; active dreaming occurs and dreams are remembered; brain is highly active and person is difficult to arouse or may wake up spontaneously; rapid eye movements and irregular muscle movements take place; muscle tone is depressed and heart and respiratory rates are irregular

sleep about 14 of every 24 hours; half of the time, infants have light sleep, and 20 to 30% is REM sleep

3. Toddlers: normal sleep–wake cycle established by 2 to 3 years; generally sleep for 10 to 12 hours, still require a mid-afternoon nap, but morning nap needs decrease; still 20 to 30% is REM sleep

4. Preschoolers: need 11 to 12 hours sleep but may fluctuate because of activity and growth spurts; older preschoolers do not need a nap; continue to have 20 to 30% of REM sleep

5. School-age: most school-age children sleep 8 to 12 hours without daytime naps; REM sleep decreases to about 20%

6. Adolescents: amount of time for sleeping declines but adolescents still need 8 to 10 hours sleep; changes in pattern occur as some adolescents have a need for daytime napping

7. Young adults: generally, young adults require 7 to 8 hours but because of lifestyle changes they may have erratic sleep patterns

8. Middle-age adults: sleep pattern established earlier is maintained and sleep 6 to 8 hours/night (about 20% is REM sleep); the amount of Stage IV NREM sleep decreases

9. Older adults: sleep about 6 hours a night with about 20 to 25% REM sleep and a marked decrease in Stage IV NREM sleep; they awaken more frequently and have difficulty returning back to sleep, hence having less restorative sleep

C. Factors affecting sleep

1. Illness: increases requirement for sleep; however, illness may cause pain, difficulty breathing, or discomfort with movement that interferes with sleep; elevated body temperature can cause a reduction in Stages III and IV NREM and REM sleep

2. Drugs and substances: excessive alcohol disrupts REM sleep, although it may accelerate onset of sleep; alcohol-tolerant individuals may have difficulty with sleep and when drug effects wear off, there may be nightmares; caffeine-containing beverages and amphetamines act as stimulants and interfere with sleep; nicotine has a stimulating effect and smokers have more difficulty falling asleep

3. Lifestyle: shift work may interfere with client's ability to adjust sleeping patterns; inactivity or boredom may contribute to sleep problems

4. Usual sleep patterns and excessive daytime sleepiness: peoples commonly refer to themselves as morning or night people, referring to their sleep patterns; excessive daytime sleepiness may be caused by night-time sleep deprivation

5. Emotional stress: anxiety can make it difficult to fall asleep; depression may result in difficulty falling asleep or premature awakening

6. Environment: any change in noise level may inhibit sleep—people are habituated to a certain noise; ventilation and environmental temperature can affect sleep

7. Various prescribed drugs: decongestants, narcotics, sedatives, beta blockers, and antidepressants may cause drowsiness and may disrupt REM sleep

8. Exercise and fatigue: moderate exercise is conducive to sleep but if excessive, may delay sleep; moderate fatigue may lead to a restful sleep

9. Food and calorie intake: weight loss is associated with reduced quantity of sleep, broken sleep, and earlier awakening, while weight gain is associated with increased total sleep time, less broken sleep, and later waking; eating a heavy meal just prior to bedtime could interfere with sleep

D. Overview of sleep disorders

1. Insomnia: inability to obtain an adequate amount or quality of sleep; can be initial (difficulty falling asleep), middle or intermittent (difficulty maintaining sleep because of frequent or prolonged waking), or terminal (early or premature awakening), which may be associated with depression or medications, such as HIV drugs;

Practice to Pass

A client tells the clinic nurse that she is having difficulty falling asleep at night. For which common factors that interfere with sleep should the nurse assess?

treatment is usually directed at developing new sleep-inducing or sleep-maintaining behaviors such as modifying environment or relaxation techniques

2. Sleep apnea: periodic cessation of breathing during sleep; episode lasts from 10 seconds to 2 minutes and incidence may range from 50 to 600 episodes per night
   a. Is suspected when person snores loudly, has frequent nocturnal awakening, excessive daytime sleepiness, fatigue, irritability, and personality changes
   b. Incidence of sleep apnea is high in older adult men
   c. Is also more common among obese clients
   d. Complications of prolonged sleep apnea may be increased BP, cardiac arrhythmias, and left-sided heart failure
   e. Treatment is directed at cause: if obstructive, enlarged tonsils or adenoids may be removed
   f. Use of a nasal continuous positive airway pressure (CPAP) device may be effective, because it keeps alveoli and small airways open, permitting better gas exchange because alveoli cannot collapse

3. Narcolepsy: sudden wave of overwhelming sleepiness during day, where person may nod off during day while involved in activities; treatment involves use of stimulants, such as amphetamines

4. Parasomnias: abnormal behavioral or physiologic events associated with the stages of sleep and interfere with sleep; treatment consists of relaxation techniques and sleep hygiene practices
   a. Somnambulism: sleepwalking that occurs in Stage III and IV NREM sleep; it is episodic and occurs 1 to 2 hours after falling asleep; sleepwalker does not notice dangers such as stairs
   b. Sleeptalking: talking occurs during NREM sleep before REM sleep
   c. Nocturnal enuresis: bedwetting, more common in male children over 3 years old; often occurs 1 to 2 hours after falling asleep when rousing from Stage III to IV of NREM sleep
   d. Bruxism: clenching and grinding teeth that occur during Stage II of NREM sleep

5. Sleep deprivation: syndrome where a prolonged disturbance results in a decrease in amount, quality, and consistency of sleep
   a. REM sleep deprivation can be caused by use of alcohol, shift work, jet lag, or extended ICU hospitalization and can result in excitability, confusion, and emotional lability; delay procedures or medications when possible to avoid waking a client during REM sleep
   b. NREM sleep deprivation can be caused by same factors as REM deprivation as well as hypothyroidism, depression, sleep apnea, and age (common in older adults), and can result in withdrawal, excessive sleepiness, and hyporesponsiveness
   c. An individual who has both REM and NREM sleep deprivation may have difficulty with concentration, judgment, and attention, marked fatigue, and perceptual distortions

E. **Health promotion to improve sleep**
1. Environmental controls: ensure appropriate lighting, ventilation, and temperature; keep noise level to a minimum
2. Promote bedtime routines: respect client's customary rituals or routines in order to promote relaxation and encourage sleep; provide hygiene routines such as washing face, brushing teeth, and voiding; listening to music or praying; children's bedtime stories; adult's conversations with their caregivers or family members if possible
3. Promote comfort: backrubs, change of linen or clothing, positioning for comfort, and medicating for pain can promote and help maintain sleep; listening to client's concerns can alleviate emotional stress and promote relaxation; avoid heavy meal 3 hours

before bedtime, decrease fluid intake 2 hours before sleep, and avoid alcohol, caffeine, or heavily spiced foods

4. Promote activity: get adequate exercise during day to reduce stress; engage in a nonstrenuous activity prior to sleep

5. Pharmacological sleep aids: may be prescribed for short-term treatment of insomnia; however, they generally should be used as a last resort and be taken on prn (as necessary) basis; clients need to be aware of their actions and desired and adverse effects; sedatives and hypnotics have different onset and duration of their actions; regular use may lead to drug tolerance and may lead to rebound insomnia

VI. MEETING NUTRITIONAL NEEDS

▶ *Practice to Pass*

The nurse is providing health teaching to a group of clients about promoting sleep. What specific instructions would be appropriate for the nurse to provide?

A. Principles of nutrition

1. Digestion: process by which food substances are changed into forms that can be a bsorbed through cell membranes

2. Absorption: taking-in of substances from GI tract into bloodstream

3. Metabolism: sum of all physical and chemical processes by which a living organism is formed and maintained and by which energy is made available

4. Storage: some nutrients are stored when not used to provide energy; e.g., carbohydrates are stored either as glycogen or as fat

5. Elimination: process of discarding unnecessary substances through evaporation, excretion

B. Nutrients

1. Carbohydrates (CHOs): primary sources of CHOs are plant foods

   a. Types of CHOs

      1) Simple CHOs (sugars) such as glucose, galactose, and fructose—all water soluble

      2) Complex CHOs, which are insoluble, include starches (**polysaccharides**) and fibers (supplies bulk or roughage to diet)

   b. Digested CHOs are absorbed in small intestines; insulin (a hormone secreted by pancreas) augments glucose transport through cell membrane of body cells

   c. Some glucose continues to circulate in bloodstream for energy, and remainder gets converted to fat or stored as glycogen in liver and skeletal muscles

2. Proteins: organic substances made up of amino acids; complete proteins are found in animal products such as eggs, milk, and meat; incomplete proteins are found in legumes, nuts, grains, cereals, and vegetables

   a. Most protein is digested in small intestine where enzymes break it down into smaller molecules and finally into amino acids, where they are actively transported into portal blood circulation

   b. The liver uses amino acids to synthesizes specific proteins

   c. Other amino acids are transported to cells and tissues to make proteins for cell structure

3. Lipids: organic substances that are insoluble in water but soluble in alcohol and ether

   a. Fatty acids are basic structural units of all lipids and are either saturated (all carbon atoms are filled with hydrogen) or unsaturated (could accommodate more hydrogen than it presently contains)

   b. Lipids are primarily digested in small intestine by bile, pancreatic lipase, and enteric lipase (enzymes) with end products of glycerol, fatty acids, and cholesterol; these products are reassembled in small intestines and then broken down into soluble compounds called lipoproteins

   c. Food sources for lipids are animal products (milk, egg yolks, and meats) and plants and plant products (seeds, nuts, oils)

4. Vitamins: organic compounds not manufactured in body and needed in small quantities to **catalyze** metabolic processes
   a. Water-soluble vitamins include C and the B-complex vitamins: B_1 (thiamine), B_2 (riboflavin), B_3 (niacin or nicotinic acid), B_6 (pyridoxine), B_9 (folic acid), B_{12} (cobalamin), pantothenic acid, and biotin; the body cannot store water-soluble vitamins, so a daily dietary supply is needed
   b. Fat-soluble vitamins include A, D, E, and K, and these can be stored in limited amounts in body
5. Minerals: compounds that work with other nutrients in maintaining structure and function of body
   a. An adequate supply of calcium, phosphorus, sodium, potassium, chloride, magnesium, and sulfur (known as *macrominerals*), and trace elements such as iron, iodine, copper, zinc, manganese, and fluoride (known as *microminerals*) are necessary for health

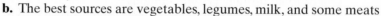

   b. The best sources are vegetables, legumes, milk, and some meats
6. Water: is body's most basic nutrient need; serves as a medium for metabolic reactions within cells and transports nutrients, waste products, and other substances

C. **MyPlate**: a graphic guide in making daily food choices; it suggests that people eat a variety of foods to obtain necessary nutrients in the proportions shown; specific food choices may be individualized to specific client needs and preferences (see Figure 7-1)

D. **Cultural factors that influence dietary practices and preferences**
   1. A client's ethnicity will often influence dietary practices and preferences
   2. The nurse should avoid the concepts of "good foods" and "bad foods"; look for variations within the culture that will support a healthy diet
   3. Universally accepted guidelines include eating a wide variety of foods and eating in moderation in order to maintain a healthy body weight
   4. Variations in nutritional practices and preference among selected cultures (see Table 7-1)

E. **Anthropometry**: noninvasive measurements that measure changes in body composition; such changes reflect chronic rather than acute changes in nutritional status
   1. Skinfold measurement: uses special calipers to measure thickness of fold in triceps (TSF—triceps skin fold) at back of upper arm
   2. Mid-arm circumference (MAC): a measure of fat, muscle, and skeleton
   3. Mid-arm muscle circumference (MAMC): estimate of lean body mass or skeletal muscle reserves; the formula is:
   [MAMC[cm] = MAC[cm] minus (3.14 multiplied by the TSF[mm] divided by 10)]

Figure 7-1

MyPlate

United States Department of Agriculture

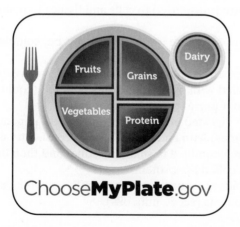

4. Body mass index: correlates weight with height using a nomogram or chart; normal range is considered to be 18.5 to 24.9; smaller number corresponds with underweight status while a larger number indicates overweight or obese status

F. Laboratory values associated with nutrition (see Table 7-2)

Table 7-1   **Variations in Nutritional Practices and Preference Among Selected Cultures**

AFRICAN AMERICAN HERITAGE
- Gifts of food are common and should never be rejected.
- Diets are often high in fat, cholesterol, and sodium.
- Being overweight may be viewed as positive.
- Many are lactose intolerant (Gaskin & Ilich, 2009).

ARAB HERITAGE
- Many spices and herbs are used such as cinnamon, allspice, cloves, mint, ginger, and garlic.
- Meats are often skewer roasted or slow simmered; most common are lamb and chicken.
- Bread is served at every meal.
- Muslims do not eat pork, and all meats must be cooked well done.
- Food is eaten (and clients fed) with the right hand.
- Beverages are drunk after the meal, not during; alcohol is prohibited.
- Muslims fast during daylight hours during the month of Ramadan (the 9th month of the year based on the lunar calendar).

CHINESE HERITAGE
- Foods are served at meals in a specific order.
- Each region in China has its own traditional diet.
- Traditional Chinese may not want ice in their drinks.
- Foods are chosen to balance *yin* and *yang* in order to avoid indigestion.
- Almost half are lactose intolerant (Gaskin & Ilich, 2009).

JEWISH HERITAGE
- Dietary laws govern killing, preparation, and eating of foods.
- Meat and milk are not eaten at the same time; dairy substitutes (e.g., margarine) are permitted.
- Pork is one meat that is forbidden to eat.
- All blood must be drained from meats.
- Always wash hands before eating.

MEXICAN HERITAGE
- Rice, beans, and tortillas are core, essential foods.
- Many are lactose intolerant. Leafy green vegetables and stews with bones provide calcium.
- Larger body size may be viewed as a positive attribute.
- Sweet fruit drinks, including adding sugar to juice, are popular.
- The main meal of the day is at noontime.
- Foods are chosen according to *hot* and *cold* theory.

NAVAJO HERITAGE
- Rites of passage and ceremonies are celebrated with food.
- Herbs are used to treat many illnesses.
- Sheep are the major source of meat.
- Squash and corn are major vegetables.
- Many are lactose intolerant.

Source: Berman, Audrey J.; Snyder, *Kozier & Erb's Fundamentals of Nursing*, 9th Ed. © 2012. Reprinted and Electronically reproduced by permission of Pearson Education, Inc., Upper Saddle River, New Jersey.

Table 7-2 Lab Values Associated with Nutritional Problems

Laboratory Test	Normal Values	Abnormal Findings
Hematocrit	Men: 40–54% Women: 36–46%	Decreased in iron deficiencies and undernutrition
Hemoglobin	Men: 13.5–18 grams/dL Women: 12–15 grams/dL	Iron-deficiency anemia
Serum potassium	3.5–5.3 mEq/L	Depletion seen in severe malnutrition
Albumin	3.5–5 grams/dL	A low serum albumin level is a useful indicator of prolonged protein depletion; altered liver function and poor hydration may lower albumin levels
Transferrin	200–430 mg/dL	Reduced numbers indicates protein deficiency, hepatitis, liver dysfunction
Total lymphocyte count	600–2,400 cells/mcL	Reduced numbers may indicate malnutrition
Blood urea nitrogen (BUN)	5 to 25 mg/dL	Elevated levels may be associated with increased protein catabolism caused by destruction or with dehydration
Urinary creatinine	Men: 20-26 mg/kg/24 h Women: 14–22 mg/kg/24 h	When skeletal muscles atrophy because of malnutrition, creatinine excretion decreases

G. Components of a diet history

1. Usual eating patterns and habits: Does client eat regularly, have snacks, and eat alone? Has client been on any diets?
2. Frequency, types, amounts, or quantities of foods consumed: How much food and what types of food has client consumed in last 24 hours? In last 7 days?
3. Food preferences, allergies, and intolerances: Does client have strong preferences for specific food groups? Are allergies and intolerances affecting amount of intake?
4. Social, economic, ethnic, or religious factors that influence nutrition: Is client suffering from economic hardship? Is there an adequate facility for food preparation? Is there an adequate food storage facility?
5. Health factors that may affect nutrition: Does client have a disease that interferes with food intake? Does client have problems complying with special diets? Has client recently gained or lost weight? Can client see, taste, or smell food? Does client have any physical disability that may affect nutrition?

H. Clinical signs of poor or altered nutrition

1. General appearance: appears tired and fatigued; listless
2. Weight: overweight or underweight
3. Posture: stooped or rigid
4. Behavior, motor, or perceptual function: slowing of reflexes; motor restlessness; confusion, disorientation
5. Gastrointestinal (GI) function: lack of appetite (anorexia), nausea, vomiting, overeating, indigestion, constipation
6. Hair: dry, dull, sparse, loss of color, brittle
7. Skin: dry, flaky, or scaly; pale or pigmented; presence of **petechiae** (pinpoint red areas) or bruising; lack of subcutaneous fat; poor skin turgor
8. Face and neck: facial edema; any swelling in neck (enlarged lymph nodes)
9. Lips: swollen, red cracks at side of mouth (angular stomatitis), vertical fissures (cheilosis)
10. Mouth and oral membranes: dry buccal cavity
11. Tongue: swollen, beefy-red or magenta-colored; coated; smooth appearance; increase or decrease in size
12. Teeth: dental caries; gums inflamed (gingivitis), spongy, bleed easily

13. Eyes: pale or red conjunctiva; dryness (xerophthalmia); soft cornea (keratomalacia); dull cornea
14. Nails: brittle; pale; ridged; spoon-shaped
15. Legs and feet: numbness, tingling, edema
16. Musculoskeletal: underdeveloped flaccid, soft, wasting muscles

I. **Therapeutic diets**: special diets prescribed for different reasons: for example, to treat a disease process or modified in texture, consistency, nutrients, or kilocalories (see Table 7-3); a regular diet is a balanced diet that supplies nutrients to meet metabolic requirements of a person who is **sedentary** (low activity); light diets have foods that are plainly cooked; DASH diet (dietary approaches to stop hypertension) for the client with hypertension

Practice to Pass

The nurse is evaluating a client for nutritional deficiencies. What are the signs of altered nutrition?

Table 7-3 **Therapeutic Diets**

Type of Diet	Purpose of Diet	Examples of Foods Allowed in the Diet and Other Recommendations
Clear liquid	Used after certain surgeries or in acute stages of GI tract infection (to minimize stimulation and prevent dehydration)	Coffee, tea, carbonated beverages, bouillon, clear fruit juices (apple, cranberry, grape), other juices (strained), popsicles, gelatin, hard candy, sugar, honey
Full liquid	Used for clients unable to tolerate solid or semisolid foods or who have GI disturbances	All foods allowed in the clear-liquid diet plus milk and milk drinks, custards, ice cream, sherbet, yogurt, vegetable juices, strained cereals (e.g., Cream of Wheat), butter
Soft	Used for clients who have difficulty chewing or swallowing	All foods in clear and full liquid plus: all lean meats chopped or shredded; scrambled or poached eggs; mashed potatoes and cooked chopped vegetables and fruits (low in fiber, without membranes or peels); rice, pasta, soft breads, cooked cereals
Pureed	See soft diet	All foods in soft diet: fluid is added to the food and blended to a semisolid consistency
Mechanical or dental	Used when clients are edentulous, have poorly fitted dentures, or have difficulty chewing	Any food that can be broken down easily
High fiber (high residue)	Used to treat constipation and diverticulosis (not with diverticulitis)	Cereals and grains such as wheat or oat bran, cooked cereals, dry cereals such as cornflakes, shredded wheat; whole grain breads; fruits such as unpeeled raw apples, peaches, or pears; oranges and berries; vegetables such as broccoli, carrots, peas, corn, beans, celery, and tomatoes
Sodium restricted	Used to manage hypertension, hepatitis, congestive heart failure, renal insufficiency or failure, cirrhosis of the liver	Allow most fresh fruits and vegetables (except beets, celery and frozen or canned vegetables with added salt); and most meats (except processed ones such as bacon, sausage, luncheon meats, cold cuts or smoked fish); restrict salt in cooking or at the table; avoid foods naturally high in sodium: brains, kidney, clams, crab, lobster, oysters, shrimp, dried fruit, spinach, carrots, cheese, buttermilk, most dry cereals
Healthy heart	Used to help control cholesterol levels and promote weight reduction; calories may be reduced	Wide variety of foods allowed; low-fat or nonfat dairy products such as yogurt, skim milk; fish, poultry; monounsaturated fats found in canola, olive, and peanut oils; all fresh fruits and vegetables; whole grain cereals, rice, and pasta
DASH diet	Dietary approaches to stop hypertension for the client with hypertension	Diet designed to help reduce hypertension or the development of hypertension; low in total and saturated fats. Dietary focus is on fruits (5 daily servings), vegetables (3 daily servings), and low-fat dairy products (2 daily servings). Diet also includes poultry and fish, whole grains, and nuts; red meat and sweets are limited

(continued)

Table 7-3	Therapeutic Diets (Continued)	
Type of Diet	**Purpose of Diet**	**Examples of Foods Allowed in the Diet and Other Recommendations**
Diabetic exchange	Structured diet to prevent hyperglycemia; exchange list diet based on person's ideal weight, activity level, age, and occupation	Distribution of foods based on exchange lists with 3 groups of foods; carbohydrates, meat and meat substitutes; and fats; 1 food portion of the list can exchanged or substituted for another with little difference in calories or amount of carbohydrates, proteins, or fats; examples of carbohydrate exchanges: ½ cup of cereal, ½ cup of pasta, ½ slice bagel, ½ hamburger bun, 1 medium pancake; examples of protein exchanges: 1 oz lean poultry no skin, 1 oz fish, ¼ cup nonfat cottage cheese, 1 egg, 1 oz cheese; examples of fat exchanges: 1 tsp margarine, 6 cashews, 2 tsp mayonnaise substitute, 1 tbsp cream cheese

  J. Enteral (tube) feeding
  1. Is a method of providing nutritional needs when oral intake is physically limited or prohibited
  2. Short-term enteral feeding is through a nasogastric tube (NG); long-term enteral feeding is through gastrostomy (G-tube), jejunostomy (J-tube), percutaneous endoscopic gastrostomy (PEG-tube), or percutaneous endoscopic jejunostomy (PEJ-tube)
  3. May be infused as continuous feedings or intermittent bolus feedings (over a short prescribed amount of time)
  4. The health care provider prescribes calories and nutrients according to specific client needs
  5. Additional water boluses (also called "free water") may be prescribed to ensure that client receives sufficient amounts of water daily, since enteral feedings tend to be hyperosmolar

VII. MEETING URINARY ELIMINATION NEEDS
  A. Normal urinary function

  1. Normal output of urine is 60 mL/hr or 1500 mL/day; should remain ≥ 30 mL/hr to ensure continued normal kidney function
  2. Urine normally consists of 96% water
  3. Solutes found in urine include the following:
      a. Organic solutes, including urea, ammonia, uric acid, and creatinine
      b. Inorganic solutes, including sodium, chloride, potassium, sulfate, magnesium, and phosphorus
  4. Table 7-4 describes characteristics of normal urine as well as possible abnormal findings
  B. Common assessment findings
  1. Urgency: strong desire to void may be caused by inflammation or infection in bladder or urethra
  2. Dysuria: painful or difficult voiding
  3. Frequency: voiding that occurs more than usual when compared to person's regular pattern or the generally accepted norm of voiding once every 3 to 6 hours
  4. Hesitancy: undue delay and difficulty in initiating voiding
  5. Polyuria: a large volume of urine voided at any given time
  6. Nocturia: excessive urination at night interrupting sleep
  7. Hematuria: red blood cells in urine
  8. Oliguria: reduced urine output between 100 and 500 mL/24 hr
  9. Anuria: urine output less than 100 mL in 24 hr

Table 7-4	Characteristics of Normal and Abnormal Urine		
Characteristic	**Normal**	**Abnormal**	**Nursing Considerations**
Amount in 24 hours (adult)	1,200–1,500 mL	Under 1,200 mL A large amount over intake	Urinary output normally is approximately equal to fluid intake. Output of less than 30 mL/hr may indicate decreased blood flow to kidneys and should be immediately reported.
Color, clarity	Straw, amber Transparent	Dark amber Cloudy Dark orange Red or dark brown Mucous plugs, viscid, thick	Concentrated urine is darker in color. Dilute urine may appear almost clear, or very pale yellow. Some foods and drugs may color urine. Red blood cells in the urine (hematuria) may be evident as pink, bright red, or rusty brown urine. Menstrual bleeding can also color urine but should not be confused with hematuria. White blood cells, bacteria, pus, or contaminants such as prostatic fluid, sperm, or vaginal drainage may cause cloudy urine.
Odor	Faint aromatic	Offensive	Some foods (e.g., asparagus) cause a musty odor; infected urine can have a fetid odor; urine high in glucose has a sweet odor.
Sterility	No microorganisms present	Microorganisms present	Urine in the bladder is sterile. Urine specimens may become contaminated by bacteria from the perineum during collection.
pH	4.5–8	Under 4.5 Over 8	Freshly voided urine is normally somewhat acidic. Alkaline urine may indicate a state of alkalosis, UTI, or a diet high in fruits and vegetables. More acidic urine (low pH) is found in starvation, with diarrhea, or with a diet high in protein foods or cranberries.
Specific gravity	1.010–1.025	Over 1.025 Under 1.010	Concentrated urine has a higher specific gravity; diluted urine has a lower specific gravity.
Glucose	Not present	Present	Glucose in the urine indicates high blood glucose levels (greater than 180 mg/dL), and may be indicative of undiagnosed or uncontrolled diabetes mellitus.
Ketone bodies	Not present	Present	Ketones, the end product of the breakdown of fatty acids, are not normally present in the urine. They may be present in the urine of clients who have uncontrolled diabetes mellitus, who are in a state of starvation, or who have ingested excessive amounts of aspirin.
Blood	Not present	Occult (microscopic) Bright red	Blood may be present in the urine of clients who have UTI, kidney disease, or bleeding from the urinary tract.

Source: Berman, Audrey J.; Snyder, Shirlee, *Kozier & Erb's Fundamentals of Nursing*, 9th Ed. © 2012. Reprinted and Electronically reproduced by permission of Pearson Education, Inc., Upper Saddle River, New Jersey.

C. Common urinary elimination problems

1. Urinary retention: occurs when bladder emptying is impaired, urine accumulates, and bladder becomes overdistended; causes include prostatic hyperplasia, surgery, and medications such as anticholinergics, antidepressants, antipsychotics, antiparkinsonian agents, and antihypertensives

2. Urinary tract infections (UTI): infectious process leads to inflammation in any portion of urinary tract

   a. Lower UTI: includes urethritis (inflammation of urethra), cystitis (inflammation of urinary bladder, most common), and prostatitis (inflammation of prostate gland); manifestations may include dysuria, pyuria, frequency, urgency, suprapubic discomfort, hematuria, or nocturia; older adult clients may also exhibit confusion, lethargy, behavior changes, or anorexia

   b. Upper UTI: pyelonephritis (inflammation of renal pelvis and parenchyma, the functional portion of kidney tissue); manifestations may additionally include flank pain or costovertebral tenderness; systemic symptoms include nausea, vomiting, diarrhea, acute fever, shaking chills, and malaise

Box 7-4	
Types of Urinary Incontinence	• Stress incontinence: involuntary loss of urine of less than 50 mL occurring with increased abdominal pressure through coughing, laughing, or lifting • Reflex incontinence: involuntary loss of urine at predictable intervals when bladder reaches a specific volume • Urge incontinence: involuntary loss of urine soon after a strong urge to void • Functional incontinence: involuntary unpredictable passage of urine because of inability to get to toilet as a result of physical or cognitive impairment • Total incontinence: continuous and unpredictable involuntary loss of urine

3. Incontinence: involuntary urination of various types based on etiology (see Box 7-4)

D. **Urinary diversion devices**: ureterostomy—a surgical rerouting of urine from kidneys to a site other than bladder, usually when bladder is removed or diseased

1. Cutaneous ureterostomy: ureters brought directly to skin surface to form small stomas; disadvantages include that stomas provide direct access for microorganisms from skin to kidneys; pouches may be difficult to fit to small stomas; stenosis of stomas may occur as a complication

2. Ileal conduit: a segment of the ileum is separated from small intestine and formed into a pouch with open end brought out through abdominal wall to form a stoma; the ureters are implanted into ileal pouch (see Figure 7-2)

3. Continent urinary reservoir: created from portion of stomach, colon, or small intestine to which ureters are attached; formation of a nipple valve prevents reflux of urine; formation of a stoma is unnecessary if pouch is attached to urethral stump; drainage collection device is not necessary

E. **Common urinary tests**

1. Urinalysis: macroscopic and microscopic analysis of urine to determine physical and chemical characteristics; refer back to Table 7-4

2. Urine culture and sensitivity: identifies an infecting organism and the most effective antibiotic; a clean-catch specimen or catheterized specimen is needed; culture requires 24 to 72 hours for organism growth and identification

3. Intravenous pyelogram (IVP) or intravenous urogram (IVU): intravenous injection of a radiopaque contrast media that concentrates in urine and facilitates visualization of kidneys, ureters, and bladder

4. Renal scan: radiotraces or isotopes injected intravenously to evaluate renal size, shape, position, and function or blood flow to kidneys; pictures are taken by a scintillation camera

Figure 7-2

An ileal conduit

Berman, Audrey J.; Snyder, Shirlee, *Kozier & Erb's Fundamentals of Nursing*, 9th Ed. © 2012. Reprinted and Electronically reproduced by permission of Pearson Education, Inc., Upper Saddle River, New Jersey.

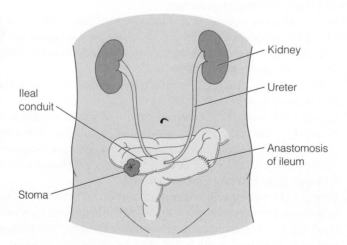

Kidney

Ureter

Ileal conduit

Anastomosis of ileum

Stoma

5. Ultrasound: high-frequency sound waves are used to create ultrasonic images of urinary system
6. Cystoscopy: direct visualization of urethra and bladder with a cystoscope that is a self-contained optical lens system and provides a magnified illuminated view of bladder
7. Bladder scan at bedside: detects amount of urine in bladder to help determine need for voiding or straight catheterization; may be done by nurses or other personnel trained to use portable device
8. Postvoiding residual (PVR) volume: determines how completely the bladder empties
9. Uroflometry: noninvasive procedure; evaluates voiding patterns
10. Cystometrography: assesses neuromuscular function of bladder; evaluates detrusor muscle function, bladder pressure, and bladder filling

F. Teaching and health promotion for urinary elimination

1. Adequate hydration: normal daily intake of 1,500 mL of measurable fluids recommended; if prone to development of stones or infections, increase fluid intake to 2,000 to 3,000 mL per 24 hours; if experiencing abnormal fluid losses, additional fluid intake is necessary
2. Personal hygiene: teach client to maintain cleanliness by washing perineal area with soap and water daily, and wiping after defecation; instruct female clients to wipe from front to back (urinary meatus toward the anus) after voiding and discard after each wipe; if recurrent infections are occurring, avoid tub baths
3. Emptying bladder completely: regular exercise increases muscle tone that helps maintain the ability to contract the detrusor muscle of the bladder for complete emptying; abdominal muscle contraction assists in bladder emptying; teach **Kegel exercises**—contract perineal muscles and hold for a count of 3 to 5 seconds and relax; do 10 contractions 5 times daily
4. Infection prevention measures
   a. Drink eight 8-ounce glasses of water daily
   b. Empty bladder at least every 2 to 4 hours while awake, avoiding voluntary retention; if client is incontinent, instruct to void according to a timetable rather than the urge to void (bladder training); void at regular intervals (habit training); or supplement habit training by encouraging and reminding client to void (prompted voiding); instruct client to practice deep, slow breathing until urge to void diminishes
   c. For women: wear cotton briefs; cleanse perineal area from front to back after voiding and defecating; void before and after sexual intercourse; avoid bubble baths, feminine hygiene sprays and douches
   d. Unless contraindicated: teach client to maintain acidity in urine by drinking at least 2 glasses of cranberry juice per day or taking vitamin C, and avoiding excess milk products and sodium bicarbonate
   e. The client should be able to identify symptoms of urinary tract infection and preventive measures, as well as reporting symptoms promptly

VIII. MEETING BOWEL ELIMINATION NEEDS

A. Factors that influence bowel elimination

Practice to Pass

A client has a urinary tract infection. What instructions are appropriate for the nurse to give the client?

1. Age
   a. Infants and toddlers: have immature control of bowel elimination; daytime control is achieved by age 2½ with toilet training
   b. School-age and adolescents: have similar bowel habits as adults; however, school-age children involved in play may delay elimination
   c. Older adults: are prone to constipation because of slowing down of GI motility and decreased food intake and activity
2. Diet
   a. Sufficient bulk is needed to provide fecal volume

      b. If a client is on low-residue or low-fiber diet, there may be insufficient volume to stimulate reflex for defecation

      c. Irregular eating can interfere with regular elimination

      d. Certain foods can affect elimination

         1) Spicy or overly sweet foods may cause diarrhea

         2) Cabbage, onions, apples, and bananas are gas producing

         3) Bran, prunes, figs, and alcohol have laxative effect

         4) Cheese, eggs, pasta, and lean meat have constipating effect

3. Position: normal bowel elimination is facilitated by thigh flexion (increases intra-abdominal pressure) and a sitting position, which increases downward pressure on rectum; using a bedpan while in a supine position is not comfortable and does not facilitate defecation, so client needs to be placed in a semi-sitting position

4. Pregnancy: there is decreased intestinal secretion; colon is displaced upward, laterally, and posteriorly; peristaltic activity is decreased, causing constipation; later in pregnancy, venous pressure increases, causing hemorrhoids

5. Fluid intake: healthy elimination requires an intake of 2,000 to 3,000 mL/day; inadequate fluid intake or excessive fluid output may lead to hard feces

6. Activity: peristalsis is stimulated by adequate activity; immobility, weak muscles from lack of exercise, or impaired neurologic functioning can lead to constipation

7. Psychological: anxiety or anger can increase peristalsis and lead to subsequent diarrhea, while depression slows intestinal activity resulting in constipation

8. Personal habits: if an individual continually ignores urge to defecate, water continues to be reabsorbed and feces harden; defecation reflex tends to be progressively weakened and may be lost

9. Pain: when pain or discomfort occurs upon defecation, clients may suppress urge to defecate to avoid pain, thereby eventually leading to constipation

10. Medications: antidepressants, antipsychotic and antiparkinsonian agents, morphine and codeine (or other opioids) may cause constipation

11. Surgery and anesthesia: general anesthetics may slow intestinal movement, resulting in constipation; abdominal surgery that involves handling of intestines may cause cessation of intestinal movement (paralytic ileus) that lasts for 24 to 48 hours

B. Characteristics of normal stool

  1. Color: varies from light to dark brown; affected by foods and medications

  2. Odor: aromatic, affected by ingested food and person's bacterial flora

  3. Consistency: formed, soft, semi-solid, moist

  4. Frequency: varies with diet; once a day is a common pattern

  5. Amount: varies with diet (about 100 to 400 grams/day)

  6. Constituents: small amounts of undigested roughage, sloughed dead bacteria and epithelial cells, fat, protein, dried constituents of digestive juices (bile pigments), inorganic matter (calcium, phosphates)

C. Common bowel elimination problems

  1. Constipation: abnormal infrequency of defecation and abnormal hardening of stools

  2. Impaction: accumulated mass of dry feces that cannot be expelled

  3. Diarrhea: increased frequency of bowel movements (more than 3 times a day) as well as liquid consistency and increased amount; accompanied by urgency, discomfort, and possibly incontinence

  4. Incontinence: involuntary elimination of feces

  5. Flatulence: expulsion of gas from the rectum

  6. Hemorrhoids: dilated portions of veins in anal canal causing itching and pain and bright red bleeding upon defecation

D. Diagnostic tests

1. Abdominal film: x-ray of the abdomen taken with client in flat and upright positions
2. Upper GI/barium swallow: fluoroscopic x-ray examination of esophagus, stomach, and small intestines after client ingests barium sulfate
3. Barium enema: fluoroscopy x-ray examination visualizing entire large intestine after client is given an enema of barium; outlines structural changes such as polyps and diverticulitis
4. Endoscopy: use of a flexible tube (fiberoptic endoscope) to visualize GI tract; images produced are transmitted to a video screen
5. Upper endoscopy: a fiberoptic endoscope connected to a telescopic eyepiece can be inserted through mouth; example is EGD—esophagogastroduodenoscopy
6. Lower endoscopy: a fiberoptic endoscope connected to a telescopic eyepiece is inserted through rectum; example is proctosigmoidoscopy

E. Health promotion for elimination problems

1. Constipation: increase fluid intake; instruct to drink fruit juices (especially prune juice) and warm liquids; encourage intake of foods high in roughage or fiber such as raw fruits and vegetables, bran products, whole grain cereals and bread
2. Diarrhea: encourage oral intake of fluids and bland foods; avoid spicy and fatty foods, alcohol, beverages with caffeine, and high-fiber foods
3. Flatulence: limit chewing gum, carbonated drinks, drinking straws, and gas-producing foods such as cabbage, cauliflower, beans, and onions

F. Bowel diversion ostomies: an ostomy is a surgical opening in abdominal wall for elimination of feces or urine; bowel diversion ostomies are classified according to status (temporary or permanent), anatomic location, and construction of stoma

1. Permanence: colostomies can be temporary (for traumatic injuries or inflammatory conditions) or permanent (birth defect or disease such as cancer)
2. Anatomic location (see Figure 7-3): identifies site from which ostomy empties
   a. Ileostomy: distal end of small intestine (ileus)
   b. Cecostomy: first part of ascending colon (cecum)
   c. Ascending colostomy: ascending colon
   d. Transverse colostomy: transverse colon
   e. Descending colostomy: descending colon
   f. Sigmoidostomy: sigmoid colon

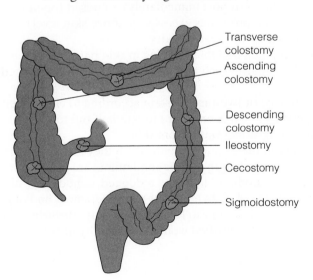

Figure 7-3

The locations of bowel diversion ostomies

Transverse colostomy

Ascending colostomy

Descending colostomy

Ileostomy

Cecostomy

Sigmoidostomy

3. Construction of stoma
   a. Single: 1 end of bowel as the opening
   b. Loop: a loop of bowel brought out into abdominal wall supported by a glass rod or a plastic bridge; has 2 openings, the proximal or active, and the distal or inactive; usually performed as an emergency procedure and situated often in right transverse colon
   c. Divided: 2 separated stomas; opening from digestive end is the colostomy and distal end is a mucus fistula (bowel continues to secrete mucus)
   d. Double-barreled: proximal and distal loops are sutured together and both ends are brought out into abdominal wall

4. Health promotion for clients with ostomies
   a. For a client with a colostomy, dietary teaching needs to include information about:
      1) Foods that cause stool odor (asparagus, beans, eggs, fish, onions, garlic)
      2) Foods that increase gas (cabbage, onions, apples, bananas)
      3) Foods that thicken stool (bananas, rice, tapioca, cheese, yogurt)
      4) Foods that loosen stool (chocolate, dried beans, fried foods, highly spiced foods, leafy green vegetables, raw fruits and vegetables)
   b. For a client with ileostomy, teaching to relieve food blockage should include the following:
      1) Drink warm fluids or grape juice if not vomiting
      2) Take a warm shower
      3) Assume a knee–chest position
      4) Massage peristomal area
      5) Remove pouch if stoma is swollen and apply one with a larger opening
      6) Eat a low-residue diet initially; avoid foods that cause blockage such as popcorn, nuts, cucumbers, celery, fresh tomatoes, figs, blackberries, and caraway seeds
      7) Limit high-fiber foods and chew them well if eaten
      8) Know signs of blockage: abdominal cramping, swelling of stoma, and absence of ileostomy output for 4 to 6 hours

5. Stoma management
   a. Stoma appearance: should be bright pink or red in color, moist and raised above abdominal skin surface, and surrounded by intact skin; abnormalities include being sunken (below level of abdominal skin), abnormal in color (dusky, pale, cyanotic, or black—report immediately), stenosed (opening is narrowed), or herniated (stoma protrudes excessively above skin level)
   b. Keep peristomal skin clean and dry
   c. Cut stoma appliance so that opening in skin barrier/wafer is no more than one-eighth to one-quarter inch larger than stoma itself in order to prevent peristomal skin irritation
   d. Use a one-piece or two-piece system according to client need
   e. Empty pouch when it is one-third to one-half full to prevent weight of pouch from separating stoma wafer from skin
   f. Pouches vary in the frequency with which they are changed; some are changed weekly (maximum length of time) and others are changed more frequently; in clients with peristomal skin that is reddened, denuded, or ulcerated, pouch should be changed every 24 to 48 hours for skin assessment and ongoing skin care
   g. Assess client's adjustment to having an ostomy (disturbed body image), and provide referrals to certified wound and ostomy nurse as needed

Practice to Pass

The nurse is taking care of a client with a colostomy. What health teaching is appropriate for this client?

Case Study

A 72-year-old female is being admitted for evaluation after a fall at home. Although x-rays revealed no fractures, the client reports severe pain in the lower back, inability to sleep at night because of the pain, difficulty breathing, and lack of appetite. You are the admitting nurse in the unit.

1. What assessments does the nurse need to make about the client's ability to meet basic needs?

2. How would the nurse ensure the safety of the client?

3. What interventions will be appropriate to promote client's sleep?

4. How would the nurse assist the client have adequate air exchange?

5. What instructions will the nurse give to promote healthy urinary elimination?

For suggested responses, see pages 307–308.

POSTTEST

① A family member of an older adult client objects that restraints are being used to prevent the client from wandering in the evening. What should the nurse consider in order to avoid the use of restraints?

1. Providing visual and auditory stimuli
2. Using antianxiety medications as prescribed
3. Assigning client to a room near the nurse's station
4. Locking the door to the client's room

② An adult client is experiencing hospitalization for the first time. What are the appropriate actions by the nurse to help promote the safety of the client? Select all that apply.

1. Maintain a clutter-free client environment.
2. Keep the client's area well lighted during the night.
3. Assure that side rails are in up position when client is in bed.
4. Examine equipment carefully before using it for client care.
5. Reorient the client to surroundings whenever necessary.

③ A client who is unconscious needs to have mouth hygiene performed. While performing this task, in what position should the nurse place the client?

1.

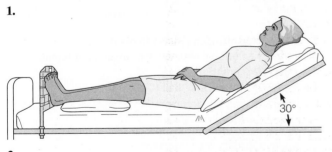

2.

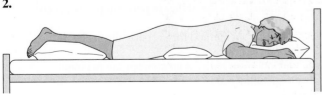

3.

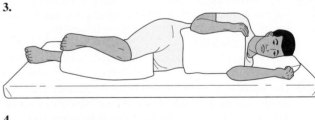

4.

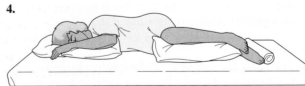

4 The nurse is providing health teaching to a client about lifestyle factors that affect oxygenation. What is the most accurate information the nurse can supply to the client? Select all that apply.

1. Epinephrine and norepinephrine released under stress increase blood pressure and cardiac rate.
2. Alcohol and opiate use will depress respirations and decrease tissue oxygenation.
3. Anemia, from an inadequate diet, can increase the risk for heart disease.
4. Physical exercise will eventually lower the need for oxygen by the tissues.
5. Smoking will cause vasoconstriction, leading to decreased oxygen to tissues.

5 A nurse is performing oropharyngeal suctioning on an unconscious client. The nurse should perform which actions? Select all that apply.

1. Insert the catheter approximately 20 cm while applying suction.
2. Allow 20- to 30-second intervals between each suction attempt and limit suctioning to a total of 15 minutes.
3. Gently rotate the catheter while applying suction.
4. Apply suction for 5 seconds while inserting the catheter and continue for another 5 seconds before withdrawing.
5. Provide oxygen to the client prior to suctioning.

6 A client with chest tubes is admitted to the nursing unit. On what action should the nurse place the highest priority during admission?

1. Measuring the client's vital signs, respiratory, and cardiovascular status regularly
2. Explaining the importance of performing deep breathing and coughing to the client
3. Reporting to the primary health care provider if drainage exceeds 100 mL/hour
4. Placing rubber-tipped clamps, sterile water, and sterile occlusive dressing at the bedside

7 After performing a physical assessment on a client, the nurse suspects that the client has poor nutritional status. Which assessment finding validates the nurse's suspicion?

1. Delayed wound healing
2. Firm, smooth pink nails
3. Moist, buccal cavity mucous membranes
4. Erect posture

8 The nurse evaluates the results of laboratory tests completed on an adult client. Which laboratory value indicates to the nurse that the client may have an abnormality related to nutritional status?

1. Blood urea nitrogen (BUN) 15 mg/dL
2. Urinary creatinine 800 mg/24 hr in an adult female
3. Albumin 5 grams/dL
4. Serum potassium 2.4 mEq/L

9 The nurse has taught a client measures to avoid complications associated with urinary elimination. Which client behavior indicates to the nurse that the client teaching has been effective?

1. Ability to identify the symptoms of and measures to prevent urinary tract infection
2. Demonstrates the ability to perform perineal care without assistance
3. Maintains a method for properly disposing of urinary output
4. Includes tub baths as an appropriate personal hygiene measure

10 A client with a colostomy asks the nurse about the effects of certain types of foods. In order to avoid loose stools or leakage, what foods should the nurse instruct the client to consume?

1. Asparagus, beans, eggs, fish, onions
2. Cheese, bananas, rice, tapioca, yogurt
3. Fried foods, highly spiced foods, raw fruits and vegetables
4. Carbonated drinks, fruit juices, oily foods, and pureed foods

➤ *See pages 184–186 for Answers and Rationales.*

ANSWERS & RATIONALES

Pretest

1 **Answer: 1** **Rationale:** A toddler is mobile and naturally curious and experiments with things in the environment; therefore, the parents need to know that supervision will be necessary. Toddlers' reflexes are not necessarily slow, and reading is not a concern. Reading is a skill not necessarily expected with a toddler; however, if the ability to read exists, it would not be a safety concern. Social and personality development is a good topic for health teaching but is not the main safety concern. **Cognitive Level:** Applying **Client Need:** Safety and Infection Control **Integrated Process:** Teaching and Learning **Content Area:** Fundamentals **Strategy:** The critical words are *parents of toddlers* and *safety education.* Recall safety risks according to developmental level to permit you to select the option that provides key information to parents. **Reference:** Berman, A. J., & Snyder, S. (2011). *Kozier and Erb's fundamentals of nursing: Concepts, process, and practice* (9th ed.). Upper Saddle River, NJ: Prentice Hall, p. 382.

2 **Answers: 2, 5** **Rationale:** One purpose for restraints should be to prevent interruption of therapy such as sutures or sterile dressings. The least restrictive restraint should be used when it is indicated; however, if the restraint is ineffective, a more restrictive restraint may be appropriate. Restraints should not be used just because a client is hyperactive or weak, or has a developmental disability. There is no reason to apply restraints to a client who is anxious about test results. **Cognitive Level:** Applying **Client Need:** Safety and Infection Control **Integrated Process:** Nursing Process: Evaluation **Content Area:** Fundamentals **Strategy:** The critical phrase is *use of restraints is appropriate.* Recall the overall objectives for restraint use to assist you in making correct decisions about the use of restraints. **Reference:** Berman, A. J., & Snyder, S. (2011). *Kozier and Erb's fundamentals of nursing: Concepts, process, and practice* (9th ed.). Upper Saddle River, NJ: Prentice Hall, p. 737.

3 **Answer: 2** **Rationale:** Because the client has been incontinent, the possibility of skin bacteria reacting with the urea in the urine can lead to ammonia dermatitis. Erythema is reddening of the skin; contact dermatitis is a possibility if a client is allergic to soaps or other substances; and petechiae are tiny pinpoints of bleeding in the skin. **Cognitive Level:** Applying **Client Need:** Basic Care and Comfort **Integrated Process:** Nursing Process: Assessment **Content Area:** Fundamentals **Strategy:** The critical words are *incontinent, pruritis,* and *lower back.* Recognize signs and symptoms of common skin problems and their underlying causes, and use knowledge of terminology to assist you in selecting the correct answer. **Reference:** Berman, A. J., & Snyder, S. (2011). *Kozier and Erb's fundamentals of nursing: Concepts, process, and practice* (9th ed.). Upper Saddle River, NJ: Prentice Hall, p. 921.

4 **Answer: 3** **Rationale:** The proper sequence for using a spirometer is to exhale completely, place the mouthpiece, inhale, remove the mouthpiece, hold breath, and exhale. A Fowler's or sitting position best allows for full chest expansion. Slower breaths are better and deeper than fast ones. The client should remove the mouthpiece, exhale through pursed lips, and not exhale into the spirometer. **Cognitive Level:** Applying **Client Need:** Basic Care and Comfort **Integrated Process:** Nursing Process: Evaluation **Content Area:** Fundamentals **Strategy:** The critical terms are *incentive spirometer* and *client understood the instructions.* Recall the correct use of the incentive spirometer to answer the question and remember the purpose of the client using it. **Reference:** Berman, A. J., & Snyder, S. (2011). *Kozier and Erb's fundamentals of nursing: Concepts, process, and practice* (9th ed.). Upper Saddle River, NJ: Prentice Hall, p. 1393.

5 **Answers: 2, 3, 4** **Rationale:** Basic measures to promote sleep in hospitalized clients include maintaining their bedtime routine, decreasing light and noise levels, and promoting relaxation and general comfort. Clients who are trying to develop a state of relaxation to enable sleep should avoid alcohol and caffeine as well as unusual exertion. **Cognitive Level:** Applying **Client Need:** Basic Care and Comfort **Integrated Process:** Nursing Process: Implementation **Content Area:** Fundamentals **Strategy:** The critical term is *difficulty sleeping*. Recall basic nursing care measures that promote rest and sleep to assist you in providing effective care to the client. **Reference:** Berman, A. J., & Snyder, S. (2011). *Kozier and Erb's fundamentals of nursing: Concepts, process, and practice* (9th ed.). Upper Saddle River, NJ: Prentice Hall, p. 1190.

6 **Answer: 3** **Rationale:** Cotton clothing limits static electricity, which could create a spark that could possibly cause a fire. Electrical equipment in good condition (with no frayed wires) is acceptable for use near oxygen. Petroleum products and most oils have the potential for being flammable when used on the body, which is a contraindication for their use. **Cognitive Level:** Applying **Client Need:** Safety and Infection Control **Integrated Process:** Teaching and Learning **Content Area:** Fundamentals **Strategy:** The critical phrase is *oxygen therapy via a nasal cannula*. Recall safety precautions needed during oxygen therapy that will help to promote client safety and improve outcomes. **Reference:** Berman, A. J., & Snyder, S. (2011). *Kozier and Erb's fundamentals of nursing: Concepts, process, and practice* (9th ed.). Upper Saddle River, NJ: Prentice Hall, p. 1389.

7 **Answer: 1** **Rationale:** Pain can often interfere with sleep. Absence of unfamiliar stimuli can assist with sleep; dealing with stress by talking about the day's events promotes relaxation and eventually sleep; moderate fatigue may lead to a restful sleep. **Cognitive Level:** Applying **Client Need:** Basic Care and Comfort **Integrated Process:** Nursing Process: Assessment **Content Area:** Fundamentals **Strategy:** The critical phrase is *negative effect on the client's sleep pattern*. Recall common factors that disrupt sleep to assist you in identifying causes of this disturbance. **Reference:** Berman, A. J., & Snyder, S. (2011). *Kozier and Erb's fundamentals of nursing: Concepts, process, and practice* (9th ed.). Upper Saddle River, NJ: Prentice Hall, p. 1195.

8 **Answer: 4** **Rationale:** Because of limited mobility, the client is already at risk for constipation. To promote bowel function, instruct clients to drink plenty of liquids, including water and fruit juices such as apple and prune. In addition, foods that are high in fiber and roughage should be encouraged to avoid constipation secondary to immobility. It is not necessary to avoid drinks with caffeine; hot caffeinated beverages such as tea or coffee can stimulate a bowel movement. **Cognitive Level:** Applying **Client Need:** Basic Care and Comfort **Integrated Process:** Teaching and Learning **Content Area:** Fundamentals **Strategy:** The critical words are *bedridden* and *constipated*. Use nursing knowledge of the common complications of immobility to allow you to select the teaching points to treat and further prevent this complication of immobility. **Reference:** Berman, A. J., & Snyder, S. (2011). *Kozier and Erb's fundamentals of nursing: Concepts, process, and practice* (9th ed.). Upper Saddle River, NJ: Prentice Hall, pp. 1348–1350.

9 **Answer: 2** **Rationale:** When a premature urge to void occurs, focused breathing exercises may assist the client to overcome the sense of urgency. The intervals between voiding should eventually lengthen, rather than voiding every hour or more often when an urge is felt. Protector pads should be worn continuously for leakage. Adult disposable briefs are used only as a last resort. **Cognitive Level:** Applying **Client Need:** Basic Care and Comfort **Integrated Process:** Teaching and Learning **Content Area:** Fundamentals **Strategy:** The critical terms are *bladder training* and *expected outcome*. Recall essential techniques of bladder training to assist in identifying appropriate client information about bladder training and the expected outcomes. **Reference:** Berman, A. J., & Snyder, S. (2011). *Kozier and Erb's fundamentals of nursing: Concepts, process, and practice* (9th ed.). Upper Saddle River, NJ: Prentice Hall, p. 1321.

10 **Answer: 2** **Rationale:** A full liquid diet allows such items as puddings, creamed soups, sherbet, strained cereals, and all items that are liquid at room temperature. Homemade clam chowder with potatoes, soft cake, and chopped vegetables are solid foods that do not liquefy at room temperature. **Cognitive Level:** Applying **Client Need:** Basic Care and Comfort **Integrated Process:** Teaching and Learning **Content Area:** Fundamentals **Strategy:** The critical words in the question are *effective* and *full liquid diet*. Recall information about the components of therapeutic diets to assist you in providing the client and family with appropriate guidance. **Reference:** Berman, A. J., & Snyder, S. (2011). *Kozier and Erb's fundamentals of nursing: Concepts, process, and practice* (9th ed.). Upper Saddle River, NJ: Prentice Hall, p. 1280.

Posttest

1 **Answer: 3** **Rationale:** The client needs to be supervised, monitored, and placed in a room that is more accessible. Assessment is needed to determine causes of wandering. Stimulation is not necessary for a client who is a wanderer. Antianxiety medications may cause more agitation. Locking the client's door will create a safety hazard; the client cannot be observed as closely and may become more agitated and susceptible to injury or harm. **Cognitive Level:** Applying **Client Need:** Safety and Infection Control **Integrated Process:** Nursing Process: Planning **Content Area:** Fundamentals **Strategy:** Recall that alternatives to restraint use include reducing noise, alarm systems, activities, family involvement, and adequate lighting. **Reference:** Berman, A. J., & Snyder, S. (2011). *Kozier and Erb's fundamentals of nursing: Concepts, process, and practice* (9th ed.). Upper Saddle River, NJ: Prentice Hall, pp. 737–739.

2 **Answers: 1, 4, 5** **Rationale:** When a client is in an acute health care setting, the nurse can promote safety by maintaining a clutter-free client environment, assuring that medical equipment is safe, and reorienting the client as needed. Lighting of the client environment should be appropriate for promoting safety while not interfering with the client's well-being. The nurse has a responsibility to understand appropriate use of side rails and how use of this equipment can actually create a safety hazard. **Cognitive Level:** Applying **Client Need:** Safety and Infection Control **Integrated Process:** Nursing Process: Implementation **Content Area:** Fundamentals **Strategy:** Consider the safety concerns when the client is admitted to the acute care setting in order to identify the correct answers. Remember that when more than one option is correct, consider each option as a true-false statement. **Reference:** LeMone, P., & Burke, K. M. (2011). *Medical-surgical nursing: Critical thinking in client care* (5th ed., Vol. Single). Upper Saddle River, NJ: Prentice Hall, p. 15.

3 **Answer: 3** **Rationale:** In the side-lying position, fluid is more likely to flow readily out of the mouth or to pool in the side of the mouth where it can be suctioned easily. Fowler's position is not appropriate since the unconscious client does not have the control to stay up in the position, and there is an increased risk for choking. The prone and Sim's positions do not provide the nurse with adequate visual or physical access to perform mouth hygiene; difficulty in protecting the client and bed linens from drainage is also a concern. **Cognitive Level:** Applying **Client Need:** Basic Care and Comfort **Integrated Process:** Nursing Process: Implementation **Content Area:** Fundamentals **Strategy:** Recall that an unconscious client always requires airway maintenance. Next, remember that side lying prevents aspiration as well as preventing the tongue from occluding the airway. Think carefully through the rationales for each option being an appropriate or inappropriate choice. **Reference:** Berman, A. J., & Snyder, S. (2011). *Kozier and Erb's fundamentals of nursing: Concepts, process, and practice* (9th ed.). Upper Saddle River, NJ: Prentice Hall, pp. 309–311.

4 **Answers: 1, 2, 5** **Rationale:** Stress, alcohol and drug use, poor dietary habits, and smoking are all lifestyle choices that can negatively impact respiratory and tissue oxygenation. Physical exercise, a healthy diet, stress management, and avoiding unhealthy life choices will promote respiratory and cardiac health, both of which are vital for adequate oxygenation of body tissues. **Cognitive Level:** Analyzing **Client Need:** Health Promotion and Maintenance **Integrated Process:** Teaching and Learning **Content Area:** Fundamentals **Strategy:** Recall general nursing knowledge related to lifestyle and its effects on the respiratory and cardiac systems, then use the process of elimination to choose the options that could be a risk factor for the client. When there is more than one correct option, consider each option as a true-false statement. **Reference:** Berman, A. J., & Snyder, S. (2011). *Kozier and Erb's fundamentals of nursing: Concepts, process, and practice* (9th ed.). Upper Saddle River, NJ: Prentice Hall, p. 1384.

5 **Answers: 3, 5** **Rationale:** Oxygenating the client before suctioning contributes to the safety and comfort of the client. Gentle rotation ensures that all surfaces are reached and prevents trauma to any one area caused by prolonged suctioning. In oropharyngeal suctioning, the catheter should be advanced to 10 to 15 cm; 20 cm is the distance for tracheal suctioning. Intermittent suctioning over 15 minutes would cause hypoxia or respiratory distress. Applying suction while inserting the catheter can cause trauma to the mucous membranes. **Cognitive Level:** Applying **Client Need:** Basic Care and Comfort **Integrated Process:** Nursing Process: Implementation **Content Area:** Fundamentals **Strategy:** Recall essentials of the suctioning procedure. Remember that airway maintenance of an unconscious client is essential. When more than one option is correct, consider each option as a true-false statement. **Reference:** Berman, A. J., & Snyder, S. (2011). *Kozier and Erb's fundamentals of nursing: Concepts, process, and practice* (9th ed.). Upper Saddle River, NJ: Prentice Hall, pp. 1410–1413.

6 **Answer: 4** **Rationale:** Although all of the actions are appropriate, the highest priority on admission is to anticipate any emergency that may take place if problems with the chest tubes occur, such as disconnection or accidental removal. **Cognitive Level:** Applying **Client Need:** Physiological Adaptation **Integrated Process:** Nursing Process: Implementation **Content Area:** Fundamentals **Strategy:** Recall that chest tubes remove air and/or fluid from the pleural space and if dislodged they could pose a threat to the client's respiratory status. Use this knowledge to select the option that prepares for a possible emergency with the chest tube. **Reference:** Berman, A. J., & Snyder, S. (2012). *Skills in clinical nursing* (7th ed.). Upper Saddle River, NJ: Prentice Hall, pp. 695–697.

7 **Answer: 1** **Rationale:** Delayed wound healing may be a sign of inadequate nutritional status. Clients need a diet rich in protein, carbohydrates, lipids, vitamins A and C, and minerals such as iron, zinc, and copper to promote adequate healing. Firm, smooth pink nails, moist buccal mucous membranes, and erect posture are consistent with adequate nutritional status. **Cognitive Level:** Analyzing **Client Need:** Basic Care and Comfort **Integrated Process:** Nursing Process: Assessment **Content Area:** Fundamentals **Strategy:** Recall that inadequate nutrition is manifested by muscle weakness, weight loss, decreased cognition, poor wound healing, and increased risk of infection. **Reference:** Berman, A. J., & Snyder, S. (2011). *Kozier and Erb's fundamentals of nursing: Concepts, process, and practice* (9th ed.). Upper Saddle River, NJ: Prentice Hall, p. 929.

8 **Answer: 4** **Rationale:** A serum potassium level of 2.4 mEq/L is indicative of potassium depletion, which occurs in severe cases of malnutrition. The blood urea nitrogen (BUN), urinary creatinine, and albumin levels are within normal limits. **Cognitive Level:** Analyzing **Client Need:** Reduction of Risk Potential **Integrated Process:** Nursing Process: Evaluation **Content Area:** Fundamentals **Strategy:** Use knowledge of normal laboratory test results to make a selection. Recall that laboratory studies can predict potential or actual nutritional deficits, but it is important not to draw a conclusion based on a single laboratory value. The potassium depletion revealed in this client's laboratory value is an indication

ANSWERS & RATIONALES

of malnutrition; because of the impact of this critical finding, immediate intervention is required. **Reference:** Kee, J. L. (2009). *Handbook of laboratory and diagnostic tests* (6th ed.). Upper Saddle River, NJ: Prentice Hall, pp. 17, 85, 138, 322.

9 **Answer: 1** **Rationale:** Symptoms of an infection and ways to prevent one are crucial for a client to understand. Performance of independent perineal care and disposal of urinary output are not essential in preventing urinary tract infections. Tub baths are to be avoided, especially for females, as tub baths may increase the possibility of developing lower tract infections. **Cognitive Level:** Applying **Client Need:** Physiological Adaptation **Integrated Process:** Teaching and Learning **Content Area:** Fundamentals **Strategy:** An important test-taking concept is to remember that the option that includes one or more of the other options is often the correct answer. When evaluating the effectiveness of client teaching, expect the client to identify appropriate preventive measures. **Reference:**

Berman, A. J., & Snyder, S. (2011). *Kozier and Erb's fundamentals of nursing: Concepts, process, and practice* (9th ed.). Upper Saddle River, NJ: Prentice Hall, p. 1309.

10 **Answer: 2** **Rationale:** Cheese, bananas, rice, tapioca, and yogurt thicken stool. Asparagus, beans, eggs, fish, and onions increase stool odor. Fried foods, highly spiced foods, raw fruits and vegetables, carbonated drinks, fruit juices, oily foods, and pureed foods can loosen the stool and increase intestinal motility. **Cognitive Level:** Applying **Client Need:** Basic Care and Comfort **Integrated Process:** Teaching and Learning **Content Area:** Fundamentals **Strategy:** To answer this question correctly, it is necessary to learn which foods loosen the stool and which foods thicken it. Memorize common foods and use the process of elimination to answer the question. **Reference:** Berman, A. J., & Snyder, S. (2011). *Kozier and Erb's fundamentals of nursing: Concepts, process, and practice* (9th ed.). Upper Saddle River, NJ: Prentice Hall, p. 1357.

References

Ball, J. W., Bindler, R. C., & Cowen, K. (2010). *Child health nursing: Partnering with children and families* (2nd ed.). Upper Saddle River, NJ: Pearson Education.

Berman, A. J., Snyder, S., & McKinney, D. S. (2011). *Nursing basics for clinical practice.* Upper Saddle River, NJ: Pearson Education.

Berman, A., & Snyder, S. J. (2012). *Kozier & Erb's fundamentals of nursing: Concepts, process, and practice* (9th ed.). Upper Saddle River, NJ: Pearson Education.

Berman, A. J., & Snyder, S. (2012). *Skills in clinical nursing* (7th ed.). Upper Saddle River, NJ: Pearson Education.

Kee, J. L. (2010). *Laboratory and diagnostic tests* (8th ed.). Upper Saddle River, NJ: Pearson Education.

LeMone, P., Burke, K. M., & Bauldoff, G. (2011). *Medical-surgical nursing: Critical thinking in patient care* (5th ed.). Upper Saddle River, NJ: Pearson Education.

Tucker, S. (2011). *Nutrition and diet therapy for nurses.* Upper Saddle River, NJ: Pearson Education.

Meeting Needs of Clients With Pain

8

Chapter Outline

Introduction
Neurophysiological
   Mechanisms of Pain
Theories of Pain
Types of Pain

Barriers to Pain Relief
Pain Assessment
Pharmacologic Therapies for
   Pain Control

Nonpharmacologic Techniques
   for Promoting Comfort
Common Nursing Diagnoses
   for Clients With Pain

Objectives

➤ Define the concept of pain.
➤ Explain various theories of pain.
➤ Identify barriers to adequate pain relief.
➤ List components of a thorough pain assessment.
➤ Compare pharmacologic and nonpharmacologic therapies for
  managing pain and discomfort.
➤ Identify common nursing diagnoses associated with pain.

NCLEX-RN® Test Prep

Use the accompanying online resource,
NursingReviewsandRationales, to test
yourself with hundreds of NCLEX®-style
practice questions.

Review at a Glance

addiction compulsive use of a substance despite negative consequences, such as health threats or legal problems

agonist a substance that when combined with the receptor produces the drug effect or desired effect

antagonist a substance that blocks or reverses the effects of the agonist (e.g., morphine) by occupying the receptor site without producing the drug effect

bradykinin amino acid that appears to be most potent pain-producing chemical

breakthrough pain additional pain that is of rapid onset and greater intensity than baseline pain

ceiling doses doses beyond which additional drug amounts do not produce additional relief

drug tolerance process by which body requires a progressively larger amount of a drug to achieve same results

endorphins naturally occurring peptides present in neurons of brain, spinal cord, and gastrointestinal tract that bind with opiate receptors on neurons to inhibit pain impulse transmission

equianalgesia equivalent analgesia

nociceptor nerve receptors for pain

non-nociceptor nerve fibers that do not usually transmit pain

opioid morphine-like compound that produces systemic effects, including pain relief and sedation

pain tolerance amount of pain or discomfort that a person is able or willing to endure; varies from person to person

patient-controlled analgesia (PCA) self-administration of intravenous analgesics by a client instructed about the procedure

physical drug dependence biologic need for a substance; if substance is not supplied, physiological withdrawal symptoms occur

prostaglandins chemical substances that increase sensitivity of pain receptors by enhancing pain-provoking effect of bradykinin

referred pain pain that is perceived in an area distant from site of stimulus

PRETEST

1 A 30-year-old client arrives at the clinic for a diagnostic work-up related to chronic right hip pain. What should the nurse include when teaching the client about chronic pain? Select all that apply.

1. It is an unusual occurrence for younger adults.
2. It lasts longer than 6 months in duration.
3. It can be difficult to treat effectively.
4. It is often associated with nerve damage.
5. It involves the parasympathetic nervous system.

2 Which technique is the most effective method for the nurse to use to validate an alert client's level of pain?

1. Ask client to use a pain scale.
2. Note physiological responses to pain.
3. Determine degree of anxiety associated with pain.
4. Observe and document client's facial expressions.

3 A client who is experiencing pain is receiving an opioid analgesic and a nonsteroidal anti-inflammatory drug (NSAID), which are given together for pain relief. Which statement made by the nurse best explains the purpose for the medication prescription?

1. "The NSAID will decrease the likelihood of respiratory depression caused by the opioid."
2. "The NSAID targets muscle pain while the opioid relieves central nervous system irritation."
3. "Giving the medications together reduces the need for additional pain medication during the night-time hours."
4. "Giving the medications together will provide better relief of pain while decreasing the amount of opioid medication required."

4 A client with chronic back pain is using transcutaneous electrical nerve stimulation (TENS). The nurse is planning client teaching regarding the therapy. What information is most appropriate for the nurse to provide for the client?

1. The TENS unit stimulates nerves and blocks the transmission of pain sensations.
2. An electrical current from the TENS unit alters cell function and stops pain.
3. The primary function of the TENS unit is to create a distraction to sensations of pain.
4. The TENS unit will decrease the amount of tissue damage associated with pain.

5 A client is placed on a patient-controlled analgesia (PCA) pump with an opioid medication following total hip replacement surgery. After the client has self-administered the initial dose of the prescribed medication, what is the nurse's highest priority?

1. Allow client to rest uninterrupted for several hours.
2. Assess the client's level of sedation.
3. Record amount of medication the client received.
4. Monitor the client for respiratory arrest.

6 A client has had chest surgery and is using patient-controlled analgesia (PCA) with morphine to manage the pain. What observation by the nurse would be considered most important for prompting the nurse to intervene?

1. Respiratory rate 24 breaths per minute
2. Respiratory rate 8 breaths per minute
3. Sleeping but arousable
4. Comfortable when reading a book but uncomfortable when ambulating to restroom

7 An adult client is receiving medication through an epidural catheter for pain resulting from metastatic cancer. The nurse should perform which essential nursing actions related to the epidural catheter in order to provide safe care to this client? Select all that apply.

1. Assist client to change position every 2 hours.
2. Aspirate catheter prior to administration of medication.
3. Label the tubing, infusion bag, and infusion pump.
4. Inspect catheter insertion site every hour.
5. Avoid use of alcohol during catheter and insertion site care.

8 A client has approached the nurse at a pain management clinic and relates an interest in trying biofeedback for pain relief. Which statement indicates to the nurse that the client understands this treatment?

1. "I have spent a lot of money on medication and look forward to a treatment that will not cost me anything."
2. "I am so tired of focusing on my pain. This treatment will allow me to concentrate on something else."
3. "I enjoy being around other people and feel certain a support group will be beneficial to my pain relief."
4. "I want to try to control how blood flows to different parts of my body in order to make some progress."

9 A male client has undergone bowel resection surgery and is given an oral analgesic for reported incision pain; he reports that the analgesic has provided an acceptable degree of relief. The client's wife states, "I had a similar procedure a few years ago. I believe he needs a stronger medicine this soon after surgery." Which statement is the nurse's best reply to this concern?

1. "He has intravenous medication ordered, too. I'll use that next time."
2. "The oral route is the preferred way for giving medications."
3. "A stronger analgesic may delay the return of his bowel functioning."
4. "I believe you are concerned for him, but it is your husband's perception of pain that I need to assess."

10 An older adult female client is admitted to the emergency department (ED) after falling on ice and sustaining a fractured hip. The client's daughter pulls the nurse aside and states, "Watch my mother carefully—she has an amazing tolerance for pain." Based on this information being accurate, the nurse will anticipate which client need? Select all that apply.

1. The client will be able to endure a great deal of pain.
2. The client will experience discomfort with the slightest movement.
3. The client will probably not experience significant pain.
4. The client will ask for pain medication more often than prescribed.
5. The client will not ask for pain medication and may need to be assessed more frequently for comfort.

➤ *See pages 209–211 for Answers and Rationales.*

I. INTRODUCTION

A. Definitions of pain
1. "Pain is an unpleasant sensory and emotional experience associated with actual or potential tissue damage, or described in terms of such damage" (American Pain Society [APS], 2003; Gordon, 2009); this definition clarifies the multiple dimensions of pain; pain is more than a change in the chemical and physiological functioning of nervous system; it also reflects a client's past pain experiences and the meaning of pain
2. "Pain is whatever the person says it is, experienced whenever they say they are experiencing it" (McCaffery, M. & Pasero, C. (1999). *Pain: Clinical manual* (2nd ed.). St. Louis, MO: Mosby.); this definition describes the subjectivity of pain; nurses cannot know when another is experiencing pain unless it is communicated; self-report is the only valid measure of pain

B. The Joint Commission (formerly known as JCAHO) Standards
1. Clients have a right to pain assessment
   a. Facility must provide pain assessment tools
   b. If a facility cannot treat a client for pain, such as providing a PCA pump, client must be referred to a facility that can
2. Clients must be treated for pain and involved in their own pain management
3. Discharge planning and teaching must include pain management strategies

C. At end of life, many clients cannot communicate pain because of delirium, dementia, aphasia, motor weakness, language barriers, and other factors; if a client has any potential physical reason for discomfort, the nurse should consider the client to have pain until proven otherwise

II. NEUROPHYSIOLOGICAL MECHANISMS OF PAIN

A. Stimuli

1. A **nociceptor** is a nerve receptor responsible for pain sensation; such receptors are located at ends of small afferent neurons and are woven throughout all body tissues except brain; they are especially numerous in skin and muscle; a **non-nociceptor** is a nerve fiber that does not usually transmit pain

2. Pain occurs when nociceptors are stimulated by a variety of factors (see Table 8-1)

3. Intensity and duration of stimuli determine the sensation; long-lasting, intense stimulation results in greater pain than brief, mild stimulation

4. Nociceptors are stimulated either by direct damage to cells or local release of biochemicals secondary to cell injury

5. Biochemical sources

   a. **Bradykinin**: an amino acid, appears to be the most potent pain-producing chemical

   b. **Prostaglandins**: chemical substances that increase sensitivity of pain receptors by enhancing the pain-provoking effect of bradykinin

   c. Histamine

   d. Hydrogen ions

   e. Potassium ions

B. Pain pathway (see Figure 8-1)

1. Pain is perceived by nociceptors in periphery of body (e.g., skin); transmitted though small afferent A-delta and C nerve fibers to spinal cord

   a. A-delta fibers are myelinated and transmit impulses rapidly producing sharp, acute pain sensations (*Learning Hint*: Afferent *A-d*elta nerve fibers carry pain *Away* from *Distant* injury to spinal cord and brain, and they are *A*cute)

   b. C fibers are not myelinated and transmit pain more slowly; impulses are from deeper structures such as muscle and viscera, and produce more aching, chronic pain sensations (*Learning Hint: C* nerve fibers carry pain from *C*ore or *C*enter of body to spinal cord and brain, and they are *C*hronic)

Table 8-1	Examples of Painful Stimuli
Causative Factor	**Example**
Microorganisms (e.g., virus, bacteria)	Pneumonia
Inflammation	Arthritis
Impaired blood flow	Angina
Invasive tumor	Adenocarcinoma
Radiation	Treatment for cancer
Heat	Sunburn
Electricity	Electrical burn
Obstruction	Gallstone
Spasm	Muscle cramp
Compression	Carpal tunnel syndrome
Decreased movement	Skeletal traction
Stretching/straining	Sprained ligament
Fractures	Any bone
Swelling	Cellulitis
Chemicals	Skin rash

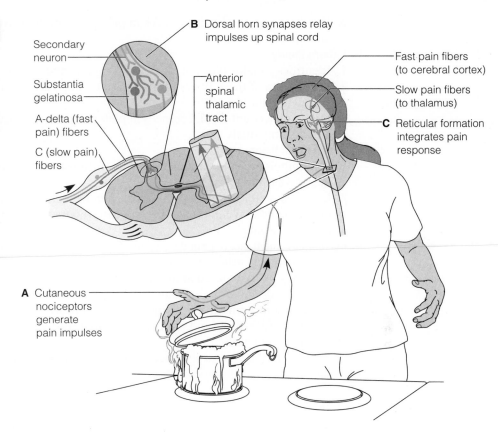

Figure 8-1

A. Cutaneous nociceptors generate pain impulses that pass via A-delta and C fibers to spinal cord's dorsal horn, B. Secondary neurons in dorsal horn pass impulses across spinal cord to anterior spinothalamic tract, C. Slow pain impulses ascend to the thalamus, while fast pain impulses ascend to the cerebral cortex. The reticular formation in the brainstem integrates the emotional, cognitive, and autonomic responses to pain.

Practice to Pass

What are 5 distinct sources of pain stimuli?

2. Secondary neurons transmit impulses from afferent neurons through dorsal horn of spinal cord; a synapse in substantia gelatinosa occurs; impulses cross over to anterior and lateral spinothalamic tracts
3. Impulses ascend anterior and lateral spinothalamic tracts and pass through medulla and midbrain to thalamus
4. Pain impulses are perceived, interpreted, and a response is generated in thalamus and cerebral cortex

C. Inhibitory mechanisms
1. Efferent fibers run from reticular formation and mid-brain to substantia gelatinosa in dorsal horns of spinal column; along these fibers, pain transmission may be inhibited, although exact process of this mechanism is not understood (*Learning Hint: E*fferent nerve fibers *E*xit brain and carry pain sensation back to involved body area.)
2. **Endorphins** (endogenous morphines) are natural occurring peptides present in neurons of brain, spinal cord, and gastrointestinal (GI) tract; they work by binding with opiate receptors on neurons to inhibit pain impulse transmission
   a. They are released in brain in response to afferent noxious stimuli
   b. They are released in spinal cord in response to efferent impulses

III. THEORIES OF PAIN

A. Specificity theory
1. Proposes that body's neurons and pathways for pain transmission are specific, similar to other senses like taste
2. Free nerve endings in skin act as pain receptors, accept input, and transmit impulses along highly specific nerve fibers

      3. Does not account for differences in pain perception or psychological variables among individuals

B. Pattern theory

      1. Identifies 2 major types of pain fibers; rapidly and slowly conducting

      2. Stimulation of these fibers forms a pattern; impulses ascend to brain to be interpreted as painful

      3. Does not account for differences in pain perception or psychological variables among individuals

C. Gate control theory

      1. Pain impulses can be modulated by a transmission blocking action within central nervous system

      2. Large-diameter cutaneous pain fibers can be stimulated (e.g., rubbing or scratching an area) and may inhibit smaller diameter fibers to prevent transmission of impulse ("close the gate")

D. Current developments in pain theory indicate that pain mechanisms and responses are far more complex than believed to be in the past

      1. Pain may be modulated at different points in nervous system

        a. First-order neurons at tissue level

        b. Second-order neurons in spinal cord that process nociceptive information

        c. Third-order tracts and pathways in spinal cord and brain that relay and process this information

      2. The role of the pain experience in developing new nociceptors and/or reducing the threshold of current nociceptors is also being investigated

IV. TYPES OF PAIN

A. Acute pain

      1. Usually temporary, sudden in onset, localized, lasts for less than 6 months; results from tissue injury associated with trauma, surgery, or inflammation

      2. Types of acute pain

        a. *Somatic*: arises from nerve receptors in skin or close to body's surface; may be sharp and well-localized or dull and diffuse; often accompanied by nausea and vomiting (N/V)

        b. *Visceral*: arises from body's organs; dull and poorly localized because of minimal nociceptors; accompanied by N/V, hypotension, and restlessness

        c. Referred pain: pain that is perceived in an area distant from site of stimuli (e.g., pain in a shoulder following abdominal laparoscopic procedure)

      3. Acute pain initiates "fight-or-flight" response of autonomic nervous system and is characterized by the signs and symptoms in Box 8-1

B. Chronic pain

      1. Prolonged, lasting longer than 6 months, often not attributed to a definite cause, often unresponsive to medical treatment

      2. Types of chronic pain

Box 8-1	Tachycardia
	Rapid, shallow respirations
Signs and Symptoms of Acute Pain	Increased blood pressure
	Sweating
	Pallor
	Dilated pupils
	Fear and anxiety

      a. Neuropathic: painful condition that results from damage to peripheral nerves caused by infection or disease; postherpetic neuralgia (shingles) is an example

      b. Phantom: pain syndrome that occurs following surgical or traumatic amputation of a limb

          1) Client is aware that the body part is missing

          2) Pain may result from stimulation of severed nerves at site of amputation

          3) Sensation may be experienced as an itching, tingling, pressure, or as stabbing or burning in nature

          4) It can be triggered by stressors (fatigue, illness, emotions, weather)

          5) This experience is limited for most clients because brain adapts to amputated limb; however, some clients experience abnormal sensation or pain over longer periods

          6) This type of pain requires treatment just as any other type of pain does

      c. Psychogenic: pain that is experienced in absence of a diagnosed physiological cause or event; client's emotional needs may prompt pain sensation

      d. Cancer pain: is associated with direct effects of disease or its treatment, or may be unrelated

          1) World Health Organization (WHO) recommends a 3-step ladder approach for management of chronic cancer pain (*Cancer Pain Relief* (2nd ed.). Reproduced by permission, The World Health Organization (WHO) Geneva, Switzerland., 2nd Edition, © 1996)

          2) WHO's 3-step ladder approach establishes a pharmacologic foundation that is applicable to management of other types of pain

      e. Other malignant pain: pain category associated with conditions such as HIV/AIDS or burns; cancer pain and malignant pain are treated more aggressively than non-malignant pain

  3. Depression is a common associated symptom for a client experiencing chronic pain; feelings of despair and hopelessness along with fatigue are expected findings

V. BARRIERS TO PAIN RELIEF

  A. Importance of discussing barriers

    1. Identify where obstacles exist; these barriers are prevalent throughout health care; nurses can work to overcome barriers through education, quality improvement efforts, and involvement in professional groups that advocate for those in pain

    2. Recognize when and what client teaching is required; clients have many of the same myths and attitudes that plague health care professionals; nurses empower clients through education

  B. Specific barriers

    1. Barriers to pain relief can be related to health care professionals, health care system, and clients (see Box 8-2)

    2. Client education

      a. Nurses can reassure clients that pain control is every client's right, health professionals rely on client to report pain, and that good pain management will improve quality of life

      b. Proactive education of clients and family or support persons is necessary, including information about addiction, drug tolerance, and physiological dependence

      c. Clients may use such terms as "hooked" when referring to **addiction** (compulsive use of a substance despite negative consequences, such as health threats or legal problems)

      d. Clients may express anxiety about becoming "immune" to a medication when discussing **drug tolerance** (process by which body requires a progressively greater amount of a drug to achieve same results)

Practice to Pass

What are the psychological symptoms generally associated with acute and chronic pain?

Practice to Pass

What are common barriers that prevent nurses from providing adequate pain relief measures to clients experiencing pain?

Box 8-2	**Barriers Related to Health Care Professionals**

Barriers to Pain Relief

Barriers Related to Health Care Professionals
- Inadequate or inaccurate information about pain management
- Inadequate or suboptimal pain assessment techniques
- Concern about overuse of controlled substances and subsequent client addiction
- Concern about excessive adverse effects
- Concern about clients developing tolerance to analgesics

Barriers Related to Health Care System
- Low priority given to pain treatment in relation to other client needs
- Inadequate reimbursement for other or costly pain management therapies
- Restrictive regulation of controlled substances
- Less than optimal availability or access to treatment; possible inadequate opioid availability in inner-city pharmacies or rural areas; nurses should work to ensure that necessary medications are available, regardless of environment

Barriers Related to Clients
- Reluctance to report pain or to take pain medications
- Fear that pain indicates the disease process is progressing
- Concern about being thought about as a "complainer"
- Cultural and ethnic background may influence client reaction to and expression of pain and can affect level of pain client is willing to tolerate
- Reluctance to take pain medications for a variety of reasons
- Concern about adverse drug effects
- Concern about developing tolerance or addiction to pain medications
- Cost; note that many pharmaceutical companies have programs that provide medications at reduced or no cost to clients with financial need

    e. Clients may worry about developing a **physical drug dependence** (a biologic need for a substance; if substance is not supplied, physiological withdrawal symptoms occur)
    f. Give clients or caregivers permission to discuss concerns and fears

VI. PAIN ASSESSMENT

A. Tools and instruments used

1. Various pain assessment tools are available to use, which provide the client and nurse with an easy method to quantify pain (see Figure 8-2 for samples of visual analog scales)
2. A verbal report using an intensity scale is a fast, easy, and reliable method that allows client to state pain intensity and, in turn, promotes consistent communication among nurse, client, and other health care professionals about client's pain status; the 2 most common scales used are "0 to 5" or "0 to 10," with 0 specifying no pain and highest number specifying worst pain
3. A visual analog scale is a horizontal pain-intensity scale with word modifiers at both ends of the scale, such as "no pain" at one end and "worst pain" at the other; clients are asked to point or mark along the line to convey degree of pain being experienced
4. A graphic rating scale is similar to a visual analog scale but adds a numerical scale with word modifiers; usually the numbers "0 to 10" are added to scale
5. Children, clients who do not speak English, and clients with communication impairments may have difficulty using a numerical pain intensity scale; alternative pain scales using pictures may be used for these clients and for children as young as 3 years old

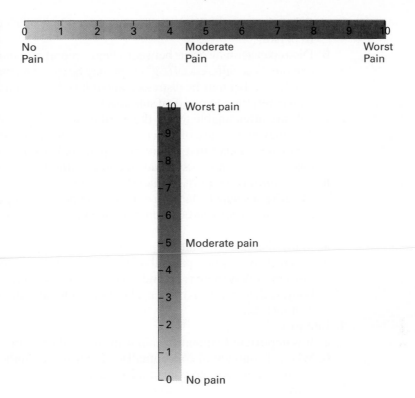

Figure 8-2

Numerical rating scale for pain assessment. A numerical rating scale for pain perception may be used verbally by asking the client to rate pain from 0 to 10 or to use a visually presented scale with both words and numbers along a vertical or horizontal line as shown here. For intensity, 0 represents no pain and the highest number represents the worst pain.

6. Physiological indicators of pain may be the only means a nurse can use to assess pain in a noncommunicating client; facial and vocal expressions may be initial manifestations of pain; expressions may include rapid eye blinking, biting of lip, moaning, crying, screaming, either closed or clenched eyes, or stiff unmoving body position

B. **PQRST assessment for pain perception**
1. This method is especially helpful when approaching a new pain problem; this method can be used to assess any symptom, not only pain
2. P = What *precipitated* the pain? Has anything *palliated* the pain? What is the *pattern* of the pain?
3. Q = What are the *quality* and *quantity* of the pain? Is it sharp, stabbing, aching, burning, stinging, deep, crushing, viselike, or gnawing?
4. R = What is the *region* of the pain? Does the pain *radiate* to other areas of the body? Does anything *relieve* or *reduce* the pain?
5. S = What is the *severity* (or intensity) of the pain?
6. T = What is the *timing* of the pain? When does it begin, how long does it last, and how is it related to other events in the client's life?

C. **COLDERR assessment for pain**
1. **C =** character of the pain
2. **O =** onset of the pain
3. **L =** location of the pain
4. **D =** duration of pain, whether constant versus intermittent
5. **E =** exacerbating factors that makes the pain worse
6. **RR =** relief of pain (what makes it better) and radiation of the pain?

D. **Pain history**
1. Involve family or caregiver when obtaining a pain history, keeping in mind client's self-report is the most valid measure of pain

a. **Pain tolerance** (ability or willingness to endure pain) varies from person to person

b. Discrepancies may occur between client's report and those of other family members; explore these differences (e.g., client may be stoic and may underreport pain or family member may be distressed about loved one's illness and overestimate client's pain in response to personal suffering)

2. People are often unable to use the word *pain*
   a. This may be because of stoicism, concern about appearing whining or a complainer, belief that admitting to pain makes it real (implying that underlying disease is real and possibly advancing), cultural biases, or other causes
   b. *Discomfort* is the most frequently used alternative
   c. Other terms may include *hurt* or *ache*; some terms suggest emotion, such as *distressing* or *horrible*; explore the meaning of pain for each client and family

3. Location
   a. Many clients have multiple pain sites
   b. When clients report "pain all over," this generally refers to total pain or existential distress (unless there is an underlying physiological reason for pain all over the body, such as myalgias); assess client's emotional state for depression, fear, anxiety, or hopelessness

4. Intensity
   a. It is important to quantify pain using a standard pain intensity scale
   b. When clients cannot conceptualize pain using a number, simple word categories can be useful (e.g., no pain, mild, moderate, severe)

5. Quality
   a. Nociceptive pains are usually related to damage to bones, soft tissues, or internal organs; nociceptive pain includes somatic and visceral pains
      1) Somatic pain is aching, throbbing pain; arthritis is an example of somatic pain
      2) Visceral pain is squeezing, cramping pain such as pain associated with ulcerative colitis
   b. Neuropathic pain is generally caused by damage to nervous system; clients describe pain as burning, tingling, electrical, or shooting; examples include diabetic neuropathy or postherpetic neuropathy (shingles)

6. Pattern
   a. Pain may be always present for a client; this is often termed baseline pain
   b. Additional pain may occur intermittently that is of rapid onset and greater intensity than baseline pain, known as **breakthrough pain**
   c. People at end-of-life often have both types of pain
   d. Aggravating and alleviating factors: those factors that make pain better or worse; these assessments can provide information about etiology of pain as well as potential treatments; for example, if massage makes pain better, it probably has a musculoskeletal origin, rather than neuropathic
   e. Medication history: it is imperative to understand which drugs the client has already tried, whether they were effective, and what adverse effects resulted; question clients regarding what has been prescribed and what is actually being used for pain control (and reasons for any disparity); also ask clients about use of over-the-counter drugs, recreational drugs, and herbal products
   f. Meaning of pain: the meaning of a client's pain can profoundly affect pain perception; many see pain as punishment for something done (or left undone) earlier in life
   g Cultural beliefs regarding meaning of pain should be examined
   h. Client's expectations for pain relief

Practice to Pass

What elements should the nurse include when taking a pain history from a client who presents with end-stage cancer?

E. Physical examination

1. Observe for nonverbal cues that might suggest pain, including withdrawal, fatigue, grimaces, moans, irritability, particularly in a client unable to verbalize pain
2. Examine sites of pain for trauma, skin breakdown, changes in bony structures, etc.
3. Palpate the areas for tenderness
4. Auscultate for abnormal breath sounds that could signal pneumonia (e.g., crackles, rhonchi, decreased breath sounds) or abnormal bowel sounds that could signal bowel obstruction (e.g., hyperactive bowel sounds) or other syndromes
5. Percuss the area for fluid accumulation or gas (especially for abdominal pain to rule out obstruction, ascites, etc.)
6. Conduct a neurologic examination to evaluate sensory and/or motor loss, as well as changes in reflexes
7. Information derived from physical examination contributes to information obtained during history to determine underlying cause of pain; this can lead to potential treatment decisions (e.g., laxatives or softeners if client is constipated, antibiotics if there is an underlying infection, or radiotherapy for bone metastasis)

F. Reassessment

1. It is critical to reassess pain regularly, with any changes in pain, or with changes in analgesic regimen; the regularity of pain assessment depends on the degree to which a client's condition or pain state is changing; more rapidly progressive disease demands more frequent assessment
2. Pain relief should be assessed using same rating scale (such as 0 to 10) that was used to determine intensity of pain prior to nursing intervention; using same scale provides more objective data about degree of relief the client obtained
3. Pain relief can be also assessed using a 0 to 100% scale, with 0 meaning no relief and 100% meaning complete relief; when clients are unable to use this scale, options include "no relief," "a little relief," "moderate relief," or "complete/total relief"
4. When attempting to determine success of a new analgesic the client may be asked, "After taking that pill (or liquid, injection, etc.), how much pain relief did it provide?"; if client is able to articulate amount of relief, then ask, "How long did you get relief?" as this provides evidence about duration of effect
5. Pain must be made visible (such as labeling it the fifth vital sign); adding pain intensity scores to same part of health record where temperature, pulse, and other vital signs are recorded has been shown to enhance pain relief efforts and effectiveness
6. A useful strategy for reassessment is asking clients or caregivers to keep a daily pain diary; nurses can teach a client or family members to record daily pain responses (e.g., intensity scores, pain relief, times and doses of breakthrough pain medications given, additional comments about activities or other factors) to determine patterns of pain

G. Clients at risk for poor pain assessment and treatment

1. Children: may be too young to verbally express pain; health care workers may fear overmedicating them
2. Older adults: may have decreased perception of sensory stimuli and a higher pain threshold; chronic disease processes (e.g., diabetes or peripheral vascular disease) may interfere with normal nerve impulse transmission; may believe pain is a normal part of growing older and as a result, attempt to ignore or self-medicate
3. Cognitively impaired or unconscious clients
4. Non–English-speaking clients
5. Persons of different cultures from health care professionals
6. Persons with a history of substance use: reports of pain in persons with a current or past history of substance use may be disregarded or discounted as attempts to obtain additional medication

Practice to Pass

A client reports pain to the right lower quadrant of the abdomen described as "aching and throbbing" and rates it numerically as an 8 on a scale of 1 to 10. What type of pain is the client experiencing?

H. Communicating assessment findings
   1. Clear objective communication (both verbally and in writing) of pain assessment findings will ultimately improve pain management
   2. It is important to describe intensity of pain, functional limitations that result from pain (e.g., client cannot tolerate radiation therapy treatments), and response from current analgesic regimen (e.g., 50% relief, no adverse effects); this gives other health care professionals essential data when modifying the treatment plan; it also allows nurse to serve as a client advocate

VII. PHARMACOLOGICTHERAPIES FOR PAIN CONTROL

A. Nonopioids
   1. Acetaminophen (Tylenol)
      a. Has analgesic and antipyretic properties

      b. Adverse effects: can cause liver dysfunction in routine doses higher than 4,000 mg/day in clients with normal liver function; acetaminophen is present in many analgesic products and may be combined with an opioid, so it is important to track total acetaminophen dosage daily
   2. Nonsteroidal anti-inflammatory drugs (NSAIDs) have anti-inflammatory, analgesic, and antipyretic effects
      a. Examples: salicylate (aspirin), ibuprofen (Motrin), naproxen (Naprosyn); these block cyclooxygenase-1 (COX-1)
      b. Mechanism of action: inhibit prostaglandins by blocking cyclooxygenase; prostaglandins are rich in periosteum of bone and in uterus, as well as other locations; thus, NSAIDs are useful in relieving bone pain and dysmenorrhea; they are also useful in many other pain syndromes
      c. A cyclooxygenase-2 (COX-2) inhibitor is celecoxib (Celebrex), which selectively blocks the COX-2 enzymatic pathway; there appears to be less risk of GI bleeding, renal dysfunction, and generalized bleeding with the continuous or prolonged use of the COX-2 NSAID
      d. Unlike opioids, NSAIDs have a ceiling effect; increasing the dose beyond a certain point will not increase analgesia and will only increase the risk of adverse effects
      e. Adverse effects
         1) COX-1 NSAIDs produce significant gastric toxicity through local effects and systemic effects; locally, they migrate through gastric mucus and into epithelial cells that line the stomach; once in these cells, they convert to their ionized form, causing hydrogen ions to be trapped within cells
         2) Systemic effects of COX-1 NSAIDs are accomplished largely by inhibiting prostaglandin synthesis, which results in decreased epithelial mucus to coat the stomach, decreased mucosal blood flow, and decreased epithelial proliferation; a reduction in mucus exposes gastroduodenal mucosal lining to injury by substances within the gut (such as acid, pepsin, and bile salts)
         3) As a result of these local and systemic factors, GI bleeding is common in COX-1 NSAIDs especially in older adults, in persons at risk for ulceration, and when used in combination with other drugs such as corticosteroids
         4) Platelet aggregation is inhibited by NSAIDs, thus bleeding is a potential risk; this effect is reversible by stopping NSAID use; however, aspirin produces an irreversible effect on platelets so should be discontinued at least 7 days prior to an invasive procedure
         5) Renal dysfunction can occur because of NSAIDs, especially when clients are dehydrated; this effect is caused by inhibition of renal vasoactive prostaglandin, altering the blood flow within arterioles of kidneys; urine output diminishes; this effect is reversible by stopping the NSAID

6) The COX-2 NSAID (celecoxib) may cause indigestion, diarrhea, and stomach pain, and could lead to ulcers and GI bleeding

7) In April 2005, the FDA required that all NSAIDs include in their safety information that they potentially increase the risk of heart attack, stroke, and stomach problems

B. Opioids and adjuvant medications

1. Opioids are morphine-like compounds that produce systemic effects including pain relief and sedation

2. They can be categorized as **agonist** (a substance that, when combined with the opioid receptor [mu, kappa, or sigma], produces the drug effect or desired effect) or as a partial agonist (agonist-antagonist), which exerts effects on some types of receptors but displaces opioids from other types of receptors

3. Use of drugs that are partial agonists (which are more likely to be used to treat chronic pain or in previous opioid abusers) is associated with less risk of dependency

4. Selected examples of opioids

a. Codeine (generic)

b. Morphine (MS Contin, Oramorph, Kadian, Roxanol)

c. Hydrocodone (Vicodin/Lortab)

d. Hydromorphone (Dilaudid)

e. Fentanyl (Duragesic)

f. Methadone (Dolophine)

g Oxycodone (OxyContin, Roxicodone, OxyFAST)

h. Meperidine (Demerol)

5. Mechanism of action: opioids block release of neurotransmitters involved in the processing of pain

6. Adverse effects

a. Allergic reactions to opioids are extremely rare; clients may state there is an allergy, especially if N/V occur when given a particular opioid; this is an opportunity to educate clients regarding allergic responses versus adverse effects; the only absolute contraindication to the use of an opioid is a history of a hypersensitivity reaction (e.g., wheezing, edema)

b. Respiratory depression is greatly feared, yet rare; it is almost always preceded by sedation, thus, in most cases, the health care professional has adequate warning

c. If a client has true opioid-induced respiratory depression, it can be reversed parenterally using naloxone (Narcan), which is classified as an opioid **antagonist** (substance that blocks or reverses effects of an agonist [e.g., morphine] by occupying receptor sites without producing drug effects); naltrexone (Vivitrol) is a different antagonist that is used orally as adjunct treatment for detoxifying opioid-dependent clients

d. Naloxone should not be given to clients with known or suspected dependency on opioids (either prescribed or procured as "street drugs") because naloxone may precipitate severe withdrawal

e. Constipation is a significant effect of opioid therapy, often leading to discontinuation or reduction in opioid dose if not well-managed

1) Opioids produce many effects that lead to constipation, such as reduced peristalsis and increased resorption of water from fecal contents that result in slow-moving, dry fecal material

2) Constipation can lead to hemorrhoids or anal fissures that are painful and potential sites for infection

3) Increased fluids, addition of fiber to diet, activity or exercise, and use of a laxative or stool softener combination help counteract these effects

f. Urinary retention is more common in opioid-naive clients and is most common with spinal delivery of medications (e.g., epidural or intrathecal); tolerance to this effect usually occurs within a few days; in the meantime a client may need an indwelling urinary catheter or intermittent bladder catheterization every 6 to 8 hours prn

g. Nausea and vomiting can occur; treatment includes antiemetics or changing to a different opioid; this side effect may diminish on its own after some days of opioid therapy

h. Pruritis occurs more commonly with spinal delivery of opioids; antihistamines may help, but sedation may occur with use of these drugs; cool packs or lotions as well as diversional activities may help; tolerance to this effect will also develop over time

i. Addiction is a primary, chronic, neurobiologic disease with genetic, psychosocial, and environmental factors influencing its development and manifestations; it is characterized by behaviors that include one or more of the following: impaired control over drug use, compulsive use, continued use despite harm, and craving

j. Mixed agonist-antagonists: selected examples of medications in this class include butorphanol (Stadol), nalbuphine (Nubain), and pentazocine (Talwin)
   1) Adverse effects: the mixed agonist-antagonists are not recommended in the treatment of chronic pain; **ceiling doses** (when increases beyond a certain dose no longer produce increased relief) create a high rate of psychotomimetic effects (e.g., hallucinations and disorientation), and can produce the abstinence or withdrawal syndrome if clients are also taking pure agonist opioids
   2) Withdrawal symptoms from opioids include agitation, abdominal cramping, diarrhea, runny nose, tearing, yawning, and "goose bumps"; withdrawal from meperidine can also lead to seizures

k. Adjuvant analgesics
   1) Tricyclic antidepressants as analgesics: the mechanism of analgesic effect appears to be related to inhibition of norepinephrine and serotonin; these agents are useful when treating neuropathic pain states; amitriptyline (Amitril) and nortriptyline (Pamelor) produce more sedation and other adverse effects than desipramine (Norpramin), therefore, the first 2 should be given at bedtime and the latter given in the morning
   2) Antiepileptics as analgesics: older antiepileptics such as carbamazepine (Tegretol) block sodium channels, which prevents conduction of pain through sensory neurons; as a result, these compounds are believed to be useful in treating neuropathic pain, especially pain described as "shooting"
   3) Local anesthetics: work in a similar manner to older antiepileptics by inhibiting movement of sodium ions across sensory nerve membrane to prevent transmission of pain along the neuron
      a) Useful in relieving neuropathic pain, local anesthetics can be given intravenously (e.g., lidocaine)
      b) Epidural or intrathecal: bupivacaine (Marcaine)
      c) Topical where skin is intact (Emla cream and Lidoderm)
   4) Corticosteroids: inhibit prostaglandin synthesis and reduce edema surrounding many types of tissues; are useful in treating neuropathic pain, bone pain, and visceral pain; dexamethasone (Decadron) produces the least amount of mineralocorticoid effect and is often preferred for use in end-of-life care
   5) Baclofen (Lioresal): a skeletal muscle relaxant useful in relieving spasm-associated pain; doses are titrated gradually based upon client response and adverse effects; weakness and confusion occur with higher doses

6) Capsaicin (Zostrix): derived from chili peppers and believed to relieve pain by releasing, then depleting, supplies of substance P, a protein released from nerve endings of pain neurons that is involved in pain transmission; when capsaicin is first administered, it causes pain (caused by substance P release), and then it may relieve pain (caused by substance P depletion)

    a) Capsaicin has been shown to be useful in treating peripheral pain syndromes; examples include pain associated with postmastectomy syndrome, shingles, and postsurgical neuropathic pain in cancer; a sensation of burning is a common reason for discontinuing therapy

    b) Clients and caregivers should wash hands immediately after application of this topical medication to prevent burning on hands or inadvertently rubbing the eyes and creating severe ocular pain

l. Routes of administration

  1) Oral: tablets and liquid

    a) Immediate-release tablets or capsules

    b) Long-acting (sustained-release) tablets (e.g., MS Contin or OxyContin), capsules; "sprinkles" (currently only available in morphine preparation as Kadian); long-acting tablets allow longer periods of time between dosing (e.g., 8, 12, or 24 hours); also allow clients to obtain more consistent relief, which also provides uninterrupted sleep

    c) Sprinkles provide long-acting relief for clients who cannot swallow a tablet but can swallow small amounts of applesauce mixed with the drug

    d) There is a misconception that intravenous (IV), intramuscular (IM), or subcutaneous (subQ) delivery is stronger than oral administration; oral delivery can provide equivalent analgesia (known as **equianalgesia**), but because of first-pass metabolism, the dose must be increased when compared to IM, IV, or subQ routes; thus, 10 mg of morphine given IV, IM, or subQ is approximately equal to 30 mg of oral morphine

    e) Enteral feeding tubes can be used to administer oral medications when clients can no longer swallow; however, size of tube should be considered, especially when placing long-acting morphine "sprinkles," to avoid tube obstruction

  2) Mucosal

    a) Oral transmucosal fentanyl citrate (Actiq, Oralet) is composed of fentanyl placed on an applicator for clients to rub against oral mucosa to provide rapid drug absorption; therapeutic serum drug levels are achieved within 5 to 15 minutes of application

    b) Two examples of appropriate use of oral transmucosal fentanyl citrate might be for relief of breakthrough pain that is of rapid onset (i.e., when traditional breakthrough medications would lead to a delay in relief) or prior to a brief, but painful, dressing change

  3) Rectal (also stomal or vaginal)

    a) Thrombocytopenia or painful anorectal lesions preclude the use of these routes; additionally, delivering medications via these routes can be difficult for family members, especially if client is obtunded or unable to assist

    b) Long-acting opioid tablets have been placed rectally when clients are no longer able to swallow

    c) Because the vagina has no sphincter, a tampon covered with a condom or an inflated urinary catheter balloon may be used to prevent early discharge of drug

  4) Transdermal

    a) Currently, the only formulation for transdermal delivery is fentanyl; the patch is placed every 72 hours over nonhairy, nonedematous skin with good capillary blood flow (often over torso, shoulders, or upper arms)

        b) There is a delay in peak onset of approximately 17 hours after applying first patch

        c) The effects of cachexia and fever are believed to accelerate drug distribution; although the precise mechanisms are unknown, altered fat stores and increased capillary flow may lead to these changes

  5) Parenteral

        a) Intravenous (IV): useful when clients cannot swallow or when absorption through GI tract is altered

        b) Subcutaneous (subQ): boluses have a slower onset and lower peak effect when compared with IV boluses; subQ infusions may be run at up to 5 to 10 mL/hr, although 1 to 3 mL is ideal

        c) Intramuscular (IM): not recommended because of wide variability in absorption, potential delays in vascular uptake of drug, and pain with administration

  6) Nasal: currently, the only nasal preparation available is the mixed agonist-antagonist butorphanol (Stadol); this is not recommended for chronic pain management

  7) Spinal

        a) Epidural or intrathecal routes allow delivery of drugs, (most often used is Duramorph, a preservative-free morphine derivative) into epidural space via a catheter inserted by an anesthesiologist

        b) Benefits: produces effective analgesia without sensory, motor or sympathetic changes

        c) Disadvantages: epidural catheter's proximity to spinal nerves and canal, along with potential for catheter migration, make correct injection technique and close assessment imperative

        d) Side effects include: generalized pruritis, nausea, urinary retention, respiratory depression, and hypotension

        e) Strict asepsis is necessary when injecting the epidural catheter; initially aspirated gently; if blood or greater than 1 mL of clear fluid is aspirated, withhold injection and notify MD

        f) Opioid-related side effects are reversed with naloxone hydrochloride (Narcan)

  8) **Patient-controlled analgesia (PCA)**: self-administration of IV analgesics by a client who has been taught about the procedure

        a) A portable PCA pump-type device delivers a preset dosage of opioid IV; an adjustable lockout interval controls frequency of dose administration, preventing another one from being administered prematurely; a sample order might read: "Morphine 1 mg with a lock-out time of 6 minutes"

        b) Client pushes a button to activate the device; client should control administration of analgesic, not family, nursing staff, or any other well-intentioned individual

        c) Monitor client's sedation level, pain rating, and vital signs while using PCA; pump records settings and amount of drug delivered, as well as number of demands (for example, client may push button 10 times in a 1-minute period when in severe pain, however, will receive bolus only every 6 minutes using above order)

        d) Allows for less sedation during waking hours with smaller, frequent doses compared to oral or IM doses given every 3 to 4 hours

        e) Provide instruction about use of PCA preoperatively whenever possible; some clients fear being overdosed by pump and require reassurance; it is always important to reinforce postoperatively any instructions given before surgery for PCA to have greatest effect

C. Principles regarding the use of analgesics

1. WHO's 3-step analgesic ladder is a guide to selecting the initial analgesic choice and dosing; continued reassessment is needed to modify treatment plan based on client's response

   a. When clients present with mild pain (approximately 1 to 3 on a 0 to 10 scale) a nonopioid is prescribed, with an adjuvant drug if client has neuropathic pain

   b. If pain is moderate (4 to 6), prescriber should add an opioid in low doses; nonopioids and adjuvants may also be continued

   c. If pain is severe (7 to 10), prescriber should add higher dose(s) of opioid; nonopioids and adjuvants may be continued; if client presents with severe pain, prescriber should not start at bottom rung; but should begin at appropriate level for that client's pain

   d. One limitation of the ladder is a belief that weak opioids (e.g., codeine) must be used in step 2; actually smaller doses of strong opioids, such as morphine, are just as effective and preclude later switching between drugs

2. Prevent and treat adverse effects

   a. Anticipate, prevent, and treat predictable adverse effects

   b. Almost all clients prescribed an opioid will also require a laxative/stool softener combination; exceptions include clients with HIV-associated diarrhea, clients with pancreatic insufficiency associated with pancreatic cancers, and other clients with preexisting diarrhea

3. Properly use long-acting and breakthrough medications

   a. Begin with immediate-release formulations available to client as needed to relieve pain; once client has achieved pain relief for 24 to 48 hours, calculate the 24-hour dose of opioid and convert to long acting formulation; for example, a client who has been taking 60 mg of liquid morphine in a 24-hour period may be converted to:
      1) MS Contin 30 mg PO q12 hours
      2) Kadian 60 mg PO daily
      3) OxyContin 20 to 30 mg PO q12 hours
      4) Duragesic patch 25 mcg every 72 hours

   b. Sustained-release formulations and around-the-clock dosing should be used for continuous pain syndromes

   c. Immediate-release formulations should be made available for breakthrough pain; the dose of immediate-release drug is usually 10 to 20% of the total 24-hour dose of the routine opioid; therefore, if a 24-hour dose of MS Contin is 200 mg, a breakthrough dose should be 20 to 40 mg; start with lower dose and titrate as needed; an immediate-release drug can be repeated as often as every hour, since the peak effect of oral opioids is 1 hour

   d. If the client is receiving a continuous infusion of an opioid (either IV or subQ), breakthrough doses are calculated as 50 to 100% of the hourly rate; therefore, if client has a rate of 2 mg/hr of morphine, breakthrough dose should begin at 1 mg IV bolus with appropriate titration; peak effect of an IV bolus dose of most opioids occurs in 15 minutes; thus, if client is still in pain after that time, a bolus should be repeated

   e. Breakthrough pain can be incident-related (e.g., movement-induced), idiopathic (etiology unknown), or because of end-of-dose failure (increased pain prior to next scheduled dose)

   f. Titrate analgesics based upon client goals, requirements for supplemental analgesics, pain intensity, severity of undesirable or adverse drug effects, measures of functionality, sleep, emotional state, and client or caregiver reports of impact of pain on quality of life

4. Converting properly from one route or drug to another involves use of an equianalgesic chart (see Table 8-2 for example)

Practice to Pass

In addition to opioids, what other drug classifications can be used for pain management?

Table 8-2 **Opioid Equianalgesic Chart**

Drug	IM Route (mg)	PO Route (mg)	IM/PO Peak (hr)	IM/PO Duration (hr)	Comments
Morphine	10	30–60	½–1 IM 1 PO	Up to 7	Morphine 10 mg IM is the analgesic dose with which all other drugs in this table are compared; PO dose varies from 3–6 times the IM dose depending on drug used; also comes in suppository form, time-released oral form, and for spinal injection
Butorphanol (Stadol)	2	NA	½–1 IM	3–4 IM	Agonist-antagonist; can produce withdrawal from opioids, more likely to produce N/V; respiratory depression rare but severe and not easily reversed by naloxone (Narcan)
Codeine	130	200	½–1 IM 2 PO	4–6 IM 3–4 PO	More toxic in higher doses than morphine; causes more N/V and is extremely constipating; adding 650 mg of acetaminophen or aspirin will significantly increase analgesic effect
Fentanyl (Sublimaze)	0.05	NA	7–15 min IM	1–2 IM	Commonly used for anesthetic; IV substituted for high-dose morphine in terminally ill clients
Hydromorphone (Dilaudid)	1.5	7.5	½–1 IM ½–1½ PO	3 IM 3–4 PO	Shorter-acting than morphine; also available as rectal suppository or high-potency injection 10 mg/mL; may be used for PCA or epidural
Levorphanol (Levo-Dromoran)	2	4	1/4 – ½ IM 1 –1½ PO	6–8 IM 6–8 PO	Longer-acting than morphine when given in repeated, regular doses; good alternative to methadone; drug accumulates so analgesic effect may increase with repeated doses; subcutaneous route better than IM
Meperidine (Demerol)	75	300	1 IM/PO	2–4 IM/PO	Oral dose of 300 mg not recommended; shorter-acting than morphine; transformed to normeperidine, a toxic metabolite that stimulates the CNS and causes seizures; effects of normeperidine not reversed by naloxone
Methadone (Dolophine)	10	20	1–2 IM/PO	6–8 IM/PO/ Subcut 24–48 w/ chronic dosing	Long plasma half-life, so regular doses lead to accumulation of drug and increased analgesia; dosage must be carefully titrated over days to weeks; use with caution in older adults or with liver or kidney failure
Nalbuphine (Nubain)	10	NA	½ IV	3–6 IV/IM/ Subcut	Agonist-antagonist; similar to butorphanol; may cause withdrawal if used in clients receiving opioids; longer-acting and less likely to cause hypotension than morphine; less respiratory depression
Oxycodone	NA	30	½ –1 PO	4–5 PO	Faster onset and higher peak effect than most oral opioids; available as single agent and in combination with acetaminophen
Pentazocine (Talwin)	60	180	1 IM	3 IM	Agonist-antagonist; similar to butorphanol but much higher incidence of psychotomimetic effects; may cause withdrawal if used in clients receiving opioids
Propoxyphene (Darvon)	NA	500	2–3 PO	4–6 PO	Never give in 500 mg dose; may be used for mild to moderate pain; doses of 65–130 mg are usual

Source: Agency for Healthcare Research and Quality, U.S. Department of Health and Human Services.

VIII. NONPHARMACOLOGIC TECHNIQUES FOR PROMOTING COMFORT

A. Cutaneous stimulation

1. Touch: place hands on client's body or 1 inch above to realign energy; is thought to initiate gate closure to pain as well as communicate caring
2. Pressure: place hands firmly on or around area where client feels pain; can provide relief of discomfort, decrease bleeding, and prevent swelling
3. Massage: gently or briskly stimulate client's subcutaneous tissues by kneading, pulling or pressing with hands; thought to initiate gate closure; promotes relaxation and sedation
   a. Use warm lubricant, such as lotion
   b. Use long, smooth strokes to achieve relaxation; maintain continuous hand contact with skin
   c. Use rapid strokes, circular motions, and gentle squeezing of tissues to stimulate increase in client's level of alertness or stimulate circulation
4. Vibration: use an electrical or battery-operated vibrator to stimulate client's subcutaneous tissues; thought to initiate gate closure
5. Heat or cold applications: are better labeled as "warm" and "cool"
   a. Indications: either heat or cold may be used as preferred for muscle aches or spasms, joint pain, or itching; heat may be used for rectal pain, while cool applications may be used for headaches or surgical incisions
   b. Equipment: heat sources typically include warm moist compresses, heating pads or bottles, immersion in water, or use of plastic wraps (to retain body heat); cold sources include ice bags, gel packs, bags of frozen vegetables that are small and fairly smooth, plastic zip-lock bags with ice/water/slush (combination of one-third alcohol with two-thirds water, or soaked towels
   c. Cautionary notes
      1) Heat or cold therapy should not be continued if pain increases
      2) Use moderation with temperature (neither too hot nor too cold)
      3) Cover heat or cold source with a towel for insulation and to protect skin surfaces
      4) Moisture increases effect or intensity of heat or cold therapy
      5) Do not use heat on areas that are bleeding, have sustained recent injury, or that have menthol or oil on them
      6) Do not use cold on areas that have poor circulation; remove cold from an area if it becomes numb
   d. Apply heat or cold source for 10 to 20 minutes at a time, but it may be used for longer periods at client's discretion if source remains comfortable and does not cause skin irritation; do not use at temperatures less than 70°F or greater than 110°F
   e. If it is not possible to apply heat or cold therapy directly to a painful area, try placing it to same point on opposite side of body, or above or below the painful site

B. Transcutaneous electrical nerve stimulation (TENS)

1. A battery-operated unit with electrodes applied to skin to produce tingling, vibration, or buzzing sensation
2. Can be used for acute or chronic pain, but is most frequently used for chronic pain (such as with arthritis)
3. Based on gate control theory; thought to decrease pain through stimulation of nonpain receptors in same area as fibers that transmit pain
4. Client adjusts placement of electrodes, and timing and intensity of stimuli to obtain best pain relief
5. TENS is most effective in clients who understand and are motivated to learn to use device
6. A client may need help with electrode placement, so it is helpful and generally beneficial to include family or other support people in client teaching sessions
7. TENS units can be attached to battery packs so the unit is portable

C. Distraction

1. Client focuses on something other than pain to decrease number of painful stimuli being transmitted to brain
2. Examples include watching television, listening to music, visiting with friends or family, playing games
3. Stimulation of several senses (sight, sound, and touch) are generally more effective in reducing pain than a single sense

D. Relaxation

1. Involves learning activities or techniques that deeply relax body and mind; provides distraction, lessens effects of stress from pain, increases effectiveness of other pain relief measures, and increases perception of pain control
2. Diaphragmatic breathing can relax muscles, improve oxygen levels, and provide a feeling of release from tension
   a. Is more effective when client sits or lies down
   b. Client should have quiet environment, closed eyes
   c. Client should inhale and exhale slowly and regularly
3. Progressive muscle relaxation may be used alone or with deep breathing to manage pain
   a. Teach client to tighten one group of muscles, hold tension for a few seconds, then relax muscle group completely
   b. Client should repeat this action for all parts of body
   c. Audio tapes may be helpful to assist with relaxation process
4. Guided imagery: uses imaginative power of the mind with assistance of nurse to create a scene or sensory experience that relaxes muscles and moves client's focus away from pain experience
   a. Client must be able to concentrate, use imagination, and follow directions
   b. Facilitate this process by using a calm, soothing voice to reinforce pleasant places or situations imagined
   c. Audio tapes may be helpful to assist with imagery process
5. Meditation: is a process whereby client empties the mind of all sensory data and concentrates on a single object, word, or idea
   a. Produces a deeply relaxed state
   b. Oxygen consumption decreases, muscles relax, and endorphins are produced

E. Acupuncture

1. Ancient Chinese technique involving stimulation of certain points on body to enhance flow of vital energy (*chi*) along pathways called meridians
2. Points can be stimulated with needles, application of heat, massage, laser or electrical stimulation

F. Biofeedback

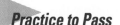

Practice to Pass

A client is interested in exploring nonpharmacologic methods of pain relief. What methods should the nurse discuss with the client?

1. Is an electronic method of measuring physiological responses with intent to condition or control these responses
2. Client's goal is to exercise voluntary control over sensations to promote relaxation, lessen anxiety, and decrease pain
3. It requires a trained facilitator to assist client and monitor physiological data such as skin temperature, brain waves, and muscle contractions
4. Client eventually learns to independently repeat actions to produce desired effect (e.g., slowing circulation to reduce heart rate and warmth of skin)

G. Nursing considerations for nonpharmaceutical pain relief techniques

1. Assess the following client variables that will affect method selected
   a. Concurrent use of analgesics (should complement, not replace their use)
   b. Attitude toward nonpharmaceutical methods in general or toward method being considered for use (based on success or lack of success in past, and on client's cultural practices)
   c. Energy level (degree of fatigue) and ability to understand and/or follow directions

2. Offer opportunities for family, friends, or significant others to be involved with therapy
3. Provide client and any helping individuals with adequate instruction and support materials (written instructions, audiotapes, films)

IX. COMMON NURSING DIAGNOSES FOR CLIENTS WITH PAIN

A. Pain
1. Applies when a client experiences discomfort or pain (either constant or intermittent) that is time-bound in that it has lasted from 1 second to less than 6 months (NANDA–I)
2. A nursing diagnostic statement for *Pain* must include the location and any etiologic or precipitating factors

B. Chronic pain
1. Applies when the client has discomfort or pain (either constant or intermittent) that has lasted for more than 6 months (NANDA–I)
2. A nursing diagnostic statement for *Chronic pain* must include the location and any etiologic or precipitating factors

C. Altered comfort: applies when client experiences some type of discomfort in response to a specific stimulus that is noxious in nature (NANDA–I)

D. Other pertinent nursing diagnoses
1. Ineffective Coping (individual and/or family) related to persistent pain that may add stress that affects client's and/or family's ability to cope
2. Deficient Knowledge related to lack of information or misinformation regarding pain treatment strategies
3. Impaired Physical Mobility related to movement limited by pain
4. Disturbed Sleep Pattern related to persistent pain
5. Anxiety related to loss of control
6. Fear related to pain
7. Powerlessness related to illness-related regimen
8. Ineffective Role Performance related to a change in health status and impaired coping
9. Ineffective Sexuality Pattern related to illness and pain
10. Activity Intolerance related to pain and/or depression
11. Self-Care Deficit (total or partial) related to pain

Case Study

A 75-year-old woman has been admitted to an orthopedic unit following a right fractured hip repair. She lives alone and fell while hanging curtains in her bedroom. Her postoperative orders include a PCA pump prescribed as morphine 1 mg every 10 minutes. She is currently alert and tells the nurse, "I am in so much pain, I'd rather be dead." Vital signs are as follows: oral temperature 99.2°F, pulse 102, respirations 20 and BP 142/92.

1. What common physiological responses are expected for a client in acute pain?
2. What are several nonopioid medications that could be used to manage pain in addition to the PCA pump?
3. What are the nursing priorities for a client using a PCA pump?
4. What additional comfort measures could be used for this client?
5. What nursing diagnoses related to pain are anticipated for this client?

For suggested responses, see page 308.

POSTTEST

1 An anxious-appearing client with AIDS tells the nurse that he has a burning sensation with shooting pain to both feet that is excruciating in nature. What condition should the nurse interpret this client's report as indicating?

1. The client is experiencing neuropathic pain to the distal lower extremities.
2. Psychogenic pain to both feet is accompanied by an anxious appearance.
3. There is referred pain described as excruciating to the bilateral feet.
4. Severe phantom pain is present to the feet and is resulting in anxiety.

2 A male client is very anxious about the pain he may experience postoperatively. Which interventions would be most effective in helping him deal with this fear? Select all that apply.

1. Teach him relaxation techniques such as deep breathing and guided imagery.
2. Explain the availability of pain medications after surgery.
3. Demonstrate various positioning techniques that promote postoperative comfort.
4. Distract the client from discussing pain by focusing on surgical preparation.
5. Encourage the client to verbalize his concerns.

3 The nurse is caring for a client receiving epidural morphine (Duramorph). For which nursing concerns would the nurse develop a care plan for this client? Select all that apply.

1. Polyuria
2. Tachypnea
3. Nausea
4. Pruritis
5. Hypotension

4 A nurse asks a client to describe the client's current pain. Using the mnemonic COLDERR, which client descriptions would the nurse document? Select all that apply.

1. Severe
2. Aching
3. Intermittent
4. Chronic
5. Area

5 The nurse would evaluate successful client teaching with regard to morphine administration via patient-controlled analgesia (PCA) when the client makes which statement?

1. "I will probably use less morphine this way than with taking injections in my hip."
2. "I will get a dose of morphine every time I push the button."
3. "Using this device will keep me comfortable at all times."
4. "If I push the control button too often, I may get more medicine than needed."

6 A hospital discharge planning nurse is making arrangements for a client (who has an epidural catheter for continuous infusion of opioids) to be placed in a skilled nursing facility in the client's neighborhood to encourage family visiting. The facility has never cared for a client with this type of need. What would be the discharge planning nurse's best action?

1. Ask the health care provider for an extension of hospitalization until epidural catheter is discontinued to allow for placement at neighborhood facility.
2. Arrange for staff at the skilled nursing facility to receive immediate in-services on pain management using epidural catheters.
3. Explain the situation to client and family and seek another skilled nursing facility for discharge from the hospital.
4. Encourage family to hire private-duty nurses skilled in epidural catheter pain management to allow for client transfer to a neighborhood facility.

7 The nurse is teaching a client with chronic pain how to use visual imagery for pain management. What is the most appropriate goal statement for this client?

1. Relaxation exercises will replace the need for analgesia.
2. Relaxation exercises will actively involve the client in pain management.
3. Relaxation exercises will decrease pain sensation.
4. Relaxation exercises will allow for better rest periods.

8 Which client would the nurse recognize as requiring the most frequent reassessment of pain after the administration of an analgesic?

1. An older adult client taking over-the-counter (OTC) medication for osteoarthritis
2. A client taking oral narcotics regularly for chronic low back pain
3. A young adult taking medication for frequent migraine headaches
4. A child with sickle cell anemia receiving IV analgesia for a painful first crisis

9 A graduate nurse is caring for a hospitalized client who is requesting medication for pain rated as "severe." The client is watching television with visitors and is eating. Which statement indicates to the nurse preceptor that the graduate nurse understands pain management?

1. "His distractions must not be very effective."
2. "He's probably anxious being in the hospital."
3. "If he says he hurts, then he must hurt."
4. "Social stimulation can increase one's pain."

10 A home health nurse is preparing to apply a fentanyl (Duragesic) transdermal patch for pain management. Under what condition would the nurse not apply the patch to the client's upper arm?

1. Had bilateral mastectomies performed one year ago.
2. Has minimal hair distribution to this area.
3. Has intravenous catheters placed in the hands.
4. Uses an overhead trapeze bar for bed mobility.

➤ *See pages 211–212 for Answers and Rationales.*

ANSWERS & RATIONALES

Pretest

1 **Answers: 2, 3, 5** **Rationale:** Chronic pain persists for 6 months or longer and can affect clients of all age groups. Chronic pain can be classified as mild, moderate, or severe, and can be constant or intermittent. The etiology is often difficult to determine, which makes it difficult to treat effectively. Nerve damage may be one of numerous causes for chronic pain. Chronic pain is characterized by signs of parasympathetic nervous system activity such as normal vital signs, dry and warm skin, and pupils that are normal or dilated. Acute pain elicits sympathetic nervous system responses such as elevated vital signs, diaphoresis, and dilated pupils. **Cognitive Level:** Analyzing **Client Need:** Basic Care and Comfort **Integrated Process:** Teaching and Learning **Content Area:** Fundamentals **Strategy:** The core issue of the question is knowledge of the characteristics of chronic pain. Recall the challenges in chronic pain management to choose correctly among the various options. When more than one option is correct, consider each option as a true or false statement. **Reference:** Berman, A., & Snyder, S. J. (2012). *Kozier & Erb's fundamentals of*

nursing: Concepts, process, and practice (9th ed.). Upper Saddle River, NJ: Pearson Education, pp. 1205–1207.

2 **Answer: 1** **Rationale:** Unless the client is cognitively impaired, the best technique for validation of pain is to use a scale to rate the intensity. Behavioral and physiological responses are not as reliable; however, they can be used to support the quantitative method of validation. **Cognitive Level:** Applying **Client Need:** Basic Care and Comfort **Integrated Process:** Nursing Process: Assessment **Content Area:** Fundamentals **Strategy:** The critical term is *most effective method.* Recall that pain assessment tools and instruments are key to effective pain assessment. **Reference:** Berman, A., & Snyder, S. J. (2012). *Kozier & Erb's fundamentals of nursing: Concepts, process, and practice* (9th ed.). Upper Saddle River, NJ: Pearson Education, pp. 1215–1217.

3 **Answer: 4** **Rationale:** When one medication is used alone, the dose must be higher to be effective. Using the opioid with the nonsteroidal anti-inflammatory drug (NSAID) decreases the opioid dose required for adequate pain relief. This method reduces, although does not eliminate, the potential side effects of the opioid analgesic.

This method does not reduce the need for additional pain medication during the night-time hours. **Cognitive Level:** Applying **Client Need:** Pharmacological and Parenteral Therapies **Integrated Process:** Teaching and Learning **Content Area:** Fundamentals **Strategy:** Knowledge of the pharmacologic effect of common analgesics is needed to select an answer. Recall general pharmacologic principles of the 2 types of analgesics and use the process of elimination to make a selection. **Reference:** Berman, A., & Snyder, S. J. (2012). *Kozier & Erb's fundamentals of nursing: Concepts, process, and practice* (9th ed.). Upper Saddle River, NJ: Pearson Education, pp. 1226–1229.

4 **Answer: 1** **Rationale:** Transcutaneous electrical nerve stimulation (TENS) is thought to be effective for chronic pain clients as a result of stimulating the nonnociceptors. This device does not provide a distraction, reduce tissue damage, or alter cell function. **Cognitive Level:** Applying **Client Need:** Basic Care and Comfort **Integrated Process:** Teaching and Learning **Content Area:** Fundamentals **Strategy:** The critical point of the question is to apply nursing knowledge in a manner that a client can comprehend. The nurse's knowledge about the anatomy of pain, the function of the nervous system and pain receptors, and methods of pain management will aid in the selection of the correct answer. **Reference:** Berman, A., & Snyder, S. J. (2012). *Kozier & Erb's fundamentals of nursing: Concepts, process, and practice* (9th ed.). Upper Saddle River, NJ: Pearson Education, pp. 1236–1237.

5 **Answer: 2** **Rationale:** Respiratory compromise is rare with opioid administration yet feared by many health care workers. Sedation precedes a fall in respiratory rate and/or depth and therefore should be noted and recorded. It may not be feasible to allow the surgical client to rest uninterrupted for a several-hour period. In addition, it is appropriate for the nurse to plan certain nursing interventions when pain medication is most effective. The infusion pump continuously records the amount of medication infused. **Cognitive Level:** Applying **Client Need:** Pharmacological and Parenteral Therapies **Integrated Process:** Nursing Process: Implementation **Content Area:** Fundamentals **Strategy:** The critical words are *highest priority*. Recall information about common side effects of patient-controlled analgesia and the administration of opioids to assist you in assuring client safety during its use. **Reference:** Berman, A., & Snyder, S. J. (2012). *Kozier & Erb's fundamentals of nursing: Concepts, process, and practice* (9th ed.). Upper Saddle River, NJ: Pearson Education, pp. 1325–1326.

6 **Answer: 2** **Rationale:** A client who is breathing 8 breaths per minute is experiencing a potentially life-threatening side effect of the analgesia. This is the highest priority for the nurse. A respiratory rate of 24 may indicate pain, and this client may need additional teaching about patient-controlled analgesia (PCA) use, but this is a lesser priority than the decreased respiratory rate. It is anticipated that postoperative discomfort may be experienced when ambulating but not at rest. A state of

sleeping but arousable indicates effective pain control. **Cognitive Level:** Applying **Client Need:** Pharmacological and Parenteral Therapies **Integrated Process:** Nursing Process: Implementation **Content Area:** Fundamentals **Strategy:** To answer this question accurately, it is necessary to understand the adverse effects of patient-controlled analgesia (PCA) use with pain medication. Use knowledge that PCA utilizes opioid or narcotic analgesics and recall their major adverse effects to make a selection. **Reference:** Berman, A., & Snyder, S. J. (2012). *Kozier & Erb's fundamentals of nursing: Concepts, process, and practice* (9th ed.). Upper Saddle River, NJ: Pearson Education, pp. 1236–1237.

7 **Answers: 2, 5** **Rationale:** Prior to administering opioid analgesics through an epidural catheter, gently aspirate to ensure there is no return of cerebrospinal fluid or blood. Alcohol is a neurotoxic substance and its use should be avoided when providing epidural catheter or site care. Changing the client's position would be an important action regardless of epidural catheter placement. However, a sign indicating the presence of an epidural should be posted so that appropriate precautions are taken during repositioning. The catheter insertion site does not require an hourly assessment; rather, it is done once a shift or each time medication is administered. Epidural tubing, infusion bag, and infusion should be carefully labeled to avoid administering IV medications through the epidural catheter. **Cognitive Level:** Applying **Client Need:** Pharmacological and Parenteral Therapies **Integrated Process:** Nursing Process: Implementation **Content Area:** Fundamentals **Strategy:** The critical term is *safe care.* Recall care measures for clients receiving spinal analgesics that are essential to client safety and use the process of elimination to make a selection. When more than one option is correct, consider each option as a true-false statement. **Reference:** Berman, A., & Snyder, S. J. (2012). *Kozier & Erb's fundamentals of nursing: Concepts, process, and practice* (9th ed.). Upper Saddle River, NJ: Pearson Education, pp. 1233–1235.

8 **Answer: 4** **Rationale:** The purpose of biofeedback in pain management is to teach the client self-control over physiological variables that relate to the pain, such as muscle contraction and circulation. The therapy requires working with a trained counselor; therefore, financial obligations are present in the early phases of training. This is a self-control treatment that does not include group therapy. **Cognitive Level:** Applying **Client Need:** Basic Care and Comfort **Integrated Process:** Teaching and Learning **Content Area:** Fundamentals **Strategy:** The critical words are *biofeedback* and *understands*. Familiarity with nonpharmacologic techniques for promoting comfort will allow you to assess client understanding of this treatment measure. **Reference:** Berman, A., & Snyder, S. J. (2012). *Kozier & Erb's fundamentals of nursing: Concepts, process, and practice* (9th ed.). Upper Saddle River, NJ: Pearson Education, p. 344.

9 Answer: 4 Rationale: A client's statement about pain intensity and pain relief should be what guides the nurse in determining medication route, dosage, and frequency. The other responses are generalizations that may not be accurate for the client's condition. **Cognitive Level:** Applying **Client Need:** Pharmacological and Parenteral Therapies **Integrated Process:** Communication and Documentation **Content Area:** Fundamentals **Strategy:** The critical term is *best reply.* Recall principles regarding the use of analgesics to assist you in assessing medication effectiveness and communicating these criteria to clients and families. **Reference:** Berman, A., & Snyder, S. J. (2012). *Kozier & Erb's fundamentals of nursing: Concepts, process, and practice* (9th ed.). Upper Saddle River, NJ: Pearson Education, pp. 1230–1231.

10 Answers: 1, 5 Rationale: Reaction to pain is very individualized and varies based on many subjective factors such as the meaning of pain and the environment of the client. The tolerance to pain reflects the amount of pain the client is willing to endure. The client may not request pain medication and may need frequent assessment. This does not mean the client will not experience pain, but may need less medication than other people in the same age group with a similar injury. Discomfort with slight movement and asking for pain medication frequently are more consistent with a low tolerance for pain. **Cognitive Level:** Applying **Client Need:** Pharmacological and Parenteral Therapies **Integrated Process:** Nursing Process: Planning **Content Area:** Fundamentals **Strategy:** The critical phrase is *amazing tolerance for pain.* Being able to identify clients that are at risk for poor pain assessment and treatment will ultimately result in more effective pain management strategies for all clients. When more than one option is correct, consider each one as a true-false statement. **Reference:** Berman, A., & Snyder, S. J. (2012). *Kozier & Erb's fundamentals of nursing: Concepts, process, and practice* (9th ed.). Upper Saddle River, NJ: Pearson Education, pp. 1219–1221.

Posttest

1 Answer: 1 Rationale: Neuropathic pain is the result of a disturbance of the peripheral or central nervous system that results in pain not necessarily associated with an ongoing tissue damage process. It is usually described as shooting, stabbing, burning, or pins and needles. It is severe in nature and is frequently seen in clients with AIDS. Psychogenic pain is emotionally based, referred pain is felt from a distant site than the actual tissue damage, and phantom pain occurs after the loss of an extremity. **Cognitive Level:** Applying **Client Need:** Basic Care and Comfort **Integrated Process:** Nursing Process: Diagnosis **Content Area:** Fundamentals **Strategy:** The critical words are *AIDS, shooting pain, and excruciating.* Recall typical client descriptions of pain quality, which can provide to valuable data on the source of the client's pain. **Reference:** Berman, A. J., Snyder, S., & McKinney, D. S.

(2011). *Nursing basics for clinical practice.* Upper Saddle River, NJ: Pearson Education, p. 477.

2 Answers: 2, 5 Rationale: The client is most likely experiencing anxiety because of fears related to the postoperative pain. The best interventions are to encourage him to verbalize his concerns and reassure him that pain medication will be available to provide relief from discomfort. Teaching relaxation techniques and discussing positioning requires concentration from the client that may not be possible because of anxiety. Promoting distraction does not address his fears and thereby may lead to increased anxiety. **Cognitive Level:** Applying **Client Need:** Basic Care and Comfort **Integrated Process:** Nursing Process: Implementation **Content Area:** Fundamentals **Strategy:** The critical phrase is *most effective;* note that multiple answers may be selected. Recall basic communication techniques and information about available pharmacologic analgesics to provide reassurance and education to the concerned client. When more than one answer is correct, consider each option as a true-false statement. **Reference:** Berman, A. J., Snyder, S., & McKinney, D. S. (2011). *Nursing basics for clinical practice.* Upper Saddle River, NJ: Pearson Education, pp. 479–482.

3 Answers: 4, 5 Rationale: Pruritis and/or development of a skin rash are commonly associated with the administration of epidural opiates. This may be due in part to histamine release. The other potential physiological problems to be anticipated include hypotension, headache, and urinary retention. Polyuria, tachypnea, and nausea are not expected with administration of epidural opiates. **Cognitive Level:** Applying **Client Need:** Pharmacological and Parenteral Therapies **Integrated Process:** Nursing Process: Diagnosis **Content Area:** Fundamentals **Strategy:** The critical words are *epidural morphine.* Recall the common side effects of various analgesics to assist you to recognizing the etiology of the stated client problem. When more than one answer is correct, consider each option as a true-false statement. **Reference:** Berman, A. J., Snyder, S., & McKinney, D. S. (2011). *Nursing basics for clinical practice.* Upper Saddle River, NJ: Pearson Education, p. 493.

4 Answers: 2, 3, 5 Rationale: Using the mnemonic of COLDERR for pain assessment is an effective way to document a client's pain. The descriptors of this tool are C for Character; O for Onset; L for Location; D for Duration; E for Exacerbation; the first R is for Relief; and the final R is for Radiation. The mnemonic COLDERR does not assess for pain intensity or distinguish if pain is chronic or acute. **Cognitive Level:** Applying **Client Need:** Basic Care and Comfort **Integrated Process:** Nursing Process: Assessment **Content Area:** Fundamentals **Strategy:** The critical term is *using the mnemonic COLDERR for the assessment of pain.* Use nursing knowledge of the range of characteristics that are part of pain assessment to choose correctly from the available options. When there is more than one correct answer, consider each option as a true-false statement.

Reference: Berman, A. J., Snyder, S., & McKinney, D. S. (2011). *Nursing basics for clinical practice*. Upper Saddle River, NJ: Pearson Education, p. 482.

5 **Answer: 1** **Rationale:** Research has shown that small, frequent doses of an opioid as administered through patient-controlled analgesia (PCA) provide better pain relief and less total medication than traditional intramuscular (IM) injections used every 3 to 4 hours prn. The goal of PCA is to provide relief of discomfort; however, with movement, stress, procedures, and so on, the client may still experience periods of pain. The pump device is regulated to avoid overdosing and will limit the amount of medication the client can receive within a given time frame. Pushing the button after a maximum dose has been infused will not result in the client receiving more medication. **Cognitive Level:** Applying **Client Need:** Pharmacological and Parenteral Therapies **Integrated Process:** Teaching and Learning **Content Area:** Fundamentals **Strategy:** Nursing knowledge of routes of analgesia administration is needed to answer this question. Recall specific information about patient-controlled analgesia (PCA) and use the process of elimination to make a selection. **Reference:** Berman, A. J., Snyder, S., & McKinney, D. S. (2011). *Nursing basics for clinical practice*. Upper Saddle River, NJ: Pearson Education, pp. 493–494.

6 **Answer: 3** **Rationale:** According to The Joint Commission's pain standards, if a facility cannot treat a client for pain, the individual must be referred to a facility that can provide the skill. The health care provider may not be able to extend hospitalization because of insurance limitations. It is the skilled nursing facility's decision and responsibility to become prepared to provide a new service. Private-duty nurses may be cost prohibitive for the client or the client's family, and the skilled nursing facility may not have the resources needed to provide safe care for this client. **Cognitive Level:** Applying **Client Need:** Management of Care **Integrated Process:** Nursing Process: Planning **Content Area:** Fundamentals **Strategy:** Recall accreditation agencies standards on pain control to allow you to plan acceptable care measures. **Reference:** Berman, A. J., Snyder, S., & McKinney, D. S. (2011). *Nursing basics for clinical practice*. Upper Saddle River, NJ: Pearson Education, pp. 28, 33, 35, 481.

7 **Answer: 2** **Rationale:** Relaxation exercises such as guided imagery enhance other pain-relief measures to promote comfort of the client. They offer the client the opportunity to participate actively in pain control. Complementary therapies for pain control should not be used as substitutes for analgesia as these measures do not decrease pain sensation. Ultimately, relaxation exercises will allow the client to experience enhanced rest periods; however, this is not the most appropriate goal in the use of this therapy. **Cognitive Level:** Applying **Client Need:** Basic Care and Comfort Integrated Process: Nursing Process: Planning **Content Area:** Fundamentals **Strategy:** Recall knowledge of nonpharmacologic techniques for managing pain to guide you in setting appropriate client outcomes. **Reference:** Berman, A. J.,

Snyder, S., & McKinney, D. S. (2011). *Nursing basics for clinical practice*. Upper Saddle River, NJ: Pearson Education, p. 497.

8 **Answer: 4** **Rationale:** The regularity of pain assessment depends on the degree to which the client's condition and/or pain status is changing. More rapidly progressive disease requires more frequent client assessment. The clients with osteoarthritis, low back pain, and migraine headaches all have recurrent, long-standing problems. Their pain should be thoroughly assessed and documented, but the client with sickle cell anemia has the most rapidly changing condition that would require the most frequent reassessment. **Cognitive Level:** Analyzing **Client Need:** Pharmacological and Parenteral Therapies **Integrated Process:** Nursing Process: Evaluation **Content Area:** Fundamentals **Strategy:** The critical term is *most frequent*. Awareness of criteria for the reassessment of pain following analgesic administration is necessary to evaluate the safety and efficacy of pain-control medications. **Reference:** Berman, A. J., Snyder, S., & McKinney, D. S. (2011). *Nursing basics for clinical practice*. Upper Saddle River, NJ: Pearson Education, pp. 486–489.

9 **Answer: 3** **Rationale:** According to McCaffery and Pasero (1999), "Pain is whatever the person says it is, experienced whenever they say they are experiencing it." Nurses must realize that individuals react very uniquely when in pain and there are no defining characteristics that are applicable to the majority of clients. Although the other statements may be accurate for this particular client, the best choice for the nurse to act upon is the client's verbal report. **Cognitive Level:** Applying **Client Need:** Basic Care and Comfort **Integrated Process:** Nursing Process: Assessment **Content Area:** Fundamentals **Strategy:** The core issue of the question is knowledge of fundamental pain assessments as they relate to the body of knowledge about the pain experience. Use knowledge of pain theory to guide you to make an accurate assessment of the client's pain. **Reference:** Berman, A. J., Snyder, S., & McKinney, D. S. (2011). *Nursing basics for clinical practice*. Upper Saddle River, NJ: Pearson Education, pp. 496–497.

10 **Answer: 1** **Rationale:** The patch is placed every 72 hours over nonhairy, nonedematous skin with good capillary flow (often over the torso, shoulders, or upper arms). Following mastectomy, the potential for lymphedema would contraindicate using the upper arms because circulation would be compromised; thus, distribution of the medication would be impaired. The presence of an IV catheter or use of a trapeze bar should not affect the site. **Cognitive Level:** Applying **Client Need:** Pharmacological and Parenteral Therapies **Integrated Process:** Nursing Process: Implementation **Content Area:** Fundamentals **Strategy:** Recall various routes of administration and principles of safe transdermal medication administration to make a selection. **Reference:** Wilson, B. A., Shannon, M. T., & Shields, K. M. (2012). *Pearson nurse's drug guide 2012*. Upper Saddle River, NJ: Pearson Education, pp. 627–630.

References

American Pain Society (APS). (2003). Principles of analgesic use in the treatment of acute pain and cancer pain (5th ed.), Glenview, IL; Author.

Berman, A., & Snyder, S. J. (2012). *Kozier & Erb's fundamentals of nursing: Concepts, process, and practice* (9th ed.). Upper Saddle River, NJ: Pearson Education.

Berman, A. J., Snyder, S., & McKinney, D. S. (2011). *Nursing basics for clinical practice*. Upper Saddle River, NJ: Prentice Hall.

Gordon, M. (2009). *The manual of nursing diagnosis* (12th ed.), St. Louis, MO: Mosby.

LeMone, P., Burke, K., & Bauldoff, G. (2011). *Medical-surgical nursing: Critical thinking in patient care* (5th ed.). Upper Saddle River, NJ: Pearson Education.

McCaffery, M., & Pasero, C. (1999). *Pain: Clinical manual* (2nd ed.). St. Louis, MO: Mosby.

Wilson, B. A., Shannon, M. T., & Shields, K. M. (2012). *Pearson nurse's drug guide 2012*. Upper Saddle River, NJ: Pearson Education.

World Health Organization (WHO). (1996). *Cancer pain relief* (2nd ed.). Geneva, Switzerland.

9 Meeting Needs of Perioperative Clients

NCLEX-RN® Test Prep

Use the accompanying online resource, NursingReviewsandRationales, to test yourself with hundreds of NCLEX®-style practice questions.

Objectives

➤ Explain the concept of perioperative nursing.
➤ Describe the purposes and types of surgical procedures and anesthesia.
➤ Identify the components of a comprehensive preoperative assessment.
➤ Explain the nurse's role in informed consent.
➤ Review the developmental needs and physical preparation of individuals undergoing surgery.
➤ Describe intraoperative factors that can affect a client's psychophysiologic functioning postoperatively.
➤ Identify assessment parameters and nursing interventions necessary to prevent and detect postoperative complications.
➤ Discuss the nursing process in the preoperative, intraoperative, and postoperative phases of care.

Review at a Glance

anesthesia partial or complete loss of sensation

conscious sedation a form of anesthesia that raises the pain threshold and provides some amnesia but allows the client to respond to verbal and physical stimuli; intravenous narcotics and antianxiety agents are used; the client can maintain a patent airway; also called moderate sedation

dehiscence partial or total rupture of a sutured wound

drain tube inserted into wound during surgery and designed to allow the removal of excessive fluids

exudate fluid and cells that accumulate in a wound

informed consent a formal process, the responsibility of the health care provider, the purpose of which is to gain permission from the client for an invasive procedure and involves an explanation of the procedure as well as the risks, benefits, and alternatives to the procedure

intraoperative phase begins when the client is transferred to the operating room table and ends when the client is transferred to the postanesthesia care unit (PACU)

moderate sedation a newer term for conscious sedation

palliative relieves or reduces pain or symptoms of a disease without curing the disease

preoperative phase begins with a determination that surgical intervention is necessary and ends with client is transferred to the operating room table

postoperative phase begins with the admission to the postanesthesia care unit (PACU) and ends when healing is complete

purulent containing pus

regional anesthesia loss of sensation in one part of the body as a result of an anesthetic agent

sanguineous bloody, refers to body fluid

serosanguineous refers to fluid composed of serum and blood

serous appearing like serum

surgical asepsis activities designed to keep operative or other sites free from the presence of microorganisms

surgical scrub a specific hand hygiene technique used by operating

room personnel that is designed to reduce microorganisms, particularly on the hands

sterile field a microorganism-free area

PRETEST

1 Which activities should the nurse carry out in the preoperative period for a client scheduled for surgery? Select all that apply.

1. Identify potential or actual health problems.
2. Verify the presence of a signed informed consent form.
3. Assess client's response to interventions.
4. Intervene to prevent complications.
5. Assess effectiveness of teaching related to postoperative recovery.

2 The nurse interprets that which client would be most likely to undergo an ablative procedure?

1. A client scheduled for breast augmentation following a mastectomy 2 years ago
2. A client scheduled for biopsy of a lung tumor
3. A client awaiting an adenoidectomy
4. A client undergoing a nerve root resection

3 A client having surgery has a degree of risk associated with the surgery. The nurse would evaluate which client-related factors as contributing to a high degree of risk associated with surgery? Select all that apply.

1. Type of institution where surgery is performed
2. Involvement of vital organs
3. Average nutritional status
4. Low likelihood of procedure complications
5. A history of respiratory disease and diabetes

4 An infant who is having surgery has a higher risk than an adult. The nurse would recognize which manifestation as the reason for the infant's increased risk?

1. Decline in functioning
2. Immaturity of vital organs
3. Increased possibility of hyperthermia
4. Volume of blood fluctuation

5 A preschool-age child is facing surgery and may have fears related to the surgery. Which type of fears would the nurse anticipate in this child?

1. The surgical procedure is punishment for being bad.
2. The child will look drastically different after surgery.
3. The child will not be able to do the things after the surgery that the child used to do.
4. The medical personnel is not competent to perform procedures correctly.

6 A client has just entered the postanesthesia care unit (PACU) from surgery. For which priority needs should the nurse immediately assess the postoperative client?

1. Vital signs, level of consciousness, and presence of pain
2. Skin coloring, surgical incision, limb movements
3. Skin temperature, blood pressure, mental status
4. Temperature, emotional status, wound drainage

7 The nurse in the postanesthesia care unit (PACU) is assessing a postoperative client. Which indicators suggest to the nurse an alteration in tissue perfusion? Select all that apply.

1. Pallor or cyanosis
2. Difficulty with mobility
3. Pain in the incision area
4. Fluid loss
5. Decreased urinary output

8 After surgery, the nurse encourages the client to move from side to side at least every 2 hours. The client questions this activity. How does the nurse explain the purpose of this intervention?

1. Assist peristalsis to return more quickly.
2. Lessen muscle weakness.
3. Increase client's ability to sleep.
4. Let the lungs alternately achieve maximum expansion.

9 The nurse is assessing the client's surgical wound in the postoperative period. Which finding indicates to the nurse that the first stage of healing is taking place?

1. Inflammation in the wound edges
2. Bleeding around the incision
3. Clot binding the wound edges
4. Collagen synthesis

10 The nurse is creating a care plan for a postoperative client. The nursing diagnosis is Acute Pain. What would be appropriate outcomes for this client? Select all that apply.

1. Balanced fluid intake and output
2. Seeks help as needed
3. Absence of nonverbal signs of pain
4. Performs leg exercises as instructed
5. Verbally rates pain as 3 on a 1 to 10 scale

➤ *See pages 232–234 for Answers and Rationales.*

I. OVERVIEW OF PERIOPERATIVE NURSING

A. Definitions

1. Perioperative nursing is defined as "those nursing activities performed by the professional nurse in the preoperative, intraoperative, and postoperative phases of the patient's surgical experience" (AORN, 2006)

   a. Association of Operating Room Nurses (AORN) is the professional organization of perioperative registered nurses, whose mission is to "promote quality patient care by providing its members with education, standards, services, and representation" (Source: Association of PeriOperative Registered Nurses (AORN) (2006).)

   b. Practice settings of perioperative nurses include hospitals, health care provider offices, and free-standing surgical settings

    c. Involves use of nursing process and includes collaboration with members of health care team, making appropriate referrals, and delegation and supervision of nursing care

2. Perioperative phases

   a. **Preoperative phase** begins with a determination that surgical intervention is necessary and ends with transfer of client to operating room (OR) table; nursing activities include:

      1) Identification of client
      2) Assessment of client
      3) Identifying potential or actual health problems
      4) Planning care based on client's specific needs
      5) Beginning postoperative teaching to client, family, and significant others

    b. **Intraoperative phase** (surgical period) begins when client is transferred to operating table and ends when client is admitted to postanesthesia care unit (PACU); nursing activities include:

      1) Participate in "time out" identification of correct surgery site according to standards and policy; especially important if surgery encompasses an anatomical bilateral organ or limb site; surgical site may be marked to ensure accuracy
      2) Preparing client for induction of anesthesia
      3) Maintaining homeostasis and asepsis throughout procedure

        4) Ensuring proper equipment functioning

        5) Assisting surgeon and team as needed by providing an aseptic environment, a hazard-free environment, and needed supplies in a timely manner

    c. Postoperative phase begins with client's admission to PACU and ends when healing is complete; nursing activities include:

        1) Assessing for physical and psychological adaptation following anesthesia and surgical intervention

        2) Performing interventions that will facilitate healing and prevent complications

        3) Teaching and providing support to client and client's support persons

        4) Assisting with planning home care

        5) Assisting client in attaining the most optimal health status possible

    d. Location of perioperative nursing care

        1) Hospital suites for inpatient and outpatient surgery, endoscopic, and laser procedures

        2) Health care provider office-based surgical suites for outpatient procedures

        3) Free-standing outpatient and ambulatory surgical centers

B. Specific nursing actions and responsibilities during the perioperative phases

  1. Preoperative

    a. Interview: current health status, allergies, current medications, previous surgical experiences, mental status, understanding of the surgical procedure and anesthesia, smoking habit, alcohol and drug use, coping strategies, social resources, and cultural considerations

    b. Arranging for pre-admission testing, consultations and education related to management of recovery from surgery and anesthesia

        1) Ordering appropriate tests, etc.

        2) Ensuring reports are available on chart

        3) Reporting to surgeon or anesthesiologist any pertinent abnormalities

    c. Day of surgery: after appropriate identification of client, nurse verifies completion of paperwork and secures valuables; if procedure is being performed as an outpatient, transportation home is verified; the nurse then proceeds with:

        1) Determining client's cognitive understanding of procedure

        2) Performing a physical assessment

        3) Planning nursing diagnoses

        4) Reinforcing preoperative teaching for postoperative care

        5) Conducting physical preparation: skin preparation, vital signs, antiembolism stockings, catheterization, and starting an IV infusion as ordered

        6) Ensuring that client has been NPO (if ordered)

        7) Ensuring that there is a signed consent form and it is placed in client record

  2. Intraoperative

    a. Administer IV infusions and medications as needed

    b. Provide safe, effective care

        1) Position client to ensure functional alignment and exposure of surgical site

        2) Apply grounding device

        3) Provide emotional and physical support if awake

        4) Account for all equipment and supplies

        5) Maintain aseptic environment

        6) Perform physiologic monitoring

        7) Assess fluid loss or gain

        8) Monitor cardiac, respiratory, and neurological status

        9) Monitor client's response to preoperative medications

       10) Prepare surgical site according to policy

    c. Nursing roles during intraoperative period (period of surgery)
       1) Circulating nurse
         a) Assist scrub nurses and surgeons
         b) Sterile scrubbing and gloving not necessary
       2) Scrub nurses
         a) Assist surgeons
         b) Maintain sterile gowns, gloves, caps
         c) Account for used sponges, needles, and instruments

3. Postoperative
  a. Immediate care
    1) Assess effects of anesthetic agents and surgical procedure
    2) Monitor vital functions
    3) Provide pain relief measures to promote comfort
  b. Ongoing care
    1) Assess for client adaptation to surgery
    2) Provide pain management
    3) Position client appropriately and reposition every 2 hours to prevent atelectasis and pneumonia
    4) Promote use of incentive spirometer and deep breathing and coughing exercises
    5) Assist with postoperative exercises, such as ankle circles, calf pumps
    6) Apply and maintain antiembolism devices such as antiembolism stockings or pneumatic compression boots as prescribed
    7) Maintain hydration and monitor fluid balance
    8) Promote urinary elimination
    9) Maintain suction to devices as needed; monitor all catheters, tubes, dressings, and drains
    10) Provide wound care and assess surgical site
    11) Continue client teaching and discharge planning
    12) Provide for safety

II. PURPOSES AND TYPES OF SURGERY AND ANESTHESIA

A. Purposes
  1. Diagnostic or exploratory: confirms or establishes a diagnosis (e.g., breast biopsy)
  2. Curative: removes pathological cause (e.g., removal of cancer)
  3. Ablative: removes a diseased body part (e.g., tonsils for tonsillitis)
  4. Reconstructive: restores function or appearance (e.g., cleft lip repair)
  5. Palliative: relieves or reduces pain or symptoms (e.g., removal of sensory nerves for intractable pain)

B. General classification of surgery
  1. According to degree of risk
    a. Major: high degree of risk; may include a prolonged intraoperative period, large loss of blood, involvement of a vital organ, or postoperative complications (e.g., liver biopsy, colectomy)
    b. Minor: lesser degree of risk to client; usually associated with few complications, may be described as "one-day surgery" or outpatient surgery (e.g., cyst removal, ingrown toenails)
    c. Degree of risk is affected by client's age, health condition, nutritional status, use of medications, and mental status
  2. Urgency classification
    a. Emergent: performed immediately to save a person's life, limb, or organ (e.g., testicular torsion)

      b. Urgent: requires prompt attention, usually within 24 hours (e.g., reduction of a broken bone)

      c. Required: necessary for client's well-being, usually within weeks to months (e.g., cholecystectomy, if not acute)

      d. Elective: surgery is necessary but not imminently life-threatening; will improve client's life (e.g., some types of plastic surgery)

      e. Optional: personal preference on part of client (e.g., gastric stapling)

C. Administration of *anesthesia* (partial or complete loss of sensation)

  1. Anesthetic agents are drugs used to affect a partial or complete loss of pain sensation; client may be conscious or unconscious

  2. Three major classifications of anesthesia

    a. Moderate sedation (also called **conscious sedation**)

      1) An anesthesia state that involves minimal depression of level of consciousness allowing client an ability to respond to verbal and physical stimuli; client can still maintain a patent airway while pain threshold is raised (which reduces pain sensation)

      2) Uses IV narcotics and antianxiety agents to maintain moderate sedation

      3) Examples: endoscopy, balloon angioplasty

    b. Regional anesthesia: loss of sensation in one part of body as a result of an anesthetic agent

      1) Local

        a) Injected in a specific area for minor surgical procedures

        b) Example of use: lidocaine for suturing a small wound

      2) Nerve block

        a) Anesthetic agent injected into and around a nerve or group of nerves

        b) Example: pudendal block used to numb perineum for an episiotomy in childbirth

      3) Epidural block

        a) Anesthetic agent injected into epidural space to anesthetize larger areas

        b) Client is awake and aware of surroundings but feels no pain

        c) Example of use: vaginal childbirth

      4) Spinal anesthesia

        a) Anesthesia is injected through a lumbar puncture into subarachnoid space

        b) Client is conscious but has no sensation or movement of lower extremities up to a specific area

        c) Example: used for hernia repairs or cesarean section deliveries

    c. General anesthesia

      1) Anesthesia that involves loss of all sensation and consciousness

      2) It is usually administered by intravenous (IV) infusion or by inhalation of gases

      3) Examples of use: major surgery, exploratory laparotomy

  3. Stages of general anesthesia

    a. Stage I

      1) Beginning anesthesia

      2) Client is drowsy and dizzy

      3) Pain sensation is depressed

    b. Stage II

      1) Excitement

      2) Client demonstrates irregular breathing and involuntary motor movements

      3) It is important to avoid stimulating client, which can trigger vomiting, holding the breath, and increased activity

      4) Ensure client's safety by proper use of safety straps

    c. Stage III

      1) Stage of anesthesia appropriate for surgical procedures

      2) Client demonstrates skeletal muscle relaxation, constricted pupils, and absence of eyelid reflex

    d. Stage IV

      1) Medullary depression

      2) Pupils are fixed and dilated, respirations are weak and pulse is rapid and thready

      3) Client is near death

  4. Preanesthesia classifications of client's physical condition: anesthesiologist reviews client's medical history as well as current findings related to diagnosis, medication use, allergies, and drug reactions (see Table 9-1 for an example of American Society of Anesthesiology Physical Status Classification System)

  5. Anesthetic agents may be administered either by inhalation or IV (see Table 9-2 for a brief overview of some anesthetic agents)

    a. Inhalation anesthetic agents are inhaled in gaseous forms

      1) Administered by mask or by endotracheal tube

      2) Induction is usually rapid

      3) Drugs are eliminated by respiratory system

      4) With normal lung function, recovery rate is predictable

    b. IV anesthesia

      1) Administered alone or in combination with inhalation anesthesia

      2) Rapid onset of unconsciousness

      3) Metabolized primarily by liver and excreted by kidneys

      4) Reversal agents may be required to stop drug's effects

> **Practice to Pass**
>
> Describe 5 purposes of surgery and include examples of each.

Table 9-1 **American Society of Anesthesiology Physical Status Classification System**

Physical Status	Findings	Examples of Accompanying Disease
I	Healthy client with no systemic disease	None
II	Mild systemic disease	Moderate obesity, mild hypertension
III	Severe systemic disease	Morbid obesity, pulmonary insufficiency
IV	Severe systemic disease that presents as a constant threat to survival	Advanced renal disease, hepatic insufficiency
V	Client who is not expected to survive without surgical procedure	Ruptured abdominal aneurysm
VI	Brain-dead client whose organs are being donated	Not applicable
E	Emergency operation of a client with a poorer physical status	Injuries sustained in motor vehicle crash

Table 9-2 **Brief Overview of Anesthetic Agents**

Anesthetic Agent	Route	Advantages	Disadvantages	Complications
Lidocaine (Xylocaine)	Topical, injected	Quick acting	May be absorbed through mucosal surfaces and open wounds	Cardiac side effects if absorbed
EMLA (Lidocaine and Prilocaine)	Topical	Very little absorption through skin	Must be done 60 minutes prior to procedure	Blanching or erythema at application site
Fentanyl (Sublimaze)	Parenteral	Moderate sedation	Prolonged use may cause myoclonus and/or tremors	Rapid infusion will cause chest wall tightening
Midazolam (Versed)	Parenteral	Promotes sedation	Pain at injection site	
Nitrous oxide	Inhalation	Quick acting	May lead to vomiting postprocedure	

III. COMPONENTS OF PREOPERATIVE ASSESSMENT

 A. Client's history

1. Medical history: current and past
   a. Current health status including any chronic disease that might affect client's response to surgery and anesthesia
   b. Past medical illnesses and treatments; previous surgical experiences including complications that occurred with any previous surgical or anesthesia experience
   c. Report of severe anxiety associated with surgery

 2. Medication use: all current medications, including prescription, over-the-counter (OTC), and herbal products

3. Allergies: food, medication, and environmental (latex, tape, soap, and antiseptic agents)

4. Tobacco use: may indicate potential problems of respiratory tract
   a. Type of product and amount and frequency used
   b. When possible, urge client to stop smoking 6 to 8 weeks prior to major surgery

5. Alcohol and controlled substance use
   a. Type of product and amount and frequency
   b. Potential for problems with withdrawal

6. Psychosocial and economic factors
   a. Occupation
   b. Financial concerns
   c. Support systems
   d. Spiritual needs
   e. Cultural beliefs
   f. Coping mechanisms used in past
   g. Fear or anxieties related to procedure (such as body image, pain, or grieving a loss of body part)

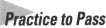

Practice to Pass

Discuss 6 issues to assess preoperatively regarding a client's history.

 B. Physical assessment

1. Assessment of factors that will affect client's response to surgery or anesthesia

2. General assessments
   a. Overall appearance, gestures, facial expression
   b. Height and weight (obesity increases risk)
   c. Vital signs (hypertension increases risk)

3. Head and neck
   a. Oral mucous membranes reveal hydration status
   b. Identify loose teeth, dentures, and orthodontic work
   c. Inspect soft palate, nasal sinuses, cervical lymph nodes
   d. Note presence of jugular venous distention

4. Integumentary
   a. Evaluate skin over entire body
   b. Note any areas where skin is thin, dry, or has poor turgor

5. Chest and lungs
   a. Auscultate for adventitious breath sounds
   b. Note degree of chest expansion, presence of cough, upper airway congestion, and/or obstructed nasal passages

6. Cardiovascular system
   a. Assess apical rate and rhythm
   b. Check color and temperature of extremities
   c. Note presence of pacemaker, arteriovenous (AV) graft

7. Gastrointestinal (GI) system
   a. Distinguish between obesity and distention of abdomen
   b. Assess baseline bowel sounds and elimination patterns

VII. INTRAOPERATIVE FACTORS AFFECTING POSTOPERATIVE PHASE

A. Principles of perioperative asepsis

1. General
   a. Keep sterile supplies dry and unopened
   b. Check package sterilization expiration date to verify sterility
   c. Maintain general cleanliness in surgical suite

   d. Maintain **surgical asepsis** (activities designed to keep sites free from presence of microorganisms) throughout procedure (refer back to Chapter 6, Table 6-2, pp. 132–133, for principles and practices for surgical asepsis)

2. Personnel
   a. Personnel with signs of illness should not report to work
   b. Surgical scrub, a specific hand hygiene technique used by operating room personnel designed to reduce microorganisms on hands and arms; is done for length of time designated by hospital policy
      1) A sensor-controlled or knee- or foot-operated faucet allows water to be turned on and off without use of hands
      2) Remove all rings and watches
      3) Use liquid soaps to prevent spread of microorganisms
      4) Keep fingernails short and well-trimmed; clean fingernails with a nail stick under running water
      5) Hold the hands higher than elbows throughout hand hygiene procedure so that run-off goes to elbows; this allows cleanest part of upper extremities to be the hands
      6) A scrub brush facilitates removal of microorganisms; clean all areas of skin on hands and arms in sequence starting at hands and ending at elbows
      7) After rinsing, dry hands with paper towels, drying first one arm from hand to elbow, then using a second towel to dry the second hand

3. Maintaining a **sterile field** (a microoganism-free area)
   a. Create a sterile field using sterile drapes
   b. Use sterile field to place sterile supplies where they will be available during procedure
   c. Drape equipment prior to use
   d. Keep drapes dry and out of contact with nonsterile objects
   e. Utilize sterile technique while adding or removing supplies from sterile fields

4. Sterile supplies and solutions
   a. Check expiration dates for sterility
   b. Do not use solutions that were opened prior to current use
   c. "Lip" solutions after initial use by pouring a small amount of liquid out of bottle into a waste container to cleanse bottle lip

B. Potential environmental health hazards during intraoperative period

1. Injuries caused by equipment
   a. Laser tools used for a surgical procedure can cause burns
   b. Improperly grounded cautery devices can cause burns
   c. Prevent by ensuring proper grounding for electrical equipment and checking equipment prior to beginning surgical procedure
   d. Latex allergy affects many people, both clients and hospital personnel
      1) Clients with spina bifida and those who have had multiple surgical procedures are at greatest risk
      2) Exposure can occur percutaneously, mucosally, parenterally, and via inhalation
      3) Symptoms can vary from contact dermatitis to anaphylaxis
      4) Symptoms in an anesthetized client would include flushing, facial swelling, urticaria, bronchospasm, hypotension, and cardiac arrest

      5) Be aware of equipment that contains latex, including tourniquets, manual resuscitation bags, balloon catheters, surgical gowns, boots, and drapes among other items

  2. Exposure to blood and body fluids

    a. Is a concern for client and staff alike

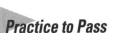

    b. Use goggles and fluid-protectant shields; gloves worn for extended period can leak and should be changed periodically

    c. Use caution with sharps

C. Potential intraoperative complications

  1. Nausea and vomiting: ensure that client is NPO for prescribed time period

  2. Hypoxia and respiratory complications

    a. Complications

      1) Aspiration of secretions or vomitus may be caused by loss of pharyngeal and cough reflexes

      2) Respiratory depression can occur from anesthetic agents

      3) Respiratory muscles become weakened or paralyzed by neuromuscular agents

      4) Positioning can negatively affect lung expansion

    b. Tissue perfusion is monitored by anesthesiologist

    c. Use of a pulse oximeter assists with monitoring of oxygenation

  3. Hypothermia

    a. Is related to room temperature of OR and exposure of internal organs

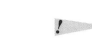

Practice to Pass

What nursing interventions will the OR nurse carry out to prevent hypothermia in the surgical client?

    b. Is minimized by preventing exposure of nonsurgical body parts, use of head covering and blankets, and warmed IV fluids and anesthetic agents

  4. Malignant hyperthermia

    a. Is defined as excessive heat production related to stress, trauma, infection; may be attributed to anesthetic agent; seen more commonly in males; there is a tendency towards development if inherited as an autosomal dominant trait

    b. Symptoms include rapid rise in body temperature, tachycardia and tachypnea, and respiratory and metabolic acidosis

    c. Skin initially appears flushed then becomes mottled and cyanotic

    d. Treatment includes administering 100% oxygen, cooling blankets and cold packs, cool IV fluids, and stomach irrigation

    e. Can be fatal

  5. Paresthesia related to positioning: use padding and proper position

  6. Excessive fluid or blood loss: monitor bleeding and intake and output

VIII. POSTOPERATIVE NURSING CARE

A. Assessments in immediate period following surgery (PACU—postanesthesia care unit) (see Box 9-1)

  1. Client is admitted from surgical suite into PACU; upon admission, the PACU nurse will:

    a. Confirm client's identity

    b. Receive report from OR or surgical nurse, which includes surgical procedure, anesthesia, drugs and IV fluids administered, and estimated blood loss

    c. Note location, types, and conditions of catheters, **drains**, or packs; drains are tubes inserted into wounds to allow removal of excessive **serosanguineous** (fluid composed of serum and blood) or **purulent** (containing pus) material from wound

  2. Nurse in PACU will:

    a. Maintain a patent airway

      1) This is a priority nursing concern

      2) Airway may be affected by continued effects of anesthetic drugs, relaxation of tongue, oropharyngeal secretions, or by vomitus

Box 9-1	

Clinical Assessment in the Immediate Postanesthetic Phase	• Adequacy of airway
	• Oxygen saturation
	• Adequacy of ventilation
	  • Respiratory rate, rhythm, and depth
	  • Use of accessory muscles
	  • Breath sounds
	• Cardiovascular status
	  • Heart rate and rhythm
	  • Peripheral pulse amplitude and equality
	  • Blood pressure
	  • Capillary filling
	• Level of consciousness
	  • Not responding
	  • Arousable with verbal stimuli
	  • Fully awake
	  • Oriented to time, person, and place
	• Presence of protective reflexes (e.g., gag, cough)
	• Activity, ability to move extremities
	• Skin color (pink, pale, dusky, blotchy, cyanotic, jaundiced)
	• Fluid status
	  • Intake and output
	  • Status of IV infusions (type of fluid, rate, amount in container, patency of tubing)
	  • Signs of dehydration or fluid overload
	• Condition of operative site
	  • Status of dressing
	  • Drainage (amount, type, and color)
	• Patency of and character and amount of drainage from catheters, tubes, and drains
	• Discomfort (i.e., pain) (type, location, and severity), nausea, vomiting
	• Safety (e.g., necessity for side rails, call bell within reach)

Source: Berman, Audrey J.; Snyder, Shirlee, *Kozier & Erb's Fundamentals of Nursing,* 9th Ed. © 2012. Reprinted and Electronically reproduced by permission of Pearson Education, Inc., Upper Saddle River, New Jersey.

    3) Position client on his or her side unless contraindicated

    4) Monitor respiratory rate, breath sounds, and suction as necessary

  b. Maintain cardiovascular stability

    1) Client is typically on a cardiac and respiratory monitor

    2) Vital signs are monitored according to hospital policy (often every 15 minutes) until stable and then every 30 minutes

    3) Changes in vital signs should be reported immediately

    4) Antiembolism stockings or pneumatic compression boots may be used to promote circulation in lower extremities

  c. Assess for hypotension or shock

    1) May be related to fluid or blood loss or as a reaction to drugs

    2) Monitor dressings and drains for amount and type of drainage

    3) Symptoms include restlessness, cool moist skin, pallor followed by cyanosis, and decreased urine output

    4) Monitor and maintain IV infusion flow rates

  d. Assess for hemorrhage

    1) Monitor dressings and drains for amount of discharge; observe appearance of urine; observe for distention of body tissues

2) A client with excessive blood loss may require a transfusion; ensure blood product and type are appropriate

    e. Assess for hypertension or dysrhythmias

    f. Relieve pain and anxiety

      1) Pain can negatively affect vital signs and recovery

      2) Assess location and cause of pain

      3) Administer analgesics as ordered

      4) Observe effectiveness of analgesics

3. Client will be discharged from PACU when:

    a. Vital signs are stable and spontaneous respirations have returned

    b. Gag reflex is present

    c. Client is easily arousable

B. Nursing management on surgical nursing unit

  1. Immediate nursing interventions

    a. Assess breathing and apply oxygen if prescribed

    b. Check vital signs and skin warmth, moisture, color

    c. Assess surgical site or wound drains; partial or total rupture of a sutured wound is termed **dehiscence**, which may be preceded by sudden straining as during coughing; when dehiscence occurs, cover wound with sterile dressings soaked in normal saline; place client in bed with the knees bent to reduce tension on wound and notify surgeon; note and record any wound **exudate** (fluid and cells that accumulate in a wound); exudate varies in appearance

      1) **Serous** (appearing like serum) exudate looks watery and clear

      2) Purulent exudate is thick and contains pus; purulent exudate varies in color and may be blue, green, or yellow tinged

      3) **Sanguineous** exudate is bloody and may be dark red or bright red depending on freshness of blood

    d. Connect tubes to drain devices or suction

    e. Perform pain assessment and utilize appropriate pain relief interventions

    f. Position client properly using support devices as necessary

    g. Monitor IV fluids and infusion pumps

    h. Monitor urine output hourly or less frequently as ordered

      1) Kidney function may have been impaired from poor perfusion during surgery; output indicates kidney response; hourly urine output should be 30 mL or more in an adult (0.5 mL/kg/hour)

      2) Bladder distention is possible for up to 24 hours following spinal anesthesia; spontaneous voiding should occur within 6 to 8 hours postoperatively

      3) If client is unable to void, catheterization may be ordered and repeated as necessary

  2. Ongoing nursing interventions

    a. Encourage deep breathing and coughing exercises

      1) Helps remove mucus that accumulates in lungs during surgery

      2) Aids in prevention of postoperative complications such as atelectasis and pneumonia

      3) Should be performed every 2 hours while awake

      4) Deep breathing frequently initiates coughing; encourage client to sit up in bed and place hands one on top of the other directly on wound dressing to reduce discomfort of coughing

      5) When increased intracranial pressure is a risk, client may deep breathe but not cough

    b. Teach and encourage leg exercises, use of support stockings, or sequential compression device

c. Keep call light; emesis basin, ice chips, bedpan, urinal within reach

d. Communicate with family or significant others

e. Monitor for infection by noting wound characteristics, temperature, and WBC test results

f. Teach self-care according to surgical procedure and client and family needs

g. Encourage activity as tolerated

h. Promote GI/GU function by providing diet/fluids once bowel sounds return; encourage early ambulation to promote bowel function; monitor voiding

i. Provide wound care as ordered (monitor incision, change dressing as ordered); document findings

j. Participate in discharge planning according to individual client needs

IX. NURSING PROCESS RELATED TO PERIOPERATIVE NURSING

A. Nursing diagnoses and expected outcomes for preoperative period

1. Diagnosis: Deficient Knowledge: operative procedure, postoperative complications, postoperative exercises, etc. (no etiology is required to explain a knowledge deficit)

2. Client outcomes: client describes operative procedure and potential complications; client demonstrates postoperative exercises

3. Diagnosis: Anxiety related to unknown outcome of surgery

4. Client outcomes: client expresses fears and identifies 2 activities that will reduce his or her fear

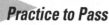

Practice to Pass

For the diagnosis Risk for Impaired Gas Exchange related to accumulation of secretions during surgery, list 1 client goal and 3 nursing interventions that will aid achievement of that goal.

B. Nursing diagnoses and expected outcomes for intraoperative period

1. Diagnosis: Risk for Impaired Gas Exchange related to depressant effect of anesthetic agents

2. Client outcome: client's respiratory rate remains between 16 and 20

3. Diagnosis: Risk for Ineffective Airway Clearance related to impaired gag reflex and unconscious state

4. Client outcome: client's breath sounds remain clear

5. Diagnosis: Risk for Ineffective Peripheral Tissue Perfusion

6. Client outcome: oxygen saturation measured by pulse oximeter remains 95–100%

C. Nursing diagnoses and expected outcomes for postoperative period

1. Nursing diagnoses related to gas exchange/airway clearance and tissue perfusion continue to be important during this period

2. Diagnosis: Risk for Infection related to loss of skin integrity

3. Client outcome: client remains free of infection as evidenced by temperature within normal range, normal WBC count, and lack of wound redness

4. Diagnosis: Impaired Skin Integrity related to surgical procedure

5. Client outcome: client's skin heals within 2 weeks

6. Diagnosis: Pain related to trauma to tissue secondary to surgical procedure

7. Client outcome: client remains pain free as evidenced by verbalization, relaxed facial expression, and participation in postoperative activities

Case Study

A 14-year-old female is admitted for an abdominal exploratory laparotomy. She has been complaining of abdominal pain intermittently for several months.

1. What ethical issues surround obtaining informed consent?

2. Discuss pertinent questions the nurse needs to ask about her history.

3. List 2 preoperative nursing diagnoses that might be appropriate for her.

4. Discuss what she needs to be taught about her postoperative care.

5. The client will have general anesthesia. Discuss what the nurse should tell her about the anesthesia.

For suggested responses, see page 308.

POSTTEST

1 A client is being admitted to the hospital on the day before a scheduled surgery. What is the most appropriate initial question for the nurse to ask this preoperative client?

1. "What did your surgeon say to you about the type of surgery you are having?"
2. "What questions do you have about your surgery?"
3. "What type of surgery are you having and why are you having it done?"
4. "What do you know about what will be done to you?"

2 A preoperative client asks the nurse for more information about the advantages of a general anesthetic. Which response would be appropriate for the nurse to include for the client?

1. Respiratory and circulatory functions are depressed.
2. Client loses consciousness and does not perceive pain.
3. Anesthetic agent is slowly excreted so that the timing of surgery can be adjusted.
4. Possibility of the client experiencing amnesia is reduced.

3 A benzodiazepine has been administered to a client preoperatively. After the drug has been administered, the nurse plans to monitor the client for which side effects? Select all that apply.

1. Anxiety
2. Hypotension
3. Hypocalcemia
4. Level of consciousness
5. Sedation

4 A preoperative client has an elevated hemoglobin and hematocrit. What would the nurse suspect regarding the significance of this increased value?

1. Immune deficiency
2. Kidney dysfunction
3. Malignancy
4. Dehydration

5 The nurse has completed preoperative teaching with a pregnant woman. During the discussion, the nurse describes the different types of anesthesia available. Which statement by the client indicates to the nurse an understanding of regional anesthesia?

1. "In spinal anesthesia, the anesthetic agent is injected into the subarachnoid space."
2. "The anesthetic agent is injected into the dura mater of the spinal cord for epidural anesthesia."
3. "The client is sedated and has some awareness of the event."
4. "Regional anesthesia produces analgesia and amnesia."

6 The client arrives in the postanesthesia care unit (PACU) in an unconscious state. In what position would the nurse place this client in the immediate postanesthesia stage?

1. Side lying with the face slightly down
2. Side lying with a pillow under the client's head
3. Semi-prone position with the head tilted to the side
4. Dorsal recumbent with head turned to the side

7 The client has been in the postanesthesia care unit (PACU) for one hour. The client is now groggy but able to respond to voice commands. While assessing the client, for what reason would the nurse check the bedclothes underneath the client?

1. Determine drainage from tubes or drains.
2. Assess for fluid balance.
3. Detect possible hemorrhage.
4. Monitor perspiration.

8 A client is in the postoperative stage and the health care provider has prescribed ambulation. The client has shown difficulty understanding the necessity for early ambulation. The nurse would formulate which appropriate nursing diagnosis for this client?

1. Self-Care Deficit
2. Deficient Knowledge
3. Ineffective Coping
4. Risk for Injury

9 The nurse is assessing a client upon return to the nursing unit from the postanesthesia care unit (PACU) and notices the presence of a drain in the surgical wound. A family member sees the drain and asks why the tube was left in the wound. What information should the nurse include in the explanation related to drains?

1. Allows drainage of excessive fluids such as blood, lymph, or pus from the surgical site
2. Promotes healing to occur at an accelerated rate
3. Prompts healing to occur from the inside out
4. Provides a means for connecting suction tubes

10 A client is being discharged following outpatient surgery. The nurse, who is providing the caregiver with instructions for wound care, would instruct the caregiver to report which findings to the surgeon?

1. Scar formation
2. Increased redness or drainage
3. Nonnoxious odor of the wound drainage
4. Thin, pale, yellow color of the drainage

➤ *See pages 234–235 for Answers and Rationales.*

See pages 234–235 for Answers and Rationales.

POSTTEST

ANSWERS & RATIONALES

ANSWERS & RATIONALES

Pretest

1 **Answers: 1, 2, 5** **Rationale:** Assessment in the preoperative phase includes anticipating any health problems that may occur during and after surgery. The nurse also has the responsibility to validate the presence of an informed consent form before the client is moved to the surgery area. The appropriate time to assess the effectiveness of preoperative teaching is before surgery. The client will need to utilize the skills during the postoperative phase in order to promote healing and prevent complications. Assessing response to interventions is a very general activity that should occur at any time. Prevention of complications occurs in the postoperative stage. **Cognitive Level:** Applying **Client Need:** Reduction of Risk Potential **Integrated Process:** Nursing Process: Implementation

Content Area: Fundamentals **Strategy:** The critical term is *preoperative period.* Recall activities associated with each phase of the perioperative period to direct you to provide care to clients in each phase. When there is more than one correct answer, consider each option as a true-false statement. **Reference:** Berman, A., & Snyder, S. J. (2012). *Kozier & Erb's fundamentals of nursing: Concepts, process, and practice* (9th ed.). Upper Saddle River, NJ: Pearson Education, pp. 962–973.

2 **Answer: 3** **Rationale:** Ablative surgery involves removal of diseased body parts. Breast augmentation following a mastectomy is classified as reconstructive surgery. A surgical procedure that involves attaining a biopsy is considered diagnostic. Nerve root resections are most frequently performed for clients with intractable pain and are considered to be palliative in nature.

Cognitive Level: Applying **Client Need:** Reduction of Risk Potential **Integrated Process:** Nursing Process: Diagnosis **Content Area:** Fundamentals **Strategy:** Knowledge of terminology related to purposes and types of surgery will enable you to recognize the accurate option and make a correct selection. **Reference:** Berman, A., & Snyder, S. J. (2012). *Kozier & Erb's fundamentals of nursing: Concepts, process, and practice* (9th ed.). Upper Saddle River, NJ: Pearson Education, p. 960.

3 **Answers: 2, 5 Rationale:** When surgery is performed on vital organs and when there is a greater likelihood for complications due to client age and condition (such as health disorders), there is a greater likelihood for complications and therefore the risk is higher. Risk is not associated with the place where surgery is performed; also, this is not a client-related factor. Risk is associated with poor nutritional status. The higher the likelihood of complications, the greater the risk. **Cognitive Level:** Applying **Client Need:** Reduction of Risk Potential **Integrated Process:** Nursing Process: Assessment **Content Area:** Fundamentals **Strategy:** The critical terms are *client-related factors* and *high degree of risk*. Being able to recall surgical risks is vital to care and client education and is the core issue of the question. Use nursing knowledge and the process of elimination to make a selection. When there is more than one correct answer, consider each option as a true-false statement. **Reference:** Berman, A., & Snyder, S. J. (2012). *Kozier & Erb's fundamentals of nursing: Concepts, process, and practice* (9th ed.). Upper Saddle River, NJ: Pearson Education, pp. 960–962.

4 **Answer: 2 Rationale:** The infant has immature vital organs that affect the infant's ability to metabolize medications such as the anesthetic and the ability to resist infection. Infants do not have declines in functioning. Hypothermia is more likely to occur than hyperthermia since the infant has an immature temperature regulation and large body surface area. The volume of blood in an infant is limited and does not fluctuate. **Cognitive Level:** Applying **Client Need:** Reduction of Risk Potential **Integrated Process:** Nursing Process: Diagnosis **Content Area:** Fundamentals **Strategy:** To answer the question correctly, it is necessary to have knowledge of surgical risk factors, which will then enable you to make an accurate selection. **Reference:** Berman, A., & Snyder, S. J. (2012). *Kozier & Erb's fundamentals of nursing: Concepts, process, and practice* (9th ed.). Upper Saddle River, NJ: Pearson Education, pp. 960–961.

5 **Answer: 1 Rationale:** Since preschool-age children have a very limited understanding of cause and effect, they often interpret illness and related procedures such as surgery as punishment for bad behavior. Appearance is not a primary concern at this age. Anticipating inability of doing things is not a concern at this developmental level. Preschool-age children are unaware of competency issues of medical personnel. **Cognitive Level:** Analyzing **Client Need:** Health Promotion and Maintenance **Integrated Process:** Nursing Process: Diagnosis **Content Area:** Fundamentals

Strategy: The critical words are *preschool-age child*. Understanding developmental stages and tasks will enable you to make the best selection using the process of elimination. **Reference:** Berman, A., & Snyder, S. J. (2012). *Kozier & Erb's fundamentals of nursing: Concepts, process, and practice* (9th ed.). Upper Saddle River, NJ: Pearson Education, pp. 960–961.

6 **Answer: 1 Rationale:** Although all the options contain aspects that need assessment, initially vital signs, level of consciousness, and presence of pain are the most important to assess because they relate to physiological needs and are more global indicators of overall functioning than the other options. **Cognitive Level:** Applying **Client Need:** Reduction of Risk Potential **Integrated Process:** Nursing Process: Assessment **Content Area:** Fundamentals **Strategy:** The critical terms are *priority needs* and *immediately*. Recall the necessary nursing responsibilities for the postoperative client and the relative importance of these responsibilities to enable you to set priorities for care. **Reference:** Berman, A., & Snyder, S. J. (2012). *Kozier & Erb's fundamentals of nursing: Concepts, process, and practice* (9th ed.). Upper Saddle River, NJ: Pearson Education, p. 976.

7 **Answers: 1, 4, 5 Rationale:** The color of the skin, nails, and lips are indicators of tissue perfusion, and pallor and cyanosis indicate alteration. Decreased urinary output related to hypovolemia is also an indicator of alteration in tissue perfusion. Fluid loss can ultimately contribute to a reduction in tissue perfusion. Mobility alterations and the presence of pain are incorrect as they are not signs of tissue perfusion. **Cognitive Level:** Analyzing **Client Need:** Reduction of Risk Potential **Integrated Process:** Nursing Process: Assessment **Content Area:** Fundamentals **Strategy:** The critical phrase is *alteration in tissue perfusion*. Recall the signs and symptoms of common postoperative complications to assist you in making accurate nursing diagnoses. When more than one answer is correct, consider each option as a true-false statement. **Reference:** Berman, A., & Snyder, S. J. (2012). *Kozier & Erb's fundamentals of nursing: Concepts, process, and practice* (9th ed.). Upper Saddle River, NJ: Pearson Education, pp. 977–978.

8 **Answer: 4 Rationale:** Turning side to side allows the lungs alternatively to expand properly. Peristalsis increases with movement even if it is not turning, and muscle weakness can be lessened with movement. Turning does not necessarily induce sleep. **Cognitive Level:** Applying **Client Need:** Reduction of Risk Potential **Integrated Process:** Teaching and Learning **Content Area:** Fundamentals **Strategy:** Knowledge of potential postoperative complications will enable you to use client education as a tool to prevent their occurrence. Recall that promoting lung expansion prevents complications. **Reference:** Berman, A., & Snyder, S. J. (2012). *Kozier & Erb's fundamentals of nursing: Concepts, process, and practice* (9th ed.). Upper Saddle River, NJ: Pearson Education, pp. 978–980.

9 **Answer: 3 Rationale:** The first sign of healing is absence of bleeding and wound edges bound by fibrin in the clot.

Inflammation at the wound edges follows the first sign, and then when the clot diminishes, inflammation decreases and collagen forms a scar. **Cognitive Level:** Analyzing **Client Need:** Reduction of Risk Potential **Integrated Process:** Nursing Process: Evaluation **Content Area:** Fundamentals **Strategy:** The critical term is *first stage of healing.* Recall the differences among the various stages of healing to make an appropriate selection. **Reference:** Berman, A., & Snyder, S. J. (2012). *Kozier & Erb's fundamentals of nursing: Concepts, process, and practice* (9th ed.). Upper Saddle River, NJ: Pearson Education, p. 988.

10 **Answers: 3, 5** **Rationale:** The absence of nonverbal signs of pain is an appropriate outcome for a postoperative client. The process of verbally rating pain as a 3 on a 1 to 10 pain scale is an appropriate outcome for a postoperative client. Balanced fluid intake and output, seeking help as needed, and performing leg exercises are useful findings in the overall management of a postoperative client but are not directly related to pain management. **Cognitive Level:** Applying **Client Need:** Basic Care and Comfort **Integrated Process:** Nursing Process: Planning **Content Area:** Fundamentals **Strategy:** The critical words are *Acute Pain.* Recall that client outcome statements must always be directly related to the problem. When there is more than one correct answer, consider each option as a true-false statement. **Reference:** Berman, A., & Snyder, S. J. (2012). *Kozier & Erb's fundamentals of nursing: Concepts, process, and practice* (9th ed.). Upper Saddle River, NJ: Pearson Education, pp. 981–982.

Posttest

1 **Answer: 3** **Rationale:** Assessing the client's understanding is the best initial action by the nurse because it is exploratory in nature and will provide a basis for further communication with the client. The incorrect responses focus on the surgeon, represent an inquiry that is too broad, or are focused initially on the surgery. **Cognitive Level:** Applying **Client Need:** Reduction of Risk Potential **Integrated Process:** Communication and Documentation **Content Area:** Fundamentals **Strategy:** The critical terms are *most appropriate* and *initial.* Recall that preoperative care responsibilities include assessment of client knowledge of the impending procedure, which will then enable client teaching that enhances postoperative outcomes. **Reference:** Berman, A., & Snyder, S. J. (2012). *Kozier & Erb's fundamentals of nursing: Concepts, process, and practice* (9th ed.). Upper Saddle River, NJ: Pearson Education, p. 964.

2 **Answer: 2** **Rationale:** General anesthetics produce central nervous system depression so that clients lose consciousness and do not perceive pain. Respiratory and circulatory depression is a disadvantage of general anesthetics because there is a greater risk for complications, especially for clients with chronic illnesses. General anesthetic agents are rapidly excreted and produce amnesia. **Cognitive Level:** Applying **Client Need:** Pharmacological and Parenteral Therapies **Integrated Process:** Teaching and Learning **Content Area:** Fundamentals **Strategy:** Recall the major classifications of anesthesia and their advantages and disadvantages and use the process of elimination to make a selection. **Reference:** Berman, A., & Snyder, S. J. (2012). *Kozier & Erb's fundamentals of nursing: Concepts, process, and practice* (9th ed.). Upper Saddle River, NJ: Pearson Education, pp. 973–974.

3 **Answers: 2, 4, 5** **Rationale:** Benzodiazepines such as lorazepam and diazepam decrease anxiety as an intended effect and produce side effects such as hypotension and sedation. After administering a benzodiazepine, the nurse should frequently assess the client's level of consciousness and monitor vital signs for changes. Hypocalcemia is not an adverse effect of this class of drugs. **Cognitive Level:** Applying **Client Need:** Pharmacological and Parenteral Therapies **Integrated Process:** Nursing Process: Evaluation **Content Area:** Fundamentals **Strategy:** The critical words are *benzodiazepine* and *side effects.* Recall common side effects of frequently used perioperative medications and use the process of elimination to make a selection. When more than one answer is correct, consider each option as a true-false statement. **Reference:** Berman, A., & Snyder, S. J. (2012). *Kozier & Erb's fundamentals of nursing: Concepts, process, and practice* (9th ed.). Upper Saddle River, NJ: Pearson Education, p. 969.

4 **Answer: 4** **Rationale:** An increased hemoglobin and hematocrit may be a result of dehydration. Immune deficiency is an indication of decreased white blood cell count, while an increase in electrolytes such as potassium, sodium, or chloride indicate kidney dysfunction. Malignancy may be suspected in increased platelet count. **Cognitive Level:** Analyzing **Client Need:** Reduction of Risk Potential **Integrated Process:** Nursing Process: Diagnosis **Content Area:** Fundamentals **Strategy:** The critical phrase is *elevated hemoglobin and hematocrit.* Recall the usual causes of common lab abnormalities and use the process of elimination to identify conditions that need to be corrected prior to surgery. **Reference:** Berman, A., & Snyder, S. J. (2012). *Kozier & Erb's fundamentals of nursing: Concepts, process, and practice* (9th ed.). Upper Saddle River, NJ: Pearson Education, p. 963.

5 **Answer: 1** **Rationale:** The anesthetic agent is injected into the subarachnoid space for spinal anesthesia and into the epidural space (which is outside the dura mater) in epidural anesthesia. Regional anesthesia can include local or topical anesthesia or nerve blocks and do not require clients to have sedation or produce amnesia. **Cognitive Level:** Applying **Client Need:** Pharmacological and Parenteral Therapies **Integrated Process:** Teaching and Learning **Content Area:** Fundamentals **Strategy:** Recall information about the basic types of regional anesthesia and use the process of elimination to make a selection. **Reference:** Berman, A., & Snyder, S. J. (2012). *Kozier & Erb's fundamentals of nursing: Concepts, process, and practice* (9th ed.). Upper Saddle River, NJ: Pearson Education, p. 973.

6 **Answer: 1** **Rationale:** Placing the client in a side-lying position with the face slightly down will utilize gravity to keep the tongue forward, which prevents aspiration. A pillow would elevate the head. The semi-prone position is unsafe in most cases as it may interfere with breathing. A dorsal recumbent position does not protect the client from risk of aspiration because secretions could pool in the back of the throat. **Cognitive Level:** Applying **Client Need:** Reduction of Risk Potential **Integrated Process:** Nursing Process: Implementation **Content Area:** Fundamentals **Strategy:** The critical words are *immediate post-anesthesia stage.* Recall interventions for airway maintenance in the postanesthetic period to enable you to provide safe care for this client. **Reference:** Berman, A., & Snyder, S. J. (2012). *Kozier & Erb's fundamentals of nursing: Concepts, process, and practice* (9th ed.). Upper Saddle River, NJ: Pearson Education, p. 976.

7 **Answer: 3** **Rationale:** Excessive bloody drainage on dressings or the bedclothes, often underneath (because of gravity) the client, indicates hemorrhage. This technique would not be useful in determining tube drainage, fluid balance in the general sense, or perspiration. **Cognitive Level:** Applying **Client Need:** Reduction of Risk Potential **Integrated Process:** Nursing Process: Assessment **Content Area:** Fundamentals **Strategy:** The critical phrase is *underneath the client.* Recall that gravity will cause blood from a wound to travel to the lowest point, which is generally beneath the client. **Reference:** Berman, A., & Snyder, S. J. (2012). *Kozier & Erb's fundamentals of nursing: Concepts, process, and practice* (9th ed.). Upper Saddle River, NJ: Pearson Education, pp. 976–977.

8 **Answer: 2** **Rationale:** The client appears unable to retain the information related to the benefits of early ambulation and therefore has a deficiency in knowledge base. There is no indication that the client is exhibiting ineffective coping or is at increased risk for injury. **Cognitive Level:** Applying **Client Need:** Reduction of Risk Potential **Integrated Process:** Teaching and Learning **Content Area:** Fundamentals **Strategy:** The critical term is *difficulty understanding.* Select the nursing diagnosis that focuses on a learning need. **Reference:** Berman, A., & Snyder, S. J. (2012). *Kozier & Erb's fundamentals of nursing: Concepts, process, and practice* (9th ed.). Upper Saddle River, NJ: Pearson Education, p. 983.

9 **Answer: 1** **Rationale:** Placement of surgical drains will allow for drainage of excessive fluid or possibly purulent material that may have accumulated during the surgery. Healing is promoted, but not necessarily at a rapid rate, and not all drains have to be shortened or connected to suction. **Cognitive Level:** Analyzing **Client Need:** Reduction of Risk Potential **Integrated Process:** Teaching and Learning **Content Area:** Fundamentals **Strategy:** The critical phrase in the correct answer option is *allows drainage of excessive fluids such as blood, edema, or pus from the surgical site.* Recall the uses of surgical site wound drains and use the process of elimination to make a selection. **Reference:** Berman, A., & Snyder, S. J. (2012). *Kozier & Erb's fundamentals of nursing: Concepts, process, and practice* (9th ed.). Upper Saddle River, NJ: Pearson Education, pp. 991–992.

10 **Answer: 2** **Rationale:** Increased redness or drainage could indicate wound infection. Scar formation, nonnoxious odor to wound drainage, and pale yellow drainage are characteristics consistent with normal wound healing. **Cognitive Level:** Analyzing **Client Need:** Reduction of Risk Potential **Integrated Process:** Teaching and Learning **Content Area:** Fundamentals **Strategy:** The core issue of the question is knowledge of which postoperative findings warrant notification of the surgeon. Recall basic nursing knowledge about postoperative care and teaching and use the process of elimination to make a selection. **Reference:** Berman, A., & Snyder, S. J. (2012). *Kozier & Erb's fundamentals of nursing: Concepts, process, and practice* (9th ed.). Upper Saddle River, NJ: Pearson Education, pp. 926–928.

References

Association of PeriOperative Registered Nurses (AORN) (2006). *Standards, recommended practices and guidelines.* Denver: AORN, Inc.

Ball, J. W., Bindler, R. C., & Cowen, K. (2010). *Child health nursing: Partnering with children and families* (2nd ed.). Upper Saddle River, NJ: Pearson Education.

Berman, A., & Snyder, S. J. (2012). *Kozier & Erb's fundamentals of nursing: Concepts, process, and practice* (9th ed.). Upper Saddle River, NJ: Pearson Education.

LeMone, P. Burke, K., & Bauldoff, G. (2012). *Medical-surgical nursing: Critical thinking in patient care* (5th ed.). Upper Saddle River, NJ: Pearson Education.

Osborn, K. S., Wraa, C. E., & Watson, A. (2010). *Medical-surgical nursing: Preparation for practice* (Vol. Combined). Upper Saddle River, NJ: Pearson Education.

ANSWERS & RATIONALES

10

Meeting Needs of Clients With Altered Skin Integrity, Sensory Perception, or Mobility

Chapter Outline

Skin Integrity and Wound Care

Alterations in Sensory or Perceptual Ability

Altered Mobility

NCLEX-RN® Test Prep

Use the accompanying online resource, NursingReviewsandRationales, to test yourself with hundreds of NCLEX®-style practice questions.

Objectives

➤ Classify types of wounds and the products used to promote skin integrity.
➤ Define the elements associated with alterations in sensory perception.
➤ Identify methods the nurse can use to promote self-care and safety for clients with sensory perception deficits.
➤ List common causes and complications of immobility.
➤ Discuss the purpose and types of exercise for individuals with mobility problems.
➤ Describe the correct and safe use of assistive devices that facilitate ambulation.

Review at a Glance

conductive hearing loss interrupted transmission of sound through ear

debridement removal of dead necrotic tissue from a wound

dehiscence an unintentional opening of a wound

evisceration bursting open of a suture line with protrusion of organs

hyperopia farsightedness

keloid scar tissue

myopia nearsightedness

orthostatic intolerance also called postural hypotension, a transient drop in blood pressure caused by a change in position that may be

accompanied by dizziness or vertigo; the client should change positions slowly

presbycusis loss of hearing related to aging process

presbyopia loss of elasticity of lens of eye related to aging process

primary intention healing of a wound without infection or scarring; wound edges are well approximated

pressure ulcers lesions involving skin and underlying tissues caused by inadequate blood supply secondary to unrelieved pressure

purulent exudate wound drainage containing pus

secondary intention wound healing by granulation or indirect union; edges are widely separated and granulation tissue fills in between the edges

sensory deficit impairment of both reception and perception of one or more senses

sensory deprivation lack of stimuli that is meaningful

sensory overload bombardment of an individual by stimuli that have no meaning to that person

wound a break in skin or mucous membranes resulting from physical means

PRETEST

1 The nurse assessing a bedridden client notes a large erythemic area on the client's buttocks. In addition, the center of the area looks like an abrasion with a shallow crater. The nurse would document this ulcer as being at which stage?

1. Stage I
2. Stage II
3. Stage III
4. Stage IV

2 A client was assessed to have a Stage I pressure ulcer on his hip despite turning and positioning every 2 hours. The nurse formulates which of the following as the appropriate nursing diagnosis for this client?

1. Impaired Skin Integrity related to infrequent turning and positioning
2. Impaired Skin Integrity related to the effects of pressure
3. Risk for Impaired Skin Integrity related to redness
4. Risk for Pressure Ulcer

3 A nurse is working in a screening clinic in an elderly housing complex. The nurse expects that the skin of a normal older adult client will have which of the following characteristics? Select all that apply.

1. Appearance of being tight and shiny with edema in distal legs
2. Moist with elastic skin turgor
3. Skin turgor showing a loss of elasticity
4. Overhydration causing the skin to wrinkle
5. Fragile skin that is wrinkled

4 A hospitalized client exhibits all of the following symptoms: excessive yawning, drowsiness, impaired memory, crying, and depression. The nurse would suspect which of the following problems?

1. Sensory deprivation
2. Sensory overload
3. Visual deficit
4. Auditory deficit

5 In planning nursing care to prevent pressure ulcers in the bedridden client, the nurse should include which of the following interventions? Select all that apply.

1. Lift the client when turning or repositioning.
2. Assess the condition of the bed linens frequently, changing whenever damp or soiled.
3. Vigorously massage bony prominences.
4. Post a turning schedule at the client's bedside.
5. Use a bed sheet that has been folded into quarters for a turning sheet.

6 A nurse preceptor overhears 2 student nurses discussing techniques for dressing changes. The nurse concludes that the student who needs to review the skill is the one who makes which statement?

1. "I will clean the wound from the center out."
2. "To remove the used dressing, I should wear sterile gloves."
3. "After I clean the wound, I should assess its appearance."
4. "While irrigating the wound, I can use a catheter, which is placed close to the open area."

7 A client with a hearing impairment is admitted to a busy hospital unit. Which intervention is most important for the nurse to employ to meet the client's needs while preventing sensory overload?

1. Encourage all of the client's family members to stay with the client at all times.
2. Address the client directly and face the client during the conversation.
3. Keep the television or radio on for the client continuously.
4. Keep the overhead light on at all times.

8 A 78-year-old client who is visually impaired is admitted to the nursing unit. Which of the following interventions selected by the nurse would be most appropriate in reducing sensory deprivation?

1. Adjust window shades to reduce glare.
2. Keep doors open to provide indirect light in the room.
3. Avoid use of overhead lighting.
4. Keep lights in the room dimmed.

9 A client uses a cane to assist with ambulation. After teaching the client how to use a cane, which statement made by the client indicates to the nurse the need for additional teaching?

1. "My elbow should be slightly flexed while using the cane."
2. "I should hold the cane on my affected side."
3. "A walker would be better to use than a cane."
4. "While walking here in the hospital, I need to wear my shoes because socks alone may cause me to slip."

10 Which of the following client wounds would the nurse expect to heal by secondary intention? Select all that apply.

1. A surgical incision that is closed with staples
2. A clean leg laceration that was closed with sutures
3. A large, open abdominal wound from a gunshot injury
4. A Stage 4 pressure ulcer
5. A puncture wound to the finger from a sewing needle

➤ *See pages 256–257 for Answers and Rationales.*

I. SKIN INTEGRITY AND WOUND CARE

A. Normal skin integrity

1. Skin is the largest organ in the body
2. Five functions of skin

   a. It is the body's first line of defense against microorganisms; as such, it serves as a barrier preventing invasion by microorganisms; this function is interrupted if skin is not intact
   b. It assists in regulating body temperature
   c. It is a sense organ transmitting sensations of pain, temperature, touch, and pressure
   d. It synthesizes vitamin D
   e. It secretes sebum that has several functions, including softening and lubricating skin and hair
3. Layers of skin vary in thickness but in places can be as thick as 1/4 in.; skin can be divided into layers of epidermis and dermis; beneath the dermis is a subcutaneous layer of tissue
   a. Epidermis: outermost layer of skin made of stratified squamous epithelial cells; epidermis can be further divided into 5 layers, the innermost of which is the basal-cell layer, the cells responsible for replacing sloughed and damaged cells
   b. Dermis: second layer of skin composed of connective tissue; is the layer that gives elasticity to skin; blood vessels, nerve fibers, glands, and hair follicles are embedded in this layer
   c. Subcutaneous tissue: consists of adipose tissue and provides support and blood flow to dermis
4. Skin glands: skin has 3 kinds of glands, sebaceous glands, sudoriferous glands, and ceruminous glands
   a. Sebaceous glands are within the dermis; they secrete an oily substance called sebum, made up of fats, cholesterol, proteins, and salts; sebum protects hair from drying, forms a protective film on skin that prevents excessive evaporation of water, and inhibits growth of certain bacteria on skin
   b. Sudoriferous glands (sweat glands) produce a watery secretion; body has up to 5 million sweat glands that are present at birth; there are 2 types: apocrine and eccrine
      1) Apocrine glands are primarily in axilla and pubic regions and begin functioning at puberty; secretions are odorous because, when decomposed by bacteria, they produce an unpleasant odor

       2) Eccrine glands are distributed throughout skin; they are chiefly found on palms of hands, soles of feet, and forehead; they produce a watery discharge to help cool body through evaporation

    c. Ceruminous glands secrete a thick, oily substance called cerumen, a waxy secretion of external ear (also known as earwax)

  5. Skin alterations related to aging: overall health status, age, nutritional status, and energy or activity level play a role in maintaining a client's skin condition; normal skin changes associated with aging include:

    a. Thinning of epidermis and an associated lower water content, leading to dry skin

    b. Elasticity and some of the fatty cushion is lost, resulting in wrinkles and fragile skin

    c. Blood vessels in skin also become more fragile with aging, leading to easy bruising

B. Classification of wounds: a **wound** is a break in skin or mucous membranes resulting from physical trauma; a wound may be superficial (affecting only skin surface) or deep (involving blood vessels, nerves, muscle, fascia, tendons, ligaments, and bones)

  1. Open versus closed: is a classification of wounds according to continuity of the surface it covers (tissue involved)

    a. An open wound is characterized by a break in skin and could be superficial or deep; examples are an abrasion, laceration, or puncture

    b. A closed wound is one in which there is no break in skin; examples are a contusion and ecchymosis; these injuries may be caused by a blow or another type of blunt force or trauma

  2. Superficial and full and partial thickness refer to depth of injury and are used most frequently to refer to burns or pressure-related injuries

    a. Superficial thickness involves only epidermis

    b. Partial thickness involves entire epidermis and part of dermis; sweat glands and hair follicles are intact

    c. Full thickness involves epidermis and dermis extending to subcutaneous tissue, possibly even muscle and bone

  3. Clean versus infected wounds

    a. A noninfected or clean wound has not been invaded by pathogenic microorganisms; a clean wound heals without infection

    b. An infected or septic wound is one in which pathogenic microorganisms have invaded the wound and clinical signs and symptoms of infection develop

  4. Surgical wound: an intentional wound made by a surgeon for therapeutic purposes using a sharp cutting instrument; it is a clean wound that is expected to heal without infection

  5. Pressure ulcers: lesions caused by unrelieved pressure; this in turn damages underlying tissues

    a. Contributing factors

      1) Pressure ulcers occur mainly in people who are chairbound, bedbound, or have an altered level of consciousness (LOC) that causes them to be immobile

      2) Older adults are at greater risk for developing pressure ulcers because of fragility of skin, loss of subcutaneous tissue, and decreased mobility

      3) Moisture on skin from sweating or incontinence can lead to skin breakdown

      4) Malnutrition contributes because of reduced nutrient stores including protein for tissue repair

      5) Shearing pressures cause injury by contributing to tissue hypoxia; this often occurs when head of the bed is elevated, when skin remains stationary while underlying tissues shift with pull of gravity

      6) Friction that occurs when a client is moved in the bed contributes to tissue damage and can be a precursor to a pressure ulcer

      7) Clients who were allowed to become hypothermic during surgical procedures are at a substantially increased risk for development of pressure ulcers

      8) Contributing factors can be assessed to determine an individual client's relative risk using scales such as Braden Scale or Norton Scale (see Table 10-1)

  b. Four stages of pressure ulcers

    1) Stage 1: skin is intact, although nonblanching erythema will be noted; blanching is done by applying and quickly releasing pressure to an area to determine color changes of skin; nonblanching erythema shows no color change, while blanching erythema is a reddened area that turns white or pale when blanched; client may report tingling or burning; darker-skinned clients may have skin discoloration, warmth, edema, and induration or hardness as indicators

Table 10-1 Pressure Ulcer Risk Assessment Scales

Norton Scale

Physical Condition		Mental Condition		Activity		Mobility		Continence		
Good	4	Alert	4	Walks	4	Full	4	Good	4	
Fair	3	Apathetic	3	Walks with help	3	Slightly limited	3	Occasional incontinence	3	
Poor	2	Confused	2	Sits in chair	2	Very limited	2	Frequent incontinence	2	
Very poor	1	Stuporous	1	Remains in bed	1	Immobile	1	Urine and fecal incontinence	1	
Total ____		Total ____		Total ____		Total ____		Total ____		

Grand total = _____

A score of 14 or less indicates risk of pressure ulcer; a score under 12 indicates high risk.

Braden Scale

Sensory Perception		Moisture		Activity		Mobility		Nutrition		Friction and Shear	
No impairment	4	Rarely moist	4	Walks frequently	4	No limitations	4	Excellent	4		
Slightly limited	3	Occasionally moist	3	Walks occasionally	3	Slightly limited	3	Adequate	3	No apparent problems	3
Very limited	2	Moist	2	Chairfast	2	Very limited	2	Probably inadequate	2	Potential problem	2
Completely limited	1	Constantly moist	1	Bedfast	1	Immobile	1	Very poor	1	Problem	1
Total ____		Total ____		Total ____		Total ____		Total ____		Total ____	

Grand total = _____

Assign a score of 1 to 4 in each category. Total the score; no risk: 19–23; at risk: 15–18; moderate risk: 13–14; high risk: 10–12; very high risk: 9 or below.
Norton Scale: Adapted from *Pressure Ulcers in Adults: Predictions and Prevention.* AHCRP Publication No. 92-0047 1992, Agency for Healthcare Research, U.S. Department of Health and Human Services.
Braden Scale: Adapted from *Pressure Ulcers in Adults: Predictions and Prevention.* AHCRP Publication No. 92-0047 1992, Agency for Healthcare Research, U.S. Department of Health and Human Services..

Source: Smith, Sandra F.; Duell, Donna J.; & Martin, Barbara C.; *Clinical Nursing Skills: Basic to Advanced Skills*, 7th Ed. Reprinted and electronically produced by permission of Pearson Education, Inc., Upper Saddle River, New Jersey.

    2) Stage 2: involves superficial or partial-thickness skin loss with blister or abrasion-like appearance; it may also look like a shallow crater

    3) Stage 3: full-thickness skin loss; necrotic tissue will be seen in subcutaneous layer that extends down to (but not through) underlying fascia; ulcer will appear as a deeper crater with or without undermining of surrounding tissue

    4) Stage 4: continuation of Stage 3 with damage to muscle, bone, and supporting structures such as tendons or joint capsule; undermining of tissue and sinus tracts may also be present

C. Wound healing

    1. The process of wound healing can be divided into 3 phases

       a. Inflammatory phase: occurs immediately after injury and lasts 3 to 4 days; a blood clot forms a fibrin matrix, which becomes the framework for cell repair; blood flow increases to area, bringing oxygen and nutrients for healing; phagocytosis occurs to remove microorganisms and cellular debris; the wound surface dries out, forming a scab that seals the skin

       b. Proliferative phase: fibroblasts synthesize collagen to add tensile strength to wound and deposit fibrin as this phase occurs (4 to 21 days), granulation tissue forms and is very friable, soft, and pinkish red in color because of new capillaries in the area; next, epithelial cells grow from edges to cover the wound; connective tissue then fills area and becomes a scar that is stronger than granulation tissue; when wound is extensive and cannot close by epithelialization, the area becomes covered with eschar, consisting of dead cells and dried plasma proteins

       c. Maturation or remodeling phase is the healing of the scar; often occurs by day 21, but can extend for 1 to 2 years after injury; this phase is characterized by reorganization of collagen fibers, wound remodeling and contraction, and tissue maturation; a fully healed wound has tensile strength that still will not exceed 80% of preinjury state, making it more susceptible to injury in the future; in some clients (particularly those with dark skin), an abnormal amount of collagen is laid down, forming a hypertrophic scar called a **keloid**

    2. Factors affecting wound healing include age, nutrition, condition of the tissue, efficiency of circulation, medication, and the relationship between rest and anxiety or stress

       a. Age: healthy children and adults heal faster than older clients; see Box 10-1 for factors that inhibit healing in older adults

---

Box 10-1 **Factors Inhibiting Wound Healing in Older Adults**	• Vascular changes associated with aging, such as atherosclerosis and atrophy of capillaries in the skin, can impair blood flow to the wound. • Collagen tissue is less flexible, which increases the risk of damage from pressure, friction, and shearing. • Scar tissue is less elastic. • Changes in the immune system may reduce the formation of antibodies and monocytes necessary for wound healing. • Nutritional deficiencies may reduce the numbers of red blood cells and leukocytes, thus impeding the delivery of oxygen and the inflammatory response essential for wound healing. Oxygen is needed for the synthesis of collagen and the formation of new epithelial cells. • Having diabetes or cardiovascular disease increases the risk of delayed healing due to impaired oxygen delivery to these tissues. • Cell renewal is slower, leading to delayed healing.

Source: Berman, Audrey J.; Snyder, Shirlee, *Kozier & Erb's Fundamentals of Nursing*, 9th Ed. © 2012. Reprinted and Electronically reproduced by permission of Pearson Education, Inc., Upper Saddle River, New Jersey.

     b. Nutrition: good physiological functioning is essential for wound healing; protein is needed to build new tissue and vitamin C for maturation of fibrous tissue; vitamin C also enhances protein synthesis; overall nutrition also affects healing; under-nourished clients may lack adequate body stores to utilize as nutrients, while obese clients tend to have decreased blood flow to tissue and have a greater risk of developing infection

     c. Condition of tissues: wound contamination and infection will slow down healing process; organisms present in wound will compete with body cells for oxygen and nutrition

     d. Efficiency of circulation: any factor that restricts blood supply to a wound will interfere with healing; blood transports the products used in healing; therefore factors such as damaged arteries, tissue edema, and dehydration impede healing; anemia and blood dyscrasias may interfere with oxygen reaching the tissue; conditions such as diabetes and liver dysfunction can also delay healing; individuals who participate in regular exercise tend to have better circulation and thus tend to heal faster; smoking is a risk factor that may limit amount of oxygen that blood can supply to tissues as well as causing vasoconstriction of peripheral vessels that will diminish blood flow to injured area

     e. Rest, anxiety, and stress: adequate rest of injured part will affect wound closure; anxiety and stress can stimulate release of hormones that will slow down healing; it is important that a client with a wound take measures to ensure adequate rest and reduce stress whenever possible

     f. Medications: anti-inflammatory drugs such as steroids or hormones slow down formation of fibrous tissue and therefore impair healing

  3. Wound healing is a natural function and occurs with primary and secondary union or as a result of surgical intervention

     a. The first type of healing is **primary intention**, characterized by return of tissues to normal with minimal inflammation and little if any scarring; wound edges are well approximated and wound heals without infection

     b. **Secondary intention** healing occurs when wound is extensive, and wound edges cannot or should not be approximated; there is greater injury and more granulation tissue is needed to close wound; healing by secondary intention is different from primary intention in a variety of ways: healing time is more prolonged, there is a deeper, more extensive scar, and risk for infection is greater since first line of defense is broken for an extended period

     c. Surgical interventions: sutures, staples, and clips are devices used to help approximate wound edges; sutures are threads used to sew tissues together; a variety of materials may be utilized, some that absorb and others that have to be removed; staples and clips are alternatives to suturing and are usually made of silver; these require removal in approximately 7 to 10 days

  4. Complications that affect wound healing

     a. Hemorrhage: after tissue damage occurs (from pressure, surgery, or trauma) bleeding usually results; this may result from rupture of small blood vessels or from trauma; internal hemorrhage may be noted by distention in wound area; external hemorrhage is noted by blood on dressing or leaking from dressing; if bleeding is severe then client may exhibit signs and symptoms of shock; risk of hemorrhage is greater within first 48 hours; if pressure dressings do not successfully stop bleeding, surgical intervention may be necessary

     b. Infection results from pathogenic microorganisms invading the wound; local clinical signs and symptoms of infection include redness, swelling, heat, and pain at the site; **purulent exudate** (consisting of leukocytes, liquefied dead tissue debris, and dead and living bacteria) may be noted; the client may be anorexic, nauseous, febrile, and have chills (systemic signs of infection); the provider may prescribe a wound culture, and antibiotics will usually be administered after culture is obtained

c. Dehiscence occurs when a wound's suture line accidently reopens; it usually involves an abdominal wound, but any wound could have this complication; layers of tissue under wound separate; this may occur because of an infected suture line or if client has any factor previously discussed that impedes wound healing; clients often state they "feel something giving way"; when abdominal dehiscence occurs, place client in bed with head of bed low to eliminate gravity and with knees bent to decrease pull on suture line; cover wound bed with large sterile dressings moistened with normal saline; notify surgeon immediately since surgical repair is usually necessary

d. Evisceration occurs when edges of a suture line separate and internal organs (viscera) protrude through incision; a number of factors contribute to this complication including infection, poor nutrition, failure of suture material, dehydration, and excessive coughing; evisceration is treated in a manner similar to dehiscence, and surgical repair will be required

D. Wound management therapies

1. Providers and certified wound care nurse consultants may choose a variety of therapies to treat wounds
2. A decision to apply or not to apply a dressing is based on several factors including location, size, and type of wound along with amount of exudate and presence or absence of infection; dressed and undressed wounds may require cleansing and irrigation to aid healing

E. Wound assessment

1. Inspect wound and gently palpate surrounding area regularly
2. Note whether wound edges are approximated; as an incision heals, a healing ridge may be noted
3. Note presence and characteristics of any drainage from wound
4. Observe for signs of infection: redness, swelling, increased tenderness, or disruption of wound edges; note body temperature and white blood cell count as other indicators
5. Purposes for dressing a wound
   a. Absorb drainage
   b. Splint or immobilize wound to provide rest
   c. Protect wound from mechanical injury
   d. Promote hemostasis
   e. Prevent contamination
   f. For client's mental and physical comfort
6. Purposes for maintaining a wound undressed
   a. Eliminate darkness and moisture that favor growth of microorganisms
   b. Allow for better observation and assessment of wound
   c. Facilitate bathing and hygiene
   d. Avoid adhesive tape reaction
   e. Avoid friction and irritation that destroy new epithelial cells
7. Wound irrigation: may be needed to cleanse or flush wound to enhance healing; normal saline and antibiotic solutions are solutions frequently used

F. Wound management products

1. Wound cleansers: all wounds need to be cleansed appropriately; in clean wounds where tissue is granulating, minimize any disruption of wound bed; use gentle cleansing techniques and rinse away debris with normal saline (see Box 10-2 for wound cleaning clinical guidelines)

Practice to Pass

The nurse is caring for a client who is 1 week postop from abdominal surgery. What would the nurse expect assessment of this wound to reveal?

Box 10-2	
Clinical Guidelines for Cleaning Wounds	• Follow standard precautions for personal protection. Wear gloves, gown, goggles, and mask as indicated. • Use solutions such as isotonic saline or wound cleansers to clean or irrigate wounds. If antimicrobial solutions are used, make sure they are well diluted. • Microwave heating is not recommended. When possible, warm the solution to body temperature before use. This prevents lowering of the wound temperature, which slows the healing process. Microwave heating could cause the solution to be too hot. • If a wound is grossly contaminated by foreign material, bacteria, slough, or necrotic tissue, clean the wound at every dressing change. Foreign bodies and devitalized tissue act as a focus for infection and can delay healing. • If a wound is clean, has little exudate, and reveals healthy granulation tissue, avoid repeated cleaning. Unnecessary cleaning can delay wound healing by traumatizing newly produced, delicate tissues, reducing the surface temperature of the wound, and removing exudate which itself may have bactericidal properties. • Use gauze squares. Avoid using cotton balls and other products that shed fibers onto the wound surface. The fibers become embedded in granulation tissue and can act as foci for infection. They may also stimulate "foreign body" reactions, prolonging the inflammatory phase of healing and delaying the healing process. • Clean superficial noninfected wounds by irrigating them with normal saline. The hydraulic pressure of an irrigating stream of fluid dislodges contaminating debris and reduces bacterial colonization. • To retain wound moisture, avoid drying a wound after cleaning it. • Hold cleaning sponges with forceps or with a sterile gloved hand. • Clean from the center of the wound in an outward direction to avoid transferring organisms from the surrounding skin into the wound. • Consider not cleaning the wound at all if it appears to be clean.

Source: Berman, Audrey J.; Snyder, Shirlee, *Kozier & Erb's Fundamentals of Nursing*, 9th Ed. © 2012. Reprinted and Electronically reproduced by permission of Pearson Education, Inc., Upper Saddle River, New Jersey.

2. Dressings: a variety of dressing materials are available, each with different purposes; some are designed to provide barrier protection from contamination; some may be impregnated with antibiotics; others are moist and aid in liquefying necrotic tissue; dressing types include:

   a. Gauze dressing: plain or impregnated with an antimicrobial; this dressing packs and fills wound; it absorbs drainage; gauze dressings are used for full- and partial-thickness wounds with drainage; may be applied dry to cover wound or as damp-to-damp dressing to pack a wound requiring debridement

   b. Transparent dressing: adhesive membrane that is occlusive to liquids and bacteria; protects wound and promotes autolytic **debridement** (removal of dead tissue from a wound); Op-site and Tegaderm are examples; transparent dressings are impermeable to bacteria

   c. Composite dressing: contains an absorbent pad and an adhesive covering; purpose is to absorb drainage; advantage of this type of wound coverage is that it only has to be changed 3 times per week

   d. Hydrocolloids: adhesive made of gelatin; Duoderm and Tegasorb are examples; this dressing is occlusive to microorganisms and liquids and promotes absorption of wound exudates; autolysis of necrotic tissue within wound bed is enhanced

   e. Hydrogel: water or glycerin is the primary component of this nonadherent dressing; hydrogel maintains a moist wound surface and provides some absorption; these products are permeable to oxygen and can fill dead spaces in a wound; a secondary nonadhesive dressing may be required

   f. Calcium alginates: a pad made of seaweed fibers; the purpose of this dressing is to absorb larger amounts of drainage

    g. Exudate absorbers, also called polyurethane foam: semipermeable polyurethane foam dressings that absorb large amounts of exudate while keeping wound moist; these dressings are nonadherent

    h. Absorptive or filler dressings: have ability to absorb moderate amounts of drainage; Duo-Derm paste is an example

3. Bandages are strips of cloth used to wrap a body part

    a. Bandages are made of gauze, which is light and porous, or of an elasticized material, which provides pressure to area

    b. Widths of bandages vary from 1 to 4 in. and are determined by part of body to be wrapped

    c. Purposes include to anchor dressings, provide support to a body part, immobilize a body part, or to promote circulatory return

    d. Guidelines for bandaging

        1) Bandage with body part in a normal or functional position

        2) Pad bony prominences

        3) Bandage from distal to proximal area to support blood return

        4) Use even pressure while applying bandage; this is especially important when using elastic bandages that could impair circulation

        5) Inspect and palpate area regularly; assess a fresher wound more frequently and an older wound less frequently; note presence of drainage from wound; assess neurovascular status of extremity including temperature, blanching, and sensation; assess for pain and evaluate its cause; assess extremity distal to bandage for evidence of edema or decreased venous return, which would be indications to loosen the bandage

4. Enzymatic debriding agents: an enzyme paste or solution that is applied to necrotic tissue; the enzyme digests necrotic tissue; for example, Elase

Practice to Pass

A 72-year-old client is admitted with a Stage 1 pressure ulcer on his sacrum. What wound care should the nurse provide for this client?

II. ALTERATIONS IN SENSORY OR PERCEPTUAL ABILITY

A. Factors affecting sensation and perception

1. Numerous factors affect sensory function; these include illness, developmental stage, medications, stress, and lifestyle

2. Illness may result in hospitalization; this change of environment may have an effect on mentation, especially for the older client; this could result from underlying disease process or simply a change in physical environment

3. Developmental stage affects sensory perception; infants have adequate sensory organs but lack an ability to conceptualize and understand sensory input; as development occurs, an individual develops understanding of sensory input; adults have many learned responses to sensory cues; with aging, sensory input diminishes because of decreased sense organ functioning

4. Medications can affect both sensory function and sensory awareness; many drugs are known to decrease LOC; others contribute to mental confusion; in older adults, polypharmacy may lead to drug interactions that result in decreased sensory functioning

5. Stress can be described as eustress or distress

    a. Eustress is stress that stimulates increased individual functioning; an example is a student who wants to do well on an exam, and stress encourages the student to study and score well on exam

    b. Distress is the presence of more stress than an individual can cope with; it depresses functioning; anxiety tends to limit amount of sensory input a client can deal with effectively; if the student in the above scenario had test anxiety, the student may be unable to score well on the exam; prolonged distress also suppresses the immune response and can lead to disease

    c. Illness and hospitalization can both cause distress; today, hospitals have made great efforts to create an aesthetic environment more conducive to healing, such as bright and cheerful walls that are hung with beautiful pictures, floors that may be carpeted, and an overall attempt to create a pleasant "homelike" environment

  6. Lifestyle influences sensory perception; one individual may thrive in a stimulating environment that may overwhelm others

B. Sensory perceptual alterations

  1. Identified factors that contribute to alterations in client's behavior include, but are not limited to, sensory deprivation, sensory overload, and sensory deficits

  2. Sensory deprivation is defined as a lack of meaningful stimuli; the actual amount of incoming stimuli is reduced because of either a decrease of environmental stimuli or impairment in one or more client senses; decreased sensory input can lead to disorientation over a period of time

    a. If client cannot derive meaning from environment, this can lead to sensory deprivation; an example is a blind client who is admitted to the hospital; the environment for this client has changed drastically because landmarks that were present at home are gone

    b. Changes in any kind of sensory input could lead to deprivation; an example is a person who has a visual impairment and loss of tactile perception as a result of a neurological illness; sensory deprivation can then lead to distortions in perception, which may then affect client's ability to perceive the environment correctly

    c. Risk factors that may lead to sensory deprivation include dysfunction of senses; medications, immobility, isolation, and language barriers

    d. See Box 10-3 for clinical signs and symptoms of sensory deprivation

    e. Hospital rooms now have clocks, calendars, and frequently boards that identify names of caregivers on that shift, all of which provide meaningful stimuli to hospitalized client and promote orientation to surroundings

  3. Sensory overload is defined as an increase in intensity of stimuli to levels beyond normal; it generally occurs when a person is unable to process the amount or intensity of stimuli or with exposure to numerous stimuli that are not meaningful (bombardment of client's senses)

    a. Two factors contribute to sensory overload

      1) Increased quantity of internal stimuli as in anxiety

      2) Increased quantity of external stimuli in environment such as noise, equipment, multiple health care personnel, bright lights, and frequent care measures

    b. Sensory overload leads to sleep deprivation; sleep deprivation diminishes client's coping abilities, increases stress levels, impairs cognition and immune responses; when overloaded with sensory stimuli, client may feel that he or she is not in control; nurse should assess environment and recognize that sights and sounds familiar to health care worker may add to overload for client

Box 10-3 **Clinical Signs of Sensory Deprivation**	• Excessive yawning, drowsiness, sleeping • Decreased attention span, difficulty concentrating, decreased problem solving • Impaired memory • Periodic disorientation, general confusion, or nocturnal confusion • Preoccupation with somatic complaints, such as palpitations • Hallucinations or delusions • Crying, annoyance over small matters, depression • Apathy, emotional liability

Source: Berman, Audrey J.; Snyder, Shirlee, *Kozier & Erb's Fundamentals of Nursing*, 9th Ed. © 2012. Reprinted and Electronically reproduced by permission of Pearson Education, Inc., Upper Saddle River, New Jersey.

      c. Contributing factors that add to overload could be pain, anxiety, and lack of sleep

      d. Clinical signs and symptoms of sensory overload include increased muscle tension, fatigue and inability to sleep, irritability and restlessness, inability to concentrate, decreased problem-solving performance, and diminished cognition (poor reasoning and problem-solving ability)

      e. Sensory overload is frequently experienced by clients in intensive care units (ICU)

        1) This syndrome was recognized in the 1960s and was named ICU psychosis

        2) It was noted that clients in ICU experienced confusion, disorientation, and memory loss after 2 to 3 days in ICU

        3) ICU syndrome served as the motivation behind changes in hospital environments; ICU and other units now have calendars, clocks, windows, and television; ICU and some nursing units' rooms are now private rooms, and to help maintain client orientation, adjusting light levels and timing of care activities may be arranged to allow for a more natural sleep cycle (see Chapter 7)

        4) **Sensory deficit**: is impairment of both reception and perception of one or more senses; when loss of sensory function is gradual, client compensates for loss; for instance, someone with impaired vision may decrease the area in which he or she travels alone

C. Common sensory deficits

    1. Visual: vision is an important sense because it allows people to interact with their environment

      a. People with visual impairment may wear glasses or contact lens to correct refraction errors of lens of eye

      b. Some of these refraction errors include

        1) **Myopia**, commonly called nearsightedness

        2) **Hyperopia**, or farsightedness

        3) **Presbyopia**, the loss of elasticity of lens of eye; as a result, there is a loss of ability to see objects that are close; presbyopia is a visual disturbance that occurs with aging, often beginning around age 45 years; bifocal or reading glasses are often used to correct this problem

      c. Cataracts are another problem that occur with aging; they are often seen in clients over age 65 years and occur when lens of eye becomes opaque; lens opacity blocks light rays and distorts and impairs visual field; surgical removal is often required as cataract progresses

      d. Glaucoma: is a painless blockage in circulation of aqueous fluid in eye that leads to an increase in intraocular pressure and possibly blindness

        1) Signs of glaucoma can include blurry or foggy vision, loss of peripheral vision, difficulty adjusting to dark rooms

        2) This eye disease can be controlled using ophthalmic medications if diagnosed and treated early; therefore, screening is important

        3) Diabetic retinopathy: leading cause of blindness among adults from 20 to 70 years old; proliferative retinopathy or neurovascular disease occurs when ischemic retinal blood vessels bleed, causing vitreous hemorrhage; this hemorrhage can be repetitive and may lead to permanent visual loss

        4) Macular degeneration: refers to degenerative changes in layer of blood vessels that arise in retina; macular blood vessels then leak and damage the macula; scarring occurs and visual loss results; signs and symptoms are blurring and distortion of visual images

    2. Hearing: difficulty with hearing may make client feel isolated; it can interfere with health teaching and even increase risk of injury for a client

Practice to Pass

An older adult client is admitted to the nursing unit. What are some of the factors that will contribute to the sensory overload the client may experience?

   a. **Conductive hearing loss** is the result of interrupted transmission of sound waves through the outer and middle ear; possible causes are a tear in eardrum (tympanic membrane), obstruction in auditory canal caused by swelling or other factors, degeneration of hammer, anvil, and stirrup from infection, or continuous low sensory input

   b. Sensorineural hearing loss results from damage to inner ear, auditory nerve, or hearing center in brain from viral infection or ototoxic medications (whose names often end with -*mycin*)

   c. **Presbycusis** is a loss of hearing ability related to aging; gradual loss of hearing is more common in men than women

3. Balance: with aging comes a gradual reduction of power and contraction of muscles; after age 50, there is a steady decrease in muscle fibers; often balance is impaired with this process as well; there may be degenerative joint changes making movement more restricted

4. Taste: a reduction in ability to taste can affect appetite and contribute to poor nutrition; if a corresponding loss of sense of smell occurs, the client's appetite will also not be stimulated by aroma of food

5. Smell: in addition to its effect on client's appetite, loss of sense of smell can be a safety issue; with a decrease in smell, client will not be aware of a gas leak, for example, from stove at home; a diminished sense of smell and/or taste may be early signs of dementia in older adults

6. Touch: tactile deprivation can occur from a disease or an injury that leads to destruction of or damage to nerve cells

   a. Children born with myelomeningocele have damage to nerves below level of neural tube defect; injuries that destroy the nerves will have same effect; a loss of tactile ability may contribute to safety issues; a client who has suffered loss of sensation of a part of the body could easily be burned or develop pressure ulcers because client cannot feel pain

   b. Peripheral neuropathy is a disease process that interferes with innervation of peripheral nerves; with aging, diabetes, or arteriosclerosis, the overall effectiveness of blood vessels decreases; the body compensates by constricting superficial blood vessels to divert blood to larger blood vessels; with constriction of peripheral blood vessels, peripheral nerve endings in area that are supplied by these blood vessels suffer effects of decreased blood flow; as a result, neuropathy develops, which results in abnormal sensation in affected regions and can be quite painful

   c. Multisensory deficit conditions: some conditions lead to damage to more than one of the senses, such as strokes or "brain attack" resulting from either thrombus, embolus, or hemorrhage into an area of brain; this process leads to ischemia in area of brain affected; the results may be decreased mobility, decreased sensation, and/or paresis or paralysis of extremities, as well as aphasia, blindness, or other visual impairment, or impaired swallowing

D. **Promoting self-care**

1. Screening and prevention: early detection of sensory deprivation is an important health screening function

   a. Routine auditory testing is done at birth

   b. Periodic vision screening of all school-age children is done

   c. Health fairs often provide a means to screen a large number of healthy people

   d. Be aware of disease processes that can lead to sensory deprivation and screen for symptoms; this can lead to early recognition of sensory problems

   e. Health measures should be taught to protect sensory organs; encourage protective eyewear and ear gear; emphasize, especially to teenagers, the risk of damage to ears from loud noises or music

    f. Teach clients general health measures such as regular eye and ear exams

    g. The Occupational Safety and Health Administration (OSHA) provides regulations and guidelines to limit hazards affecting senses to those in the workplace; OSHA guidelines are carefully followed in health care settings also

2. Assistive aids: assist clients who have a sensory deficit by encouraging use of specific aids to support their sensory function; promote use of other senses and communicating effectively; and work to ensure client's safety

    a. Visual and hearing aids are available to client with visual and hearing deficits; these aids can be used in hospital and home settings

    b. For clients with smell and taste deficits, supply diets that include a variety of flavors, temperatures, and textures that may then stimulate taste buds

    c. Each client with a sensory deficit should be evaluated to determine need for assistive devices

    d. Encourage clients to utilize aids available and promote their use; for example, if a client who has limited mobility also wears glasses, offer client his or her eyeglasses upon awakening; see Box 10-4 for information on possible visual and auditory aids

3. Communication

    a. Communication is the exchange of information; a client with a sensory deficit is at risk for not accurately interpreting communication

    b. It is important to convey respect to client and enhance his or her self-esteem

    c. A person with a hearing deficit needs to concentrate at all times during a conversation

    d. When speaking to a client with a hearing deficit, face client and speak directly to him or her without large numbers of people around; too many people in environment or high level of background noise will be a distraction

    e. A client with visual deficits may miss nonverbal clues during conversation

    f. See Box 10-5 for further information about communicating with clients who have visual or hearing deficits

Box 10-4 **Aids for Clients With Visual and Auditory Deficits**	The nurse can help a client select aids that are appropriate for that client. **For Clients With Visual Deficits** • Prescription eyeglasses • Proper lighting in rooms and use of nightlights • Shades on windows to reduce glare • Large-print books • Color-code or textured appliances and medicine containers • Books on tape • Seeing-eye dog • Red-tipped cane or laser cane • Magnifying glass • Phone and clock with large numbers **For Clients With Auditory Deficits** • Hearing aids • Closed caption for television • Telephone with amplifiers • Flashing alarms in the home for smoke detectors, doorbells, etc. • Telecommunication device for the deaf (TDD) phone • Telephone with light that flashes when ringing • Vibrating or flashing alarm clock • Wireless page, phone, and email service

Box 10-5

Communicating With Clients Who Have a Visual or Hearing Deficit

Visual Deficit

- Always announce your presence when entering the client's room and identify yourself by name.
- Stay in the client's field of vision if the client has a partial vision loss.
- Speak in a warm and pleasant tone of voice; some people tend to speak louder than necessary when talking to a blind person.
- Always explain what you are about to do before touching the person.
- Explain the sounds in the environment.
- Indicate when the conversation has ended and when you are leaving the room.

Hearing Deficit

- Before initiating a conversation, convey your presence by moving to a position where you can be seen or by gently touching the person.
- Decrease background noises (e.g., radio) before speaking.
- Talk at a moderate rate and in a normal tone of voice; shouting does not make your voice more distinct and in some instances makes understanding more difficult.
- Address the person directly; do not turn away in the middle of a remark or story; make sure the person can see your face easily and that it is well lighted.
- Avoid talking when you have something in your mouth, such as chewing gum; avoid covering your mouth with your hand.
- Keep your voice at about the same volume throughout each sentence, without dropping the voice at the end of each sentence.
- Always speak as clearly and accurately as possible; articulate consonants with particular care.
- Do not "over articulate"; mouthing or overdoing articulation is just as troublesome as mumbling; pantomime or write ideas, or use sign language or finger spelling where appropriate.
- Use longer phrases, which tend to be easier to understand than short ones; for example, "Will you get me a drink of water?" presents much less difficulty than "Will you get me a drink?"; word choice is important: "Fifteen cents" and "fifty cents" may be confused, but "half a dollar" is clear.
- Pronounce every name with care; make a reference to the name for easier understanding, for example, "Joan, the girl from the office" or "Sears, the big downtown store."
- Change to a new subject at a slower rate, making sure that the person follows the change to the new subject; a key word or two at the beginning of a new topic is a good indicator.

> *Source:* Berman, A., & Snyder, S. J. (2012). *Kozier & Erb's fundamentals of nursing: Concepts, process, and practice* (9th ed.). Upper Saddle River, NJ: Pearson Education, p.1012.

Practice to Pass

An 80-year-old client has a hearing impairment (presbycusis). What would be the nurse's best approach when communicating with this client to ensure client understanding?

III. ALTERED MOBILITY

A. Activity develops and maintains the proper functioning of the body

1. Inactivity will lead to physical deterioration; clients can have impaired mobility because of advancing age, paralysis, hemiplegia, muscle weakness, poor balance or poor coordination, spinal cord injuries, or because they wear a cast
2. In general, any client who is weakened by illness or surgery will have some degree of impaired mobility
3. The musculoskeletal system is one of the body's largest systems and accounts for 50% of body weight; muscle strength peaks at age 25 to 30 and is maintained through the fifth decade; after the fifth decade musculoskeletal strength diminishes and becomes noticeably weaker after the seventies

B. Common causes of immobility

1. Common causes that place a client at risk for immobility are pain, motor function impairment, structural problems, generalized inactivity, psychological problems, and medically induced problems such as surgery (especially orthopedic surgery)

2. Pain: clients who are in pain will reduce spontaneous movement in an attempt to decrease painful stimuli; pain will also cause client to refuse to participate in rehabilitative activities including coughing and deep breathing

3. Motor and nervous system impairment: disorders of musculoskeletal and nervous systems can limit mobility; certain neurological diseases can cause muscles to become stiff or lose function

   a. Arthritis and amputations are obvious examples of musculoskeletal conditions that would impair mobility

   b. Multiple sclerosis and Parkinson's disease are neurological conditions that may render muscles unable to function normally

   c. Alterations in LOC and stroke or cerebrovascular accident (CVA) could also leave client with mobility impairments

4. Functional problems: some chronic conditions that limit supply of oxygen and nutrients to body will affect activity tolerance, such as chronic obstructive lung disease (COPD), congestive heart failure (CHF), angina, and obesity; these conditions increase heart's workload and thus restrict or impair client's activity

5. Generalized weakness

   a. A client's age affects body strength; as a client ages, muscle tone and bone density decrease; flexibility and reaction time decline; osteoporosis (demineralization of bone) begins; changes associated with aging will affect posture, balance, and gait

   b. Chronic illness may also cause bodily changes that affect client's energy level and ability to be active; for example, anemia and low hemoglobin, which lower the oxygen-carrying capacity of blood, will cause client to experience fatigue; this, in turn, will reduce mobility

6. Psychological problems: emotional disorders such as depression or stress can reduce a client's desire to be active

   a. Depression may cause client to lack motivation and energy to participate in activities of daily living

   b. A client who is under prolonged stress can also be depleted of energy

   c. Fear may also prevent client from going outside or leaving the home

7. Medically induced immobility

   a. Health care providers may place clients on bed rest or restricted activity to facilitate healing

   b. Orthopedic devices can also restrict mobility; traction, casts, splints, and braces can all lead to inactivity of some part(s) of body

C. Major effects of immobility

1. Psychological effects: powerlessness and loss of self-concept

2. Atrophy and contractures

3. Disuse osteoporosis

4. Pressure ulcers

5. **Orthostatic intolerance** (also known as postural or orthostatic hypotension)

6. Deep vein thrombosis

7. Pneumonia

8. Decrease in gastrointestinal peristalsis

9. Kidney stones

D. Nursing interventions for impaired mobility

1. Exercise: a repetitive, planned body movement performed to either improve or maintain physical movement; activity is essential in preventing complications of immobility

2. Exercise is necessary for healthy functioning of body
3. The American Heart Association recommends that for a healthy heart and cardio-vascular system, exercise should be performed most days of the week for 30 minutes
4. Benefits of exercise
   a. Exercise improves muscle tone and strength; it also improves joint flexibility and range of motion
   b. Exercise promotes good pulmonary ventilation; this, in turn, prevents pooling of secretions in lungs and reduces risk of pneumonia
   c. Gastrointestinal motility and tone are improved, thereby improving digestion and elimination
   d. Since exercise decreases bone loss of calcium, the urine maintains acidity and thus decreases risk for renal calculi
5. Types of exercise
   a. Isometric: produces tension or resistance in a muscle without a change in muscle length; are helpful for immobilized clients because they strengthen muscle groups that will be used later in ambulation; teach client to push or pull against a stationary object as a form of isometric exercise; the muscles exercised here are the abdominal, gluteus, and quadriceps
   b. Isotonic: shortens muscle to produce contraction and active movement; there is no significant change in resistance during movement, so the force of contraction stays stable; increases muscle tone and maintains joint flexibility; using a trapeze to lift body or pushing body into a sitting position are examples of isotonic exercises for bedridden client
   c. Passive range of motion: exercises accomplished with assistance of another person who will support client's body part while moving it
   d. Active range of motion: exercises performed independently; these are isotonic exercises of each joint in body and can maintain or improve muscle strength; they prevent deterioration of joint movement and subsequent contractures

E. **Assistive ambulation devices**
   1. There are many devices available to assist the client in mobility; these devices include crutches, canes, and walkers
   2. Crutches: devices used to assist client in moving and ambulating unassisted; all crutches require rubber tips to prevent slipping on slippery floors
      a. There are various types of crutches (see Figure 10-1)
         1) An axillary crutch is the most frequently used type of crutch
         2) A Lofstrand or forearm crutch is used as a substitute for a cane; it consists of a single tube of aluminum with a handle and a cuff for the forearm; it allows the user to release the hand bar because the metal cuff maintains crutch placement and prevents it from falling
         3) A Canadian or elbow extensor crutch is used for a client whose forearm extensor muscles are weak; it allows upper arm to provide stability to crutch
      b. Proper fit: it is critical that a client be fitted correctly for chosen crutch
         1) Measure client who is lying supine from anterior fold of axilla to heel of foot and add 1 in. (2.5 cm)
         2) Also measure placement of hand on crutch while client stands and adjust crutch so that it maintains elbow at a 30-degree angle
         3) With client standing erect, ensure that shoulder rest of the crutch is 3 fingerwidths (2.5 to 5 cm, or 1 to 2 in.) below axilla
      c. Safety: in addition to the rubber tip on end of crutch, client needs to know appropriate gait; prior to gait training, assist client in preparing for crutch walking by encouraging client to push body off bed with hands and arms; while utilizing crutches, the client's weight is borne by arms, not axillae, as continued pressure in this area can cause nerve damage

Figure 10-1

Three types of crutches.
A. Axillary crutch,
B. Lofstrand crutch,
C. Canadian or elbow
extension crutch.

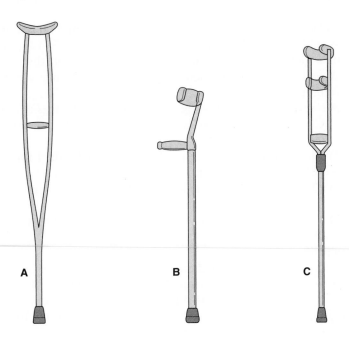

A   B   C

   d. Gaits used: there are 5 crutch-walking gaits; choice depends upon client's ability to bear weight and maintain balance on both legs or 1 leg; while using a crutch, the client alternates body weight between 1 or both legs and the crutches; the 5 gaits and their uses include:

   1) Four-point gait: partial weight bearing
     a) Client must be able to bear weight on both legs
     b) It is the safest gait and provides 3 points of support at all times
     c) It requires constant shifting of weight and coordination of movement of legs and crutches

   2) Three-point gait: requires 1 leg to be able to bear weight of entire body
     a) Non–weight bearing on affected leg
     b) Alternates between good leg and affected leg with both crutches

   3) Two-point gait: requires partial weight bearing on both feet
     a) Client can move at a faster gait than with the 4-point gait
     b) Two points are used to support body at all times
     c) Crutch movement is similar to the swinging of the arms while walking

   4) Swing-through gait: weight-bearing gait that requires strength and coordination
     a) Client moves both crutches forward together
     b) Then the client lifts his or her body weight and swings through

   5) Swing-to gait: weight bearing on both feet
     a) Similar to swing-through gait except body motion is only to level of crutches
     b) Useful for clients with paralysis of legs and hips

3. Cane: assists a client to walk with greater balance and support
   a. Three types of canes are available depending on the number of feet
     1) Quad cane: 4 feet
     2) Tripod: 3 feet
     3) Straight cane
   b. Canes are adjustable; length should allow elbow to bend slightly
   c. Canes allow clients to ambulate with faster speed and without getting fatigued as quickly

d. Clients may use 1 or 2 canes; a single cane is used on unaffected side

e. A rubber cap is fitted at tips of foot (feet) to prevent slipping

4. Walker: device that provides client with more support than a cane

    a. A walker is useful for clients who have poor balance, cardiac problems, or who cannot use crutches

    b. A standard walker has 4 legs with rubber tips on legs and plastic grips for hands

        1) Client needs to be partial weight bearing and have strength in his or her wrists and arms

        2) Client uses his or her upper body to propel walker forward

    c. Another type of walker is the 3- or 4-wheeled walker

        1) Clients who are too weak or not stable enough to move a walker by lifting it use these walkers

        2) They may contain a seat at the back to allow client to sit and rest while walking

    d. Walkers can have their height adjusted

F. Hydraulic lift

1. This apparatus is used for clients who are not able to stand and are too heavy for health care workers to lift safely; for example, Hoyer Lift

2. Lift has 3 parts: the sling, arm, and base; a pressure release valve is on base

3. Sling is placed under client; arm of the device has a hook that hooks into sling; the lift is raised to elevate the client

4. The lift is then moved and aligned with the chair; the pressure release valve is released, and the client is lowered to the chair

5. Sling can be removed from the hooks but left under client to facilitate returning client to bed

Practice to Pass

The nurse wants to assist the client in strengthening his arm muscles in preparation for crutch walking. Describe the exercises the nurse would teach.

Case Study

A 30-year-old client came to the emergency department with a swollen ankle. The nurse notes swelling over the ankle extending down to the toes. X-rays are negative for a fracture. A sprained ankle is diagnosed. The doctor orders a compression (Ace) bandage for the ankle and the use of crutches with no weight bearing on the right ankle.

1. Describe how to apply the compression bandage and give a rationale.

2. Describe how the nurse will teach the client to use the crutches without bearing weight on the right foot.

3. Describe the process for measuring the client for crutches.

4. What type of wound did this client have? How long will it take to heal?

5. What safety concerns would you include in discussions about crutch use?

For suggested responses, see page 309.

POSTTEST

1 A client has been on bed rest with cervical traction for 2 weeks. The traction is discontinued and the client is to ambulate. Prior to getting the client out of bed, it is important for the nurse to take which of the following initial actions? Select all that apply.

1. Raise the head of the bed slowly.
2. Assess lower leg muscle strength.
3. Assist the client in sitting on the side of the bed for several moments before standing.
4. Get a neck brace for the client.
5. Take the client's blood pressure while the client is sitting upright prior to ambulation.

2 A 76-year-old client is admitted to the hospital. In planning for client teaching, the nurse would assess for which condition that is often associated with aging and might interfere with the client's ability to participate in education activities? Select all that apply.

1. Presbyopia
2. Conductive hearing loss
3. Presbycusis
4. Tinnitus
5. Rheumatoid arthritis

3 A client who visits the optometrist for an eye exam is told that he has myopia. The client asks the nurse what the treatment will be. The nurse's reply would include information about which standard treatment?

1. Surgical removal
2. Eye drops or ointment
3. Glasses or contact lenses
4. Oral antibiotics

4 The nurse is performing wound care on a pressure ulcer. The doctor orders a wet-to-damp dressing. A family member asks why the dressing is put on wet. The nurse explains that which of the following is the purpose of this type of dressing?

1. Protect the wound.
2. Dilute thick exudate.
3. Promote collagen deposit.
4. Debride the wound.

5 The nurse assesses a wound of a client and finds that a scab has formed. The nurse concludes that this wound is at what point in the phases of wound healing?

1. End of the inflammatory phase
2. End of the proliferative phase
3. Midpoint of the reparative phase
4. Beginning of the maturation phase

6 A client has a large pressure ulcer on his lower extremity. The nurse instructs the client about nutrients needed for healing, especially vitamin C and protein. While evaluating intake, the nurse determines that the instruction was successful after noting that the client is eating which of the following breakfasts?

1. Coffee, buttered toast with jelly, and bacon
2. Milk, scrambled eggs, and cantaloupe
3. Pancakes with butter and syrup and hot tea
4. Oatmeal with milk, diet soda, and bacon

7 The nurse is using the Braden scale to assess a client's risk for developing a pressure ulcer and calculates a score of 7. The nurse should interpret that this client has which level of risk for development of pressure ulcers?

1. High risk
2. Moderate risk
3. Low risk
4. Unlikely to develop pressure ulcers

POSTTEST

8 During an exercise session with a client who had vascular surgery to the leg, the nurse dorsiflexes and then plantar flexes the foot. The client looks surprised and asks why the nurse is performing this activity. What should the nurse include in a response?

1. "Active range of motion will allow the fastest recovery for your leg."
2. "Passive range of motion will help maintain muscle tone until you can participate more actively in the exercises."
3. "Isometric exercise such as this will use muscles to push against resistance and build up the muscles in your leg."
4. "Isotonic exercise lets me do the work and your muscles get the benefit."

9 Which assessment of the immobilized client would prompt the nurse to take further action?

1. Client reports fatigue
2. Urinary output of 50 mL/hour
3. White blood cell count of 9,500/mm³
4. Diminished bowel sounds

10 The nurse is assessing several clients with different types of injuries. The nurse would conclude that the client who is least likely to develop a wound infection would be the client with which of the following?

1. A contusion
2. A wound healing by second intention
3. A septic wound
4. A wound with purulent exudate

➤ *See pages 258–259 for Answers and Rationales.*

ANSWERS & RATIONALES

Pretest

1 **Answer: 2 Rationale:** Stage I ulcers have nonblanchable, erythematous skin that is intact. Stage II ulcers have reddened, broken skin, giving the appearance of a broken blister. Stage III ulcers are deep with necrotic tissue, while Stage IV ulcers involve tissue necrosis and extend to underlying tissue such as muscle and bone. **Cognitive Level:** Analyzing **Client Need:** Physiological Adaptation **Integrated Process:** Nursing Process: Assessment **Content Area:** Fundamentals **Strategy:** The critical word in the question is *document.* Recall the various stages of pressure ulcer, visualize each stage, and then compare them to the ulcer description in the question to make a selection. **Reference:** Berman, A., & Snyder, S. J. (2012). *Kozier & Erb's fundamentals of nursing: Concepts, process, and practice* (9th ed.). Upper Saddle River, NJ: Pearson Education, p. 923.

2 **Answer: 2 Rationale:** Impaired skin integrity is a result of constant shearing force and pressure. The client was turned and positioned frequently enough; in addition, this type of statement is incorrectly written as it implies that the staff is to blame for the client's condition. Risk for Impaired Skin Integrity and Risk for Pressure Ulcer are incorrect because the client has an actual diagnosis, not a risk diagnosis, and Risk for Pressure Ulcer is not a valid nursing diagnosis. **Cognitive Level:** Analyzing **Client Need:** Basic Care and Comfort **Integrated Process:** Nursing Process:

Diagnosis **Content Area:** Fundamentals **Strategy:** The critical phrase is *appropriate nursing diagnosis.* Discriminate between actual and risk diagnoses. **Reference:** Berman, A., & Snyder, S. J. (2012). *Kozier & Erb's fundamentals of nursing: Concepts, process, and practice* (9th ed.). Upper Saddle River, NJ: Pearson Education, p. 934.

3 **Answers: 3, 5 Rationale:** A loss of elastic skin turgor and increased fragility with wrinkling is part of the normal aging process of the skin. Tight, shiny skin with edema and overhydration are not expected assessment findings of the older adult client's skin. **Cognitive Level:** Applying **Client Need:** Health Promotion and Maintenance **Integrated Process:** Nursing Process: Assessment **Content Area:** Fundamentals **Strategy:** The core issue of the question is knowledge of age-related changes in the older adult client. Use knowledge of how skin changes with aging and the process of elimination to make a selection. **Reference:** Berman, A., & Snyder, S. J. (2012). *Kozier & Erb's fundamentals of nursing: Concepts, process, and practice* (9th ed.). Upper Saddle River, NJ: Pearson Education, p. 922.

4 **Answer: 1 Rationale:** Symptoms of sensory deprivation, in addition to those listed in the question, would include preoccupations with somatic complaints, hallucinations, and apathy. Sensory overload symptoms would include sleeplessness, irritability, disorientation, and reduced problem-solving ability. Visual and hearing deficits would relate to the involved sense. **Cognitive Level:** Analyzing **Client Need:** Psychosocial Integrity

Integrated Process: Nursing Process: Diagnosis **Content Area:** Fundamentals **Strategy:** Note that the client in the question is hospitalized and review the client's manifestations. Consider how the hospital environment could affect the client to make a selection. **Reference:** Berman, A., & Snyder, S. J. (2012). *Kozier & Erb's fundamentals of nursing: Concepts, process, and practice* (9th ed.). Upper Saddle River, NJ: Pearson Education, p. 1003.

5 **Answers: 1, 2, 4** **Rationale:** Sliding the client may create shearing forces that can further damage the skin and lead to the development of pressure ulcers, so the client should be lifted to avoid skin shear. Bed linens must be kept clean and dry to minimize risk for development of pressure ulcers. Many clients will need the linens changed more than once per day. Massaging bony prominences is a therapeutic intervention; however, doing it vigorously may damage capillaries in the area, so gentle massage is indicated. Posting a turning schedule with a sign sheet will help ensure the client is turned. A single-thickness pad or sheet will create fewer wrinkles and reduce the risk for pressure ulcers. **Cognitive Level:** Applying **Client Need:** Basic Care and Comfort **Integrated Process:** Nursing Process: Planning **Content Area:** Fundamentals **Strategy:** The critical words are *bedridden* and *planning nursing care*. Recall the major complications of immobility and common nursing interventions to prevent those complications to eliminate the incorrect options. **Reference:** Berman, A., & Snyder, S. J. (2012). *Kozier & Erb's fundamentals of nursing: Concepts, process, and practice* (9th ed.). Upper Saddle River, NJ: Pearson Education, p. 921.

6 **Answer: 2** **Rationale:** Sterile gloves are not required to remove contaminated dressings. Cleaning the wound from the center out is correct wound care technique. It is important to assess the wound after cleaning, when the wound characteristics will be most visible. A catheter can be used for wound irrigation and it would be placed close to the open area. **Cognitive Level:** Applying **Client Need:** Safety and Infection Control **Integrated Process:** Nursing Process: Evaluation **Content Area:** Fundamentals **Strategy:** The critical phrase is *the student who needs to review the skill*. This tells you the correct answer is the statement that contains incorrect information. Use knowledge of wound management techniques and the process of elimination to make a selection. **Reference:** Berman, A., & Snyder, S. J. (2012). *Kozier & Erb's fundamentals of nursing: Concepts, process, and practice* (9th ed.). Upper Saddle River, NJ: Pearson Education, pp. 942–944.

7 **Answer: 2** **Rationale:** Having the conversation directed to the client meets the client's needs while creating fewer disturbances and increases the likelihood that the client will be able to understand what is said to them. This will help decrease overstimulation, especially for the client who is hearing impaired. Having too many family members or continuous radio or television will only add to the overwhelming stimuli that the client may have trouble processing and will contribute to sensory

overload. Lights in the room should be dimmed to reduce visual overload. **Cognitive Level:** Applying **Client Need:** Basic Care and Comfort **Integrated Process:** Nursing Process: Implementation **Content Area:** Fundamentals **Strategy:** The critical words in the question are *hearing impairment* and *preventing sensory overload*. Use knowledge of techniques for communicating with clients who have sensory deficits and the process of elimination to make a selection. **Reference:** Berman, A., & Snyder, S. J. (2012). *Kozier & Erb's fundamentals of nursing: Concepts, process, and practice* (9th ed.). Upper Saddle River, NJ: Pearson Education, pp. 1012–1013.

8 **Answer: 1** **Rationale:** Reducing glare can help improve vision for the older client. Indirect light may not be sufficient to maximize visual acuity in older clients. The quality of the light source is more important than its location (overhead). Dim lights reduce the client's perception of the environment. **Cognitive Level:** Applying **Client Need:** Basic Care and Comfort **Integrated Process:** Nursing Process: Implementation **Content Area:** Fundamentals **Strategy:** The critical terms are *visually impaired* and *reducing sensory deprivation*. Recall basic information about aids for clients with visual deficits and use the process of elimination to make a selection. **Reference:** Berman, A., & Snyder, S. J. (2012). *Kozier & Erb's fundamentals of nursing: Concepts, process, and practice* (9th ed.). Upper Saddle River, NJ: Pearson Education, p. 1012.

9 **Answer: 2** **Rationale:** The client should use a cane on the unaffected side. The elbow is held in a slight degree of flexion. There are reasons to choose a walker over a cane, but neither is "better." Clients are all at greater risk when they wear socks but no shoes. **Cognitive Level:** Applying **Client Need:** Basic Care and Comfort **Integrated Process:** Teaching and Learning **Content Area:** Fundamentals **Strategy:** The critical phrase is *indicates to the nurse the need for additional teaching*. This tells you that the correct answer is an incorrect statement by the client. Use nursing knowledge of assistive ambulation devices to make a selection. **Reference:** Berman, A., & Snyder, S. J. (2012). *Kozier & Erb's fundamentals of nursing: Concepts, process, and practice* (9th ed.). Upper Saddle River, NJ: Pearson Education, p. 1170.

10 **Answers: 3, 4** **Rationale:** Healing by secondary intention occurs in large, open wounds that do not have closely approximated wound edges. Pressure ulcers must heal by secondary intention since they cannot be closed. A surgical incision, a clean suture line, and a minor puncture wound have wound edges that are approximated and are expected to heal by primary intention. **Cognitive Level:** Analyzing **Client Need:** Basic Care and Comfort **Integrated Process:** Nursing Process: Implementation **Content Area:** Fundamentals **Strategy:** Recall the types of wound healing and the characteristics of each to make the correct choices. **Reference:** Berman, A., & Snyder, S. J. (2012). *Kozier & Erb's fundamentals of nursing: Concepts, process, and practice* (9th ed.). Upper Saddle River, NJ: Pearson Education, pp. 922, 925.

ANSWERS & RATIONALES

Posttest

1 **Answers: 1, 3, 5** **Rationale:** Raising the head of the bed slowly will reduce the risk of orthostatic intolerance (or hypotension). Assisting the client in sitting on the side of the bed for several moments before standing will allow the client's blood pressure to stabilize prior to standing and reduce the risk of orthostatic intolerance. Taking the client's blood pressure while the client is sitting upright will insure that the client's BP is stable in an upright position prior to standing. Assessing the strength of the leg muscles is not something that would be done directly before getting a client up to ambulate. There is no information in the question to support the need for a neck brace. **Cognitive Level:** Applying **Client Need:** Safety and Infection Control **Integrated Process:** Nursing Process: Implementation **Content Area:** Fundamentals **Strategy:** The critical phrases are *bed rest with cervical traction for 2 weeks* and *ambulate.* Recall the major complications of immobility and related nursing actions and use the process of elimination to determine the options that will reduce the client's risk and increase client safety when getting out of bed after prolonged bed rest. **Reference:** Berman, A., & Snyder, S. J. (2012). *Kozier & Erb's fundamentals of nursing: Concepts, process, and practice* (9th ed.). Upper Saddle River, NJ: Pearson Education, p. 1167.

2 **Answers: 1, 3** **Rationale:** Presbyopia is the inability to focus on close objects; this condition normally accompanies aging. Presbycusis is the hearing loss associated with aging. A conductive hearing loss involves an obstruction in the ear canal and is not associated with normal aging. Tinnitus is ringing in the ears and is not a normal finding at any age. Rheumatoid arthritis could limit hand movement needed for psychomotor skills but this is not an age-related change. **Cognitive Level:** Applying **Client Need:** Health Promotion and Maintenance **Integrated Process:** Nursing Process: Assessment **Content Area:** Fundamentals **Strategy:** The critical word is *aging.* Recall sensory deficits that occur with advancing age and use the process of elimination to make a selection. **Reference:** Berman, A., & Snyder, S. J. (2012). *Kozier & Erb's fundamentals of nursing: Concepts, process, and practice* (9th ed.). Upper Saddle River, NJ: Pearson Education, pp. 1010–1011.

3 **Answer: 3** **Rationale:** Myopia or nearsightedness is a condition in which light rays come into focus in front of the retina. It is treated with eyeglasses or contact lenses. Surgical removal is incorrect because there is no "removal," although the condition could be treated surgically. Eye medication and oral antibiotics are of no use in improving the vision of the client with myopia. **Cognitive Level:** Applying **Client Need:** Health Promotion and Maintenance **Integrated Process:** Teaching and Learning **Content Area:** Fundamentals **Strategy:** The critical term is *myopia.* Recall information about common refractory errors to discriminate among the options and make a correct selection. **Reference:** Berman, A., & Snyder, S. J.

(2012). *Kozier & Erb's fundamentals of nursing: Concepts, process, and practice* (9th ed.). Upper Saddle River, NJ: Pearson Education, p. 596.

4 **Answer: 4** **Rationale:** A wet-to-damp dressing debrides the wound. As the dressing partially dries, necrotic debris will adhere to the dressing. When the dressing is removed, dead tissue will be removed also. Although a gauze dressing provides some protection for the wound, this is not its primary purpose. A wet-to-wet dressing, not wet-to-damp, would dilute a thickened or viscous exudate. A wet-to-damp dressing would not promote collagen deposit. **Cognitive Level:** Applying **Client Need:** Basic Care and Comfort **Integrated Process:** Teaching and Learning **Content Area:** Fundamentals **Strategy:** The critical term is *wet-to-damp dressing.* Recall the uses this type of dressing to select the option that provides accurate information to the client and family. **Reference:** Berman, A., & Snyder, S. J. (2012). *Kozier & Erb's fundamentals of nursing: Concepts, process, and practice* (9th ed.). Upper Saddle River, NJ: Pearson Education, p. 944.

5 **Answer: 1** **Rationale:** Near the end of the inflammatory phase of wound healing, protein dries out at the top of the wound, forming a scab. This scab provides safety for the wound because the first line of defense, the skin, is again covered. The end of the proliferative phase occurs after scab formation. The reparative phase is not a current term associated with phases of wound healing. The maturation phase is the final phase of wound healing marked by healing of the scar tissue. **Cognitive Level:** Applying **Client Need:** Basic Care and Comfort **Integrated Process:** Nursing Process: Diagnosis **Content Area:** Fundamentals **Strategy:** The critical word in the question is *scab.* Recall the phases of wound healing and visualize what the wound will look like in each phase to make the correct selection. **Reference:** Berman, A., & Snyder, S. J. (2012). *Kozier & Erb's fundamentals of nursing: Concepts, process, and practice* (9th ed.). Upper Saddle River, NJ: Pearson Education, pp. 925–926.

6 **Answer: 2** **Rationale:** Milk and eggs are high in protein and cantaloupe is a good source of vitamin C. A meal consisting of coffee, buttered toast with jelly, and bacon contains virtually no vitamin C and very little protein. A meal consisting of pancakes with butter and syrup and hot tea has no significant vitamin C or protein. Although the milk has some protein, no source of vitamin C is included in a meal consisting of oatmeal with milk, diet soda, and bacon. **Cognitive Level:** Analyzing **Client Need:** Basic Care and Comfort **Integrated Process:** Nursing Process: Evaluation **Content Area:** Fundamentals **Strategy:** The core issue of the question is knowledge of foods that are high in vitamin C and protein for wound healing. Use information related to nutrition and the process of elimination to make a selection. **Reference:** Berman, A., & Snyder, S. J. (2012). *Kozier & Erb's fundamentals of nursing: Concepts, process, and practice* (9th ed.). Upper Saddle River, NJ: Pearson Education, p. 929.

7 **Answer: 1 Rationale:** The Braden scale evaluates 6 factors: sensory perception, moisture, activity, mobility, nutrition, and friction or shear. Each factor can receive a score from 1 to 4 except friction or shear, which is scored 1 to 3. Low numbers indicate factors that are likely to contribute to the development of an ulcer. Overall scores above 19 indicate that the client has a low risk of pressure ulcer development. **Cognitive Level:** Analyzing **Client Need:** Reduction of Risk Potential **Integrated Process:** Nursing Process: Diagnosis **Content Area:** Fundamentals **Strategy:** The critical words in the question are *Braden scale* and *score of 7.* To answer this question correctly, it is necessary to be familiar with common pressure ulcer risk assessment scales (such as the Braden or Norton scales). **Reference:** Berman, A., & Snyder, S. J. (2012). *Kozier & Erb's fundamentals of nursing: Concepts, process, and practice* (9th ed.). Upper Saddle River, NJ: Pearson Education, p. 924.

8 **Answer: 2 Rationale:** Passive range of motion is exercise conducted with the assistance of another individual, while active range of motion is done by the client alone. Isometric exercises involve resistance while isotonic exercises involve no resistance; however, neither of these applies to the current client situation. **Cognitive Level:** Applying **Client Need:** Basic Care and Comfort **Integrated Process:** Teaching and Learning **Content Area:** Fundamentals **Strategy:** The core issue of the question is knowledge of the rationales and benefits for passive range of motion exercises. Use this knowledge and the process of elimination to make a selection. **Reference:** Berman, A., & Snyder, S. J. (2012). *Kozier & Erb's fundamentals of nursing: Concepts, process, and practice* (9th ed.). Upper Saddle River, NJ: Pearson Education, p. 1164.

9 **Answer: 4 Rationale:** Absence of bowel sounds is a complication of immobility. It could be followed by constipation and other gastrointestinal problems. Fatigue is a symptom that any client may experience in the hospital. Urinary output is within normal range as well as the white blood count. **Cognitive Level:** Analyzing **Client Need:** Basic Care and Comfort **Integrated Process:** Nursing Process: Diagnosis **Content Area:** Fundamentals **Strategy:** The critical words are *immobilized client* and *further action.* Recall the major complications of immobility and use the process of elimination to make a selection. **Reference:** Berman, A., & Snyder, S. J. (2012). *Kozier & Erb's fundamentals of nursing: Concepts, process, and practice* (9th ed.). Upper Saddle River, NJ: Pearson Education, p. 1142.

10 **Answer: 1 Rationale:** A contusion is a crushing of the tissues; there is no break in the skin. Therefore, this wound is less likely to become infected. A wound healing by second intention is a wound in which there is extensive injury and the edges of the wound are not well approximated. Because of this factor, this type of wound has a risk of infection. A septic wound is one that has been invaded by pathogenic microorganisms. Purulent exudate also is an indicator of infection. **Cognitive Level:** Analyzing **Client Need:** Physiological Adaptation **Integrated Process:** Nursing Process: Diagnosis **Content Area:** Fundamentals **Strategy:** The critical words in the question are *least likely.* This tells you that the correct option is one that has the data that is the nearest to normal of the options presented. Use nursing knowledge and the process of elimination to make a selection. **Reference:** Berman, A., & Snyder, S. J. (2012). *Kozier & Erb's fundamentals of nursing: Concepts, process, and practice* (9th ed.). Upper Saddle River, NJ: Pearson Education, pp. 922, 925.

References

Berman, A., & Snyder, S. J. (2012). *Kozier & Erb's fundamentals of nursing: Concepts, process, and practice* (9th ed.). Upper Saddle River, NJ: Pearson Education.

LeMone, P. Burke, K., & Bauldoff, G. (2012). *Medical-surgical nursing: Critical thinking in patient care* (5th ed.). Upper Saddle River, NJ: Pearson Education.

Smeltzer, S. & Bare, B. (2010). *Brunner and Suddarth's textbook of medical-surgical nursing* (12th ed.). Philadelphia, PA: Lippincott Williams & Wilkins.

Smith, S., Duell, D., & Martin, B. (2012). *Clinical nursing skills: Basic to advanced skills* (8th ed.). Upper Saddle River, NJ: Pearson Education, p. 935.

ANSWERS & RATIONALES

11

Administering Medications and Intravenous Fluids

 Test Yourself

Are you ready for the NCLEX-RN® or
course exams? Use the practice tests
on the companion website to check.

Objectives

➤ Classify the legal responsibilities of the nurse related to medication
administration.
➤ Analyze drug pharmacokinetics in relation to medication
administration.
➤ Examine the use of the nursing process to the skill of medication
administration.
➤ Analyze the procedures and techniques for safely administering
medications via all routes.
➤ Classify the purpose and types of intravenous solutions and
guidelines for administering them safely.
➤ Compare and contrast the various intravenous catheters and
solutions available, their indications, maintenance, and methods
for evaluation of potential complications.

Review at a Glance

absorption process by which a drug
moves from site of administration into
bloodstream

adverse effects more severe side
effects

allergic reaction an antigen–
antibody or immunologic reaction to
subsequent exposure to an allergen

apothecary system oldest system
of measurement, uses Roman numerals;
units of measure are represented by
special symbols; the unit of liquid
measure is the minim and the unit for
weight is the grain

aseptic free from germs

biotransformation conversion of
a drug by enzymatic action of liver into a
less active and harmless substance that
is easily excreted; also called metabolism
or detoxification

bolus direct injection of a medication
intravenously

brand name name given by each
manufacturer resulting in various names
for same drug; trade name

buccal pertaining to cheek

classification grouping drugs by
pharmacologic and therapeutic categories

conjunctival sac mucosal membrane
that lines the eye

distribution movement of drug from
site of absorption to site of action

excretion elimination of drug and
metabolites from body primarily
through kidneys but also through feces,
respiration, perspiration, saliva, and
breast milk

generic more useful drug name that
reflects its chemical family

half-life period of time after which
50% of a medication administered has
lost its effectiveness

idiosyncratic effect unexpected and unpredictable individual response to a drug manifested as an under response, over response, or completely different response

inhalation administering a drug into respiratory tract through a mist, spray, or positive pressure

intradermal into dermal layer of skin (dermis) just under outside layer of skin

intramuscular (IM) into a muscle

intravenous (IV) into a vein

irrigation cleansing of a body cavity by flushing with a solution or medication; also known as lavage

lavage cleansing of a body cavity by flushing with a solution or medication; also known as irrigation

lipodystrophy atrophy or hypertrophy of subcutaneous tissue

medication a drug administered for treatment, mitigation, diagnosis, or prevention of disease

metric a decimal system of measurement based upon units of 10 using gram as the unit of weight and liter as the unit of liquid volume

narcotic strong analgesic that in moderate doses depresses central nervous system

nonadherence failure or refusal to take medications according to instructions

ophthalmic pertaining to the eye

parenteral injection of drugs administered by any route other than alimentary canal (gastrointestinal tract)

pharmacokinetics study of metabolism and action of drugs

side effects secondary effects of a drug that are not intended; they are

usually predictable and may be harmless or life threatening

subcutaneous third layer of skin

sublingual under the tongue

sustained release drugs manufactured in a manner to delay absorption

therapeutic effect the desired effect or primary intended effect; the reason a drug is prescribed

topical applied externally

toxic effects harmful effects of a drug on body, usually resulting from excessive dose, improper route of administration, or cumulative effects resulting from impaired excretion or metabolism

trade name name given by each manufacturer resulting in various names for same drug; brand name

transdermal refers to application of a medication for absorption through skin

PRETEST

1 The nurse risk manager is reviewing a medication error involving a known diabetic client. The nurse administered 10 units NPH insulin IV stat per the provider's prescription. The client had an anaphylactic reaction and died. Based on the legal aspects of medication administration, what conclusion should the risk manager make regarding the nurse's error?

1. The nurse is not legally liable because the nurse administered the medication as prescribed by the provider.
2. The nurse is not liable because it was not an insulin reaction.
3. The nurse is legally liable for the medication administered even though the prescription was written incorrectly.
4. The nurse is not legally liable because the nurse gave the correct medication, regardless of the route.

2 While the nurse administers a client's dose of sublingual nitroglycerin, the client asks why it is administered under the tongue instead of swallowed. Which of the following is the best response by the nurse?

1. "It is absorbed more rapidly when placed under your tongue than when swallowed."
2. "It is absorbed more rapidly when swallowed than sublingually."
3. "The absorptions are the same so it really doesn't matter."
4. "Sublingual provides a sustained release of the medication."

3 A nurse is administering flu vaccines at the local walk-in clinic. When administering an intramuscular flu vaccine in the deltoid of an obese client, what size needle is appropriate?

1. 0.5 inch
2. 1 inch
3. 1.5 inches
4. 2 inches

4 The nurse is preparing an intramuscular (IM) injection of hydroxyzine (Vistaril), which is especially irritating to subcutaneous tissue. To prevent tracking of the medication and irritation to the tissues, it would be best for the nurse to take which action?

1. Use a small-gauge needle.
2. Administer at a 45-degree angle.
3. Apply ice to the injection site.
4. Use the Z-track technique.

5 A pediatric client has been diagnosed with conjunctivitis. The nurse is to administer eyedrops 4 times per day. The nurse should administer the medication by gently dropping the medication onto which of the following areas?

1. Center of the cornea
2. Sclera by the inner canthus
3. Sclera by the outer canthus
4. Lower conjunctival sac

6 A client received a severe burn in a house fire. On the second day of hospitalization, the provider prescribes the client to receive albumin. What information should the nurse provide to the client regarding the rationale for the administration of albumin?

1. Increase the level of clotting factors and prevent bleeding.
2. Provide fluid resuscitation to prevent dehydration.
3. Replace the lost red blood cells and reduce the anemia.
4. Provide proteins to increase the osmotic pressure in the blood.

7 The nurse is to administer ranitidine (Zantac) 50 mg intravenously (IV) in 50 mL of 5% dextrose in water. The nurse should set the IV infusion pump to administer the dose how many mL per hour over a 30-minute time period?

_____mL/hour

8 The provider has prescribed a hypotonic intravenous (IV) solution for a newly admitted client. The nurse obtains which of the following solutions based on the prescription and the likely type of dehydration?

1. 0.9% sodium chloride for hypotonic dehydration
2. 5% dextrose in normal saline for isotonic dehydration
3. Lactated Ringer's solution for hypovolemic dehydration
4. 0.45% sodium chloride for cellular dehydration

9 The client has been receiving total parenteral nutrition (TPN) for several days. The central venous access device became dislodged and the nurse notes that the client's IV has not been running for the last few hours. The nurse would monitor the client for which complication related to the stopped infusion?

1. Hypocalcemia
2. Hypoglycemia
3. Sepsis
4. Hyperkalemia

10 The nurse has a prescription to administer 10 grains of aspirin. The tablets that are available contain 325 mg aspirin per tablet. The nurse would administer how many tablets?

_____tablets

➤ *See pages 295–296 for Answers and Rationales.*

I. APPLICATION OF PHARMACOLOGY IN NURSING PRACTICE

A. Drug
1. A term that is sometimes used interchangeably with **medication**
2. Substance administered for treatment, mitigation, diagnosis, or prevention of disease

B. Names of drugs
1. Each drug can have 3 types of names
2. Chemical
   a. Chemical derivation of a drug that describes ingredients of that drug
   b. An example is 1-methyl-4-phenyl-4-piperidinecarboxylic acid ethyl ester hydrochloride
3. **Generic**
   a. A more useful name that reflects the chemical family
   b. An example is meperidine hydrochloride (1-methyl-4-phenyl-4-piperidinecarboxylic acid ethyl ester hydrochloride)

    4. Brand name or **trade name**

       a. A name given by each manufacturer resulting in various names for same drug

       b. An example is Demerol (1-methyl-4-phenyl-4-piperidinecarboxylic acid ethyl ester hydrochloride; meperidine hydrochloride)

C. Classification

    1. The Pharmacologic-Therapeutic Classification of the American Hospital Formulary Service (AHFS) groups drugs by pharmacologic and therapeutic categories

    2. Prototypes are listed under each classification that are representative of the actions and characteristics of the other drugs in that drug classification (e.g., Demerol is classified as a central nervous system [CNS] agent, narcotic [opiate] agonist analgesic)

D. Forms/preparation

    1. Drugs are prepared in a variety of forms

    2. See Table 11-1 for types of drug preparations

E. Federal regulations

    1. In the United States and Canada, the federal government regulates the drug industry

    2. This includes production, prescription, distribution, and administration of drugs

---

Table 11-1 **Types of Drug Preparations**

Type	Description
Aerosol spray or foam	A liquid, powder, or foam deposited in a thin layer on skin by air pressure
Aqueous solution	One or more drugs dissolved in water
Aqueous suspension	One or more drugs finely divided in a liquid such as water
Caplet	A solid form, shaped like a capsule, coated and easily swallowed
Capsule	A gelatinous container to hold a drug in powder, liquid, or oil form
Cream	A nongreasy, semisolid preparation used on the skin
Elixir	A sweetened and aromatic solution of alcohol used as a vehicle for medicinal agents
Extract	A concentrated form of a drug made from vegetables or animals
Gel or jelly	A clear or translucent semisolid that liquefies when applied to skin
Liniment	A medication mixed with alcohol, oil, or soapy emollient and applied to skin
Lotion	A medication in a liquid suspension applied to skin
Lozenge (troche)	A flat, round, or oval preparation that dissolves and releases a drug when held in mouth
Ointment (salve, unction)	A semisolid preparation of one or more drugs used for application to skin and mucous membrane
Paste	A preparation like an ointment, but thicker and stiff, that penetrates skin less than an ointment
Pill	One or more drugs mixed with a cohesive material, in oval, round, or flattened shapes
Powder	A finely ground drug or drugs; some are used internally, others externally
Suppository	One or several drugs mixed with a firm base such as gelatin and shaped for insertion into body (e.g., rectum); the base dissolves gradually at body temperature, releasing the drug
Syrup	An aqueous solution of sugar often used to disguise unpleasant-tasting drugs
Tablet	A powdered drug compressed into a hard small disc; some are readily broken along a scored line; others are enteric-coated to prevent them from dissolving in stomach
Tincture	An alcohol or water-and-alcohol solution prepared from drugs derived from plants
Transdermal patch	A semipermeable membrane shaped in the form of a disc or patch that contains a drug to be absorbed through skin over a long period of time

F. State and local regulations

1. Each state legislates a Nurse Practice Act for RNs and LVN/LPNs
2. Local health care facilities are responsible for establishing and implementing policies and procedures that conform to their state's regulations
3. When laws or regulations of a community, state, or institution differ from federal laws, the stricter law generally prevails

G. Nurse Practice Acts

1. Define nurses' boundaries and responsibilities regarding medications
2. It is a nurse's responsibility to know the state Nurse Practice Act
3. Under law, nurses are responsible for their own actions (e.g., if a medication order is written incorrectly, the nurse who administers the incorrect prescription is also responsible for the error)
4. Law also governs nursing practice involving use and management of controlled substances

H. Nontherapeutic medication use

1. Consist of chemicals that often are derived from folklore or various cultures
2. These have not passed Federal Drug Administration (FDA) approval process (e.g., ginseng)

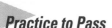

Practice to Pass

How do Nurse Practice Acts relate to federal and state laws?

II. PHARMACOKINETICS

A. Study of how drugs enter body, reach their site of action, are metabolized or biotransformed, and exit body

1. **Absorption**: process by which a drug moves from administration site into bloodstream; drugs are absorbed through gastrointestinal (GI) tract, respiratory tract, or skin and are dependent upon correct form or preparation of drug to be administered by correct route
2. **Distribution**: movement of drug from site of absorption to site of action; it depends upon vascularity for speed of onset and upon chemical and physical drug properties to attract drug to a certain area of the body where it will exert its effect
3. **Biotransformation**: conversion of a drug by enzymatic action of liver into a less active substance called a metabolite; can be affected by a variety of factors including disease states; also called detoxification or metabolism; active metabolites still exert a pharmacological effect, while inactive metabolites do not
4. **Excretion**: elimination of drug and metabolites from body primarily through kidneys but also through feces, respiration, perspiration, saliva, and breast milk; prescriber will determine frequency of drug dosing by noting drug's **half-life** (time it takes total amount of drug to be diminished by one half); a drug's half-life provides information about accumulation of drug in body with repeated doses

B. Types of medication effects

1. **Therapeutic effect**: desired effect or primary intended effect for which drug is prescribed
2. **Side effect**: an unintended secondary effect of a drug; usually predictable and may be harmless or life threatening; some side effects can have a beneficial action such as sedative effect of morphine when used for pain management during postoperative period
3. **Adverse effects**: more severe side effects that often require discontinuing drug and might require reversal of drug
4. **Toxic effects**: harmful effects of a drug on body, usually resulting from drug overdose, ingestion of a drug intended for external use, or cumulative effects resulting from impaired excretion or metabolism
5. **Idiosyncratic effect**: unexpected and unpredictable individual response to a drug manifested as an underresponse, overresponse, or completely different response

6. **Allergic reaction**: an antigen/antibody or immunologic reaction to a drug; allergic reaction can be as mild as a rash or as severe as anaphylaxis

7. Medication interactions: inhibition or enhancement of drug's action or effects as a result of interacting with foods, drugs, or other substances; results in an improved, exaggerated, or diminished response

C. **Routes of administration**

1. Refer to Table 11-2 for a summary of routes of administration and onset of action

2. Oral routes: drugs administered through mouth

   a. **Oral**: drug is swallowed and drug is absorbed from GI system; common forms of oral drugs include tablets, capsules, and liquid preparations

   b. **Sustained release** formulations (drugs manufactured in a manner to delay their absorption) are used to slow drug absorption in a controlled and planned manner; care should be taken when administering sustained release formulations to avoid breaking or opening the formulation, which alters the predictable dosage and response; most oral drugs are administered in a bolus dosing pattern

   c. **Sublingual**: drug is placed under tongue and absorbed through mucous membranes of mouth into blood vessels; uncoated tablets dissolve in mouth and are absorbed quickly

   d. **Buccal**: drug is held against mucous membranes between cheek and teeth and absorbed through mucous membranes of mouth; both buccal and sublingual administration bypass GI tract and liver, thus eliminating first-pass loss when drugs are metabolized before they have reached the site of action

3. **Parenteral** routes: injection of drugs administered by any route other than alimentary canal (gastrointestinal tract)

   a. **Subcutaneous**: injection into subcutaneous tissue, which is the third layer of tissue below skin; can be bolus or continuous infusions; volumes to be administered must be limited

Practice to Pass

One hour ago the nurse administered 2 mg of lorazepam (Ativan) orally to a client for anxiety. The client is now reporting restlessness and increased anxiety. What response is the client experiencing, and what should the nurse do?

Table 11-2	**Routes of Administration and Onset of Action**
Routes	**Onset and Action of Drugs**
Oral Routes	
Oral	Slow and irregular absorption from gastrointestinal (GI) tract
Sublingual	Rapidly absorbed into bloodstream (systemic effect) Can be administered for local effect Bypasses liver and is therefore more potent than oral route
Buccal	Pertains to the cheek and is the same as sublingual
Parenteral Routes	
Subcutaneous	Faster onset than oral Slower than intramuscular Abdomen has most rapid rate of absorption of all subcutaneous sites
Intramuscular	Rapidly absorbed: deltoid is 7% faster than vastus lateralis and 17% faster than gluteal muscles
	1½-inch needle absorbs 2½ times faster than when injected through a 1-inch needle
Intravenous	Faster onset than intramuscular, within one or more minutes
Intradermal	Slow absorption
Intrathecal	Into the spinal canal
Topical Routes	
Transdermal	Prolonged systemic effect
Inhalation	Rapid localized absorption

    b. Intramuscular (IM): injection into a muscle for rapid absorption into bloodstream; some drugs may contain a substance to delay absorption (as in procaine penicillin); most IM dosing patterns are bolus dosing

    c. Intravenous (IV): injection into a vein; the onset of action is more rapid than oral or IM; various dosing patterns are available such as bolus and continuous infusions; requires close monitoring due to immediacy of effect

    d. Intradermal: injection into dermal layer of skin (dermis), just under surface of skin; this method is primarily used to evaluate sensitivity to different agents (e.g., PPD skin test)

4. Topical routes: drugs administered on body surface that are intended for surface use only and are not meant for ingestion or injection; creams, lotions, ointments, powders, and patches are drug formulations used by topical route

    a. Transdermal: surface application of a medication designed to provide a slow release of drug; usually applied as a patch (e.g., nitroglycerine, estrogens, and nicotine)

    b. Inhalation: administered into respiratory tract using a mist, spray, or positive pressure

    c. Ophthalmic: administered to the eye

    d. Otic: administered in the ear

    e. Nasal: administered in the nose for local or systemic effect

5. Medication measurement systems

    a. Metric: a decimal system of measurement based upon units of 10 with the gram as the unit of weight and the liter as the unit of liquid volume

    b. Apothecary system: oldest system of measurement that uses Roman numerals and special symbols; the unit of liquid measure is the minim and the unit for weight is the grain

    c. Household: a less accurate system of measurement based upon drops, teaspoons, tablespoons, cups and glasses (see Table 11-3 for approximate weight equivalents and Table 11-4 for volume equivalents)

    d. Medications are prescribed in a specific weight per volume; for instance, a single tablet may have 100 mg of drug and the volume of that tablet is 1; a drug that comes in 80 mg per 2 mL of liquid has a volume of 2; a few liquid drugs are prescribed by volume alone and come in only one strength; when the provider orders a weight of medication, the nurse determines how much drug to give based on volume (solid or liquid) needed to include that weight

    e. Calculations: a variety of formulas are utilized in calculating drug doses; one is called ratio and proportion; in this calculation, the weight of a prescribed drug dose is compared to the weight and volume of available forms of the drug; if 40 mg of furosemide (Lasix) is prescribed, and the drug comes in 80 mg per 2 mL, the nurse would calculate the volume to be administered as $80/2 = 40/x$ or 1 mL

Practice to Pass

The client is experiencing a hypertensive crisis and is receiving nitroprusside (Nipride) IV drip at 0.5 micrograms/kg/min. The client weighs 160 pounds. How much nitroprusside should the client receive per minute?

Table 11-3 **Approximate Weight Equivalents**	
Metric System	**Apothecary System**
1 mg (milligram)	1/60 grain
60 mg	1 grain
1,000 mg = 1 gram	15 grains
1,000 grams = 1 kg	2.2 lb (pounds)

Table 11-4	Approximate Volume Equivalents	
Metric	**Apothecary**	**Household**
1 mL	15 minims	15 drops (gtt)
4–5 mL	1 fluid dram	1 teaspoon
15 mL	4 fluid drams	1 Tbsp (tablespoon)
30 mL	1 fluid ounce	2 Tbsp
250 mL	8 fluid ounces	1 cup
500 mL	16 fluid ounces	1 pint
1,000 mL	32 fluid ounces	1 quart
4,000 mL	64 fluid ounces	1 gallon

III. NURSE'S ROLE IN ADMINISTERING MEDICATIONS

A. Standards

1. In administering medications, the nurse must check the 10 "rights" of drug administration: right medication, right dose, right client, right route, right time, right documentation, right client education, right to refuse, right assessment, right evaluation
2. Right medication: compare drug container label to the medication administration record (MAR) 3 times; note expiration date of drug; check the drug name (many drugs have very similar names) and correctness of therapy; be knowledgeable about any medications administered, if unsure of a specific medication, review information in an appropriate drug resource
3. Right dose: check recommended dose for drug and appropriateness of dose for client, confirm calculations, and verify laboratory results or serum levels that could alter drug dose; check heparin, insulin, and digitalis doses with another nurse; validate medication prescriptions requiring multiple unit doses to be administered at one given time
4. Right client: have client state name and often date of birth and check room and bed number and client's identification band before administering medication
5. Right route: confirm route of administration with MAR and note on medication label that the specific medication preparation can be administered by the prescribed route and that it is the correct route for client's condition
6. Right time: confirm time of day with time of administration noted on MAR and when last dose was given; verify that drug dosing schedule is consistent with maintaining therapeutic levels; if not on military time, validate the time as either a.m. or p.m.
7. Right documentation: chart each medication completely and correctly
   a. Record in client's chart the administration details
   b. Include exact time of administration, name and dosage of drug, along with route of administration
   c. Record any pertinent information associated with drug such as heart rate with digoxin (Lanoxin) or blood pressure with methydopa (Aldomet)
   d. Sign the administration record; if an electronic MAR is used, the nurse's login provides the electronic signature
   e. Each agency will have specific policies regarding where and how medications are documented
   f. If a drug is a prn medication for a specific symptom, note follow-up assessment data indicating success or failure of medication effects
8. Right client education: explain to client the drug's purpose, rationale for receiving it, what the client should expect from the drug, and any precautions such as client safety

9. Right assessment: implement specific client assessments prior to administering drug, and identify specific parameters related to assessments; for example, digoxin (Lanoxin) should not be administered to a client who has an apical pulse rate below 60 per minute

10. Right evaluation: assess client after drug administration to determine if desired effect has been attained or if adverse effects or adverse reactions have occurred

B. Maintaining client's rights in relation to medications

1. Clients have the right to have medications administered safely
2. The nurse is responsible to ensure drug administration safety
3. Right of client to refuse medication
   a. Nurse needs to inform client of drug name, its intended action, and possible side and adverse effects so that client can make an informed decision about whether to take dose
   b. If client refuses drug, note this information on the medical record indicating client's rationale and attempts by nurse to correct any misinformation and allay fears

C. Nursing process

1. Assessment: psychosocial and biophysical parameters are used to assess clients' needs for medication and response to drug therapy
   a. History: general, allergies, medication use, and diet history
      1) A general history provides baseline information essential to safe drug administration
      2) The database reveals information concerning potential contraindications, drug incompatibilities, client knowledge deficits, and physical or psychological conditions that could affect drug **pharmacokinetics**
      3) Allergies: includes client's allergic responses to drugs, food, products, or environmental allergens; obtain specific information about type of reaction; an allergy to one prototype drug may cause an allergic reaction with other drugs within same class as prototype
      4) Medication use: includes information on frequency, amount, and duration of current and recent drug use including prescription drugs, over-the-counter drugs, herbal preparations, alcohol, tobacco products, illegal drugs, and drug dependencies; question client about effectiveness, side effects, and if client knows purpose for medications
      5) Diet: obtain data about normal eating habits through a typical 24-hour dietary recall of types and amounts of all foods and beverages consumed; this assists in determining potential food and medication incompatibilities and need to adjust medication schedule with mealtimes or specific food items
   b. Client's perceptual or coordination problems
      1) Perception and coordination are important elements in assessing client's reaction to medication as well as ability to self-administer medications
      2) Baseline data including client's orientation to time, place and person, memory, attention span, equilibrium, muscle control, and movement
      3) This information assists in assessing central nervous system (CNS) responses to medications and client's ability to self-administer drugs
      4) Assess for visual, tactile, or neuromuscular disabilities that would affect client's ability to manage necessary equipment or route of administration (e.g., using syringes, opening medication bottles, administering a suppository)
   c. Client's experience with medications
      1) Clients with previous allergic reactions to other medications are more likely to have an allergic reaction to new medications than those who have had none
      2) In addition, clients who have demonstrated idiosyncrasies to medications should also be monitored closely when new medications are added

Practice to Pass

Upon entering a client's room to administer her daily dose of enalapril maleate (Vasotec) for hypertension, the client tells the nurse that she does not want to take the medication. What are the nursing actions and why?

          3) Previous experience with medication may affect client's attitude toward a new medication

      d. Client's knowledge and understanding of medications

          1) Is client able to understand action, side effects, dosage, and administration schedule?

          2) Determine whether client can afford drugs and if client knows what to do should he or she encounter a side effect

      e. Client's learning needs

          1) Assessment of client's knowledge and understanding of medications provides insight into what client teaching is necessary

          2) Assessing educational background assists nurse in determining optimal client education approach

          3) Determine: What is the education level? Can client read and write English, or is another language preferred? What learning style is best—written materials, oral explanation, or demonstration?

2. Planning: the following goals and expected outcomes must be met:

      a. Client and family state understanding of medication regimen

          1) Information obtained in history assists nurse in individualizing the client teaching plan

          2) Using teaching methods specific to client's learning style, physical, emotional, and psychological abilities, and finances are crucial to compliance and favorable outcomes

      b. Client achieves therapeutic effect of medication without complications or discomfort

          1) Understanding specific purpose for which client receives the drug is crucial to evaluating its effectiveness (e.g., propanolol [Inderal] is prescribed for hypertension, angina, migraine headaches, and supraventricular arrhythmias)

          2) The plan of care includes appropriate assessments to evaluate effectiveness and to minimize potential side effects of drugs (e.g., one action of propanolol [a beta blocker] is reduction of heart rate, therefore measuring apical pulse before and after drug administration should be included in the nursing care plan)

      c. Client has no complications related to route of medication

          1) Understanding pharmacokinetics of drugs ensures proper route of administration, preparation of drug, and appropriate assessments to monitor client's response

          2) The route of administration alters absorption, distribution, and excretion of drugs

          3) Validate that route and preparation of drug is appropriate for medication as well as for client's physical condition (e.g., evaluate swallowing ability of a client admitted for a stroke prior to administering an oral medication; do not crush enteric-coated, or extended-release drugs)

      d. Client safely self-administers medications

          1) Develop teaching methods that include evaluation of client's ability to self-administer medications

          2) Cognitive, psychomotor, and affective learning are all aspects impacting successful outcomes

          3) Direct observation, tests, oral questioning, and monitoring through follow-up contacts with client can evaluate effectiveness of cognitive learning

          4) Psychomotor skills are best evaluated by direct observation

          5) Affective learning relates to client's values or attitudes and can significantly affect client's follow-through with treatment plan; evaluation of client's attitudes or values can be inferred by listening to client's responses to your questions and attentiveness to client's behavior and feelings

3. Implementation

      a. Receive medication order

          1) A medication must have a provider or nurse practitioner prescription prior to administration

    2) The prescription can be written or computerized

    3) A written prescription is recorded in client's chart or file

    4) A telephone prescription is recorded by nurse as a "telephone order" in client's chart for signature by prescriber, usually within 24 hours

    5) Orders can be prescribed as one-time-only, prn (as needed), or routine (according to instructions until prescription is cancelled)

b. Correctly transcribe or communicate order: in noncomputerized medical records, medications are transcribed from client's chart or file onto a MAR; it is the nurse's responsibility to ensure accuracy of transcription and that all essential parts of drug order are present:

    1) Client's name and room number

    2) Name of drug

    3) Date and time prescription was written

    4) Dosage

    5) Route

    6) Frequency

    7) Signature of prescriber

c. Accurate dose calculation or measurement

    1) Drug dosage includes amount and also strength (if drug is available in varying strengths)

    2) If a fractional dose is administered, accuracy depends upon correct calculations using metric or apothecary system and matching dosage with appropriate administration device (e.g., insulin requires a syringe that measures in units, liquid oral medications may require measurement in a syringe that is calculated by tenths)

    3) When pouring liquid medications into a medication cup, read solution at eye level using bottom of meniscus (crescent-shaped upper surface of a column of liquid)

d. Correct administration

    1) Use the 10 rights

    2) During preparation of medications for administration the nurse should not be interrupted by anyone

    3) Organize supplies (e.g., IV pump, alcohol swabs, medicine cups)

    4) Compare drug label with MAR—if they are not identical, check prescription in client's chart; if there is still a discrepancy, check with pharmacist

    5) Prepare dose using **aseptic** technique, free from germs, and according to guidelines for specific drug (e.g., proper diluent solution and amount)

    6) Separate **narcotics**, strong opioid analgesics that in moderate doses depress the central nervous system, from other medications requiring specific assessments (e.g., pulse or blood pressure)

    7) If administering insulin, it should be witnessed with another nurse at time dose is drawn up and again when scanned before administering to client

    8) Administer only the medications you prepare

    9) Identify the client; ask the client his/her name and, if part of agency policy, also ask date of birth, check identification bracelet; if hospital utilizes a bar coding system, scan medication's bar code, enter nurse's identification, and scan client's wristband

    10) Do not leave medications at bedside with certain exceptions such as nitroglycerine when there is a corresponding prescription to do so

    11) Ensure that client takes dose using direct observation

    12) If a medication error is made, report it immediately according to agency policies

e. Record administration

    1) Document drug name, time, dose, route, and relevant data such as pulse with digoxin (Lanoxin) on MAR

2) Initial the drug and identify your initials with your signature

3) Circle the time of withheld or refused drugs, document the reason, and report this to the health care provider

4) If agency has an electronic medical record (EMR) document medication administration as determined by agency's EMR program

5) Assess and record client's response to drug, particularly related to prn medications

f. Special considerations

1) Infants and children: children metabolize many drugs differently than adults and have immature systems for handling drugs; many drugs list recommended pediatric dosages, others can be converted to pediatric dosages based on age, weight, or body surface area; oral preparations are usually prepared as elixirs (sweetened, aromatic liquids); do not mask taste of medications in foods such as milk because child may develop an unpleasant association with the food; be truthful to child about painful procedures such as injections

2) Older adults: undergo many physical changes that may result in responses that are different from typical pharmacokinetics:

a) Less effective absorption

b) Less efficient distribution

c) Retention of fat-soluble drugs and increased potential for toxicity due to increased proportion of fat to lean body mass

d) Altered biotransformation because of liver changes

e) Less effective excretion due to reduced renal functioning

f) Older adults frequently have chronic diseases resulting in polypharmacy, which increases risk for drug interactions

3) Over-the-counter (OTC) medications

a) Products that are available without prescription for self-treatment or are recommended by health care provider

b) Clients may not consider OTC drugs to be medications and not include them in their medication history; therefore, ask specifically about OTC drug use and use of herbal therapies when obtaining a medication history

c) Some drugs previously approved as prescription drugs were found to be safe and useful for clients without need for a prescription when provided in smaller doses

d) Some of these drugs were not rigorously screened and tested according to current drug evaluation protocols because they were developed and marketed before current laws were put into effect

e) Taking these drugs could mask the signs and symptoms of underlying disease

f) Taking these drugs with prescription medications may result in drug interactions and could interfere with drug therapy

4) Misuse of medications

a) Improper use of OTC and prescription drugs can lead to acute and chronic toxicity

b) Frequently overused drugs include cough and cold medications, laxatives and antacids, which could cause harmful effects or delay the diagnosis of more serious problems

c) Drug abuse that can lead to drug dependence and illicit drugs (street drugs) are forms of misuse

5) **Nonadherence**: failure or refusal to take medications according to instructions; may also be called noncompliance; can be related to many factors, such as finances, values or attitudes, cognitive and physical ability, and knowledge and understanding of medication

4. Evaluation
   a. Monitor response: continually evaluate client for therapeutic response, and occurrence of adverse effects and drug–drug or drug–food interactions
   b. Use various evaluation measures (e.g., direct observation, checklist, BP); use psychosocial and biophysical parameters to assess client's need for and response to drug therapy (see Table 11-5)

D. Procedure for administering medications (See Box 11-1)
   1. Oral medications
      a. Break only scored tablets
      b. Crush only medications approved for crushing or chewing
         1) Extended-release medications are designed to be released over an extended period of time; some scored formulations can be broken without affecting the release mechanism; some mixed-release capsules can be opened and contents sprinkled on food
         2) Abbreviations used in brand names identifying drugs as extended-release include CR (controlled release), CRT (controlled-release tablet), LA (long acting), SR (sustained release), TR (timed release), SA (sustained action), and XL or XR (extended release)
         3) Enteric-coated drugs are designed to allow drug to pass through stomach intact with drug being released in intestines

Table 11-5	Biophysical Evaluation Parameters of Response to Drug Therapy
Parameter	**Evaluation Measures**
Cardiovascular	Blood pressure, cardiac rate and rhythm Presence or absence of chest pain Presence and strength of peripheral pulses Skin color, temperature, and turgor; presence or absence of edema Serum laboratory results: cardiac enzymes, electrolytes, complete blood count, serum concentrations of cardiac-related drugs
Respiratory	Respiratory rate, rhythm, and effort Lung sounds, especially presence or absence of adventitious sounds Dyspnea, use of accessory muscles Need for supplemental oxygen Cyanosis or clubbing Cough and sputum production Arterial blood gases, oxygen saturation obtained by pulse oximetry
Renal	Adequacy of urinary output (30 mL/hr) Urine color and clarity, specific gravity, culture and sensitivity Presence of flank pain Serum laboratory results: blood urea nitrogen (BUN), creatinine, electrolytes, serum and urine protein
Central nervous system	Glasgow Coma Scale Level of cognitive functioning in comparison to baseline level of alertness and orientation Intactness of cranial nerves Motion and sensation in extremities Serum laboratory results: blood glucose levels, serum metabolic toxin levels, arterial blood gases Analysis of cerebrospinal fluid (CSF)
Laboratory studies	Those listed under specific parameters; white blood cell count (WBC)

Box 11-1	1. Validate the medication prescription for consistency of drug, dose, time intervals, and route of administration.
General Medication Preparation Procedures	2. Compare the prescriber's most recent medication prescriptions with the medication administration record (MAR).
	3. Wash your hands.
	4. Start at the top of the MAR and compare each medication with the drug label, checking for dose, time, and route of administration. Recheck information 3 times.
	5. Prepare medication as indicated.
	6. Ask client to state name and check identification band.
	7. If a bar code system is in place scan the medication, enter the administering nurse's identification, and scan the medication.
	8. Assist client to appropriate position for the administration route.
	9. Explain the medication to the client.
	10. Perform appropriate assessments if indicated.
	11. Using aseptic technique, administer the medication. If the medication is dispensed in the unit-dose package, open the package at the client's bedside and place in a medication cup. The packaging allows identification and keeps the medication clean.
	12. Properly dispose of medication equipment.
	13. Perform hand hygiene.
	14. Document the name, dose, time, and route of the drug, and other assessments as indicated in the MAR or the electronic medical record.

2. Enteral tube
   a. Position client in semi-Fowler's position
   b. Determine correct placement (it may not be possible to reliably determine placement of small-bore enteral tubes by any technique other than radiography, which is also most reliable)
      1) Nasogastric tube: aspirate stomach contents and check pH (should be 4 or less) or auscultate air insufflation; secretions should be greenish, tan to clear
      2) Nasointestinal tubes: aspirate stomach contents and check for pH greater than 6; duodenal secretions should be deep yellow in color
      3) Percutaneous endoscopic gastrostomy (PEG) and percutaneous endoscopic jejunostomy (PEJ) tubes do not require placement verification prior to each medication administration
   c. Flush enteral tube with approximately 30 mL of water
   d. Administer medication in solution or elixir forms when available; crush tablets to a fine powder and mix in warm water to make a solution or suspension; do not mix medications—administer each medication separately; flush well between medications
   e. If client is receiving enteral feeding, ensure that medication and feeding solution are compatible; if they are not, turn off tube feeding for 30 to 60 minutes before and after drug administration; if tube is connected to suction, disconnect from suction for at least 30 minutes after administering drug
   f. Flush enteral tube with approximately 30 mL of water after each drug
   g. Maintain client in semi-Fowler's position for at least 30 minutes after drug administration

3. Skin

   a. Put on gloves—prevents absorption of drug through fingertips

   b. Remove prior applications remaining on skin unless otherwise specified

   c. Remove ointments and creams from their containers and apply to skin with tongue depressors or cotton tipped applicators in thin layers unless otherwise specified

   d. Transdermal patch or premeasured paper—read package insert for application directions

      1) Remove previously applied patch or paper and cleanse skin

      2) Record date and time of application and your initials directly onto transdermal patch and remove protective covering

      3) Place prescribed amount of medication directly on premeasured paper and apply immediately; secure paper with tape

      4) Rotate application areas to prevent skin irritation and apply to clean, dry, intact, and hairless skin

4. Respiratory medications

   a. Nose drops

      1) Tilt client's head back

      2) Fill dropper with prescribed amount of medication

      3) Place dropper just inside nare and instill correct number of drops

      4) Wipe excess medication with tissue

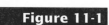

      5) Instruct client not to sneeze or blow nose and to keep head tilted back for 5 minutes until drug is absorbed

   b. Metered-dose inhaled medication (MDI) (see Figure 11-1)

      1) Shake canister before each puff to mix medication and propellant

      2) Instruct client to hold inhaler 2 inches away from mouth

Figure 11-1

Metered dose inhaler with device positioned away from the opened mouth

© Jenny Thomas

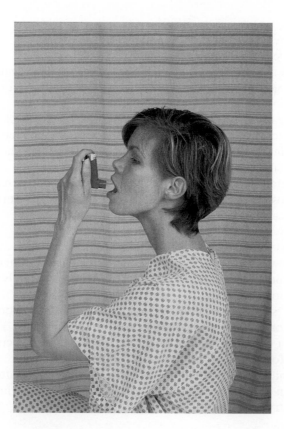

   3) Instruct client to exhale through pursed lips
   4) Instruct client to depress inhalation device, inhaling slowly and deeply through mouth
   5) Instruct client to hold breath for 10 seconds and slowly exhale through pursed lips
   6) Instruct client to wait 2 minutes (or longer if drug literature recommends) between puffs
   7) Clean device according to manufacturer's instructions
  c. Spacer with MDI (see Figure 11-2)
   1) Insert MDI mouthpiece into spacer
   2) Remove mouthpiece cover from spacer
   3) Shake MDI with spacer
   4) Hold MDI and spacer with drug canister upright
   5) Instruct client to exhale slowly through pursed lips
   6) Instruct client to close lips around spacer mouthpiece
   7) Activate MDI canister by pushing it further into plastic adapter
   8) Instruct client to inhale slowly and deeply through mouth
   9) Instruct client to hold breath 10 seconds
   10) Instruct client to exhale and relax
   11) Wipe mouthpiece after use
   12) Remove rubber end of spacer, rinse with warm water and dry thoroughly
 5. Optic medications
  a. Eye abbreviations (O.S.—left eye, O.D.—right eye, and O.U.—both eyes) should no longer be used; instead the correct eye(s) should be written or typed out

Figure 11-2

Metered-dose inhaler with extender attached to a mouthpiece placed in the mouth

© Jenny Thomas

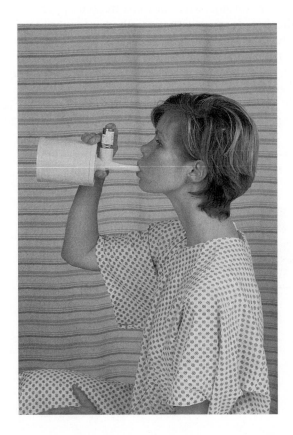

    b. Ophthalmic drops

      1) Tilt client's head slightly backward and ask client to look up

      2) Give tissue to client so that client can wipe off excess medication

      3) Hold eyedropper one-half to three-quarters of an inch above eyeball

      4) Expose lower **conjunctival sac** (mucosal membrane that lines eye) by pulling down on cheek, creating a "cup"

      5) Drop prescribed number of drops into center of conjunctival sac while applying pressure to inner canthus to reduce systemic absorption of medication

      6) Instruct client to close eyelids and move eyes

      7) Gently massage closed lid

      8) Remove excess medication with tissue

    c. Ophthalmic ointment

      1) Give tissue to client so that client can wipe off excess medication

      2) Put on gloves

      3) Gently separate client's eyelids with 2 fingers, grasping lower lid immediately below lashes; exert pressure downward over bony prominence of cheek to form a trough

      4) Instruct client to look upward

      5) Apply eye medication along inside edge of entire lower eyelid, from inner canthus to outer canthus (angles formed by upper and lower eyelids)

      6) Instruct client to close eyelids and move eyes to spread ointment under lids and over eye surface

      7) Remove excess medication with a tissue

      8) Instruct client that vision may be blurred temporarily following administration of an ointment

6. Otic (ear) medications

    a. Position client on side, with ear to be treated uppermost

    b. Fill medication dropper with prescribed amount of medication

    c. Put on gloves

    d. Straighten ear canal

      1) Infant: pull pinna, the projected part of upper exterior ear, gently downward and backward

      2) Adult: pull pinna gently upward and backward (see Figure 11-3)

      3) Instill medication drops, holding medication slightly above ear

      4) Insert cotton loosely into ear canal, if ordered

      5) Instruct client to remain on side for 5 to 10 minutes

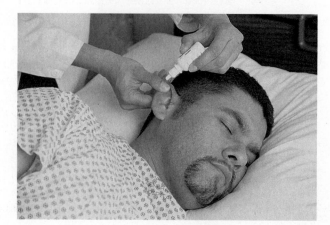

Figure 11-3

Instilling ear drops. Gently pull pinna up and back to instill medication in an adult or older child.

7. Vagina
   a. Position client in dorsal recumbent or Sims' position
   b. Put on gloves
   c. Suppository: remove foil wrapper and insert suppository into applicator
   d. Cream: attach tube of medication to applicator and squeeze tube to fill applicator with prescribed amount of medication; remove tube
   e. Insert applicator into vaginal canal at least 2 inches, push plunger until all of medication is released, and remove applicator (see Figure 11-4)
   f. Instruct client to lie quietly for 15 minutes until suppository or cream is absorbed
   g. Wash applicator and return it to appropriate place in client's room
8. Rectal
   a. Place client in Sims' (left lateral) position
   b. Wash hands and put on gloves
   c. Remove foil wrapper from suppository
   d. Apply small amount of water-soluble lubricant to suppository
   e. With index finger, insert suppository flat end first (studies indicate this promotes better retention than tapered end first) beyond internal sphincter to ensure retention
      1) Adult: insert approximately 10 cm or 4 inches (see Figure 11-5)
      2) Child or infant: insert approximately 5 cm or 2 inches
   f. Instruct client to lie quietly for 15 minutes while medication is absorbed
9. Administering medications by **irrigation (lavage)**, cleansing of a body cavity by flushing with medication (see Table 11-6)
   a. Surgical asepsis is required when there is a break in skin (e.g., wound irrigation) or when entering a sterile body cavity (e.g., bladder)

Figure 11-4

Using an applicator to instill vaginal cream

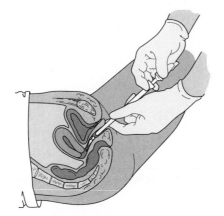

Figure 11-5

With a gloved finger, insert the rectal suppository approximately 4 inches beyond the internal sphincter in an adult and 2 inches in a child

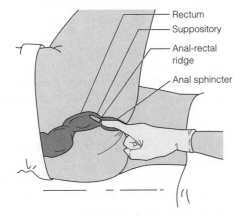

Rectum
Suppository
Anal-rectal ridge
Anal sphincter

Table 11-6 **Irrigation Syringes**

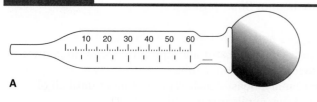

Asepto syringe is calibrated allowing for accurate measurements of irrigating solutions and produces less pressure than the piston syringe and comes in a range of sizes

A

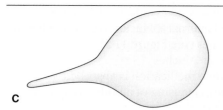

Piston or Toomy syringe is calibrated allowing for accurate measurements of irrigating solutions and produces more pressure than the asepto and comes in a range of sizes

B

Bulb comes in a variety of sizes

C

Pomeroy syringe is metal and is commonly used for ear irrigations. It has a shield near the tip to prevent solutions from spraying outward

D

Source: Berman, Audrey J.; Snyder, Shirlee, *Kozier & Erb's Fundamentals of Nursing*, 9th Ed. © 2012. Reprinted and Electronically reproduced by permission of Pearson Education, Inc., Upper Saddle River, New Jersey.

   b. Medical asepsis is used for vaginal, rectal, or gastric irrigation; the type, strength, amount, and temperature of the irrigant are prescribed

   c. Eye

     1) Wash hands and put on gloves

     2) Supply client with a receptacle to catch irrigation returns (emesis basin)

     3) Gently separate client's eyelids with 2 fingers, grasping lower lid immediately below lashes; exert pressure downward over bony prominence of cheek to form a trough

     4) Instruct client to look upward

     5) Fill and hold eye irrigator approximately 1 inch above eye to ensure safe pressure of irrigation solution

     6) Irrigate eye, directing solution on lower conjunctival sac from inner canthus to outer canthus so that irrigation returns run into collecting basin

     7) Dry around eye with cotton balls or tissues

      d. Ears
         1) Wash hands and put on gloves
         2) Straighten ear canal
         3) Supply client with a receptacle to catch irrigation returns (emesis basin)
         4) Fill and insert ear irrigator into auditory canal (do not obstruct canal with syringe, solution must be able to escape during irrigation) and gently direct solution upward against top of canal
         5) Dry outside of ear
         6) Position client on affected side and place an absorbent material under ear to collect drainage

10. Injections
      a. See Box 11-2 for withdrawing medications from a vial
      b. See Box 11-3 for withdrawing medications from an ampule
      c. Maintain sterility while assembling syringe and needle; select appropriate size needle and syringe based on volume and type of medication, desired site, client's size, and viscosity of medication
      d. See Table 11-7 for a summary of syringes, needles, and uses
      e. Using anatomical landmarks, select site of injection appropriate for type of injection and medication (e.g., intramuscular, intradermal, or subcutaneous); see Table 11-8 for a summary of injection sites
      f. Wash hands and put on gloves
      g. Cleanse area with an alcohol swab and wait for it to dry
      h. Inject medication

> **Practice to Pass**
>
> The nurse is to administer heparin by the subcutaneous route. What supplies will the nurse need and how will the nurse administer the medication?
>
> !

Box 11-2	
Withdrawing Medications From a Vial	**1.** Remove vial cap.
	2. Cleanse rubber top of the vial with alcohol.
	3. Tighten needle on syringe or use needleless syringe.
	4. Fill plunger with an amount of air equal to the amount of solution to be withdrawn.
	5. Inject air into vacant area of vial keeping the needle above the surface of medication.
	6. Invert the vial touching only the syringe barrel and plunger tip. Withdraw medication.
	7. While the syringe remains attached to the vial, expel any air bubbles from syringe by tapping the side of syringe sharply.
	8. Recheck amount of medication in syringe.
	9. Remove syringe from vial and recap needle.

Box 11-3	
Withdrawing Medications From an Ampule	**1.** Tap the neck of the ampule to move solution to the body of the ampule.
	2. Using a pad, break ampule away from you.
	3. Use a filter needle to withdraw solution. Solution can be withdrawn from either an upright or inverted position—insert needle without touching sides of neck with the bevel down and touching the bottom of the ampule (do not add air).
	4. Return ampule to upright position.
	5. Tap barrel below bubbles to dislodge air in the syringe.
	6. Eject air with syringe in an upright position.
	7. Recheck amount of medication in syringe.
	8. Remove filter needle and replace with appropriate needle.

Table 11-7 Summary of Syringes, Needles, and Uses

Use/Purpose	Site	Maximum Volume	Syringe	Needle Size	Needle Angle
Insulin					
Slow absorption to produce a sustained effect	Abdomen, lateral and posterior aspects of upper arm or thigh, scapular area, upper ventrodorsal gluteal areas	1 mL	Insulin—calibrated on 100 unit scale 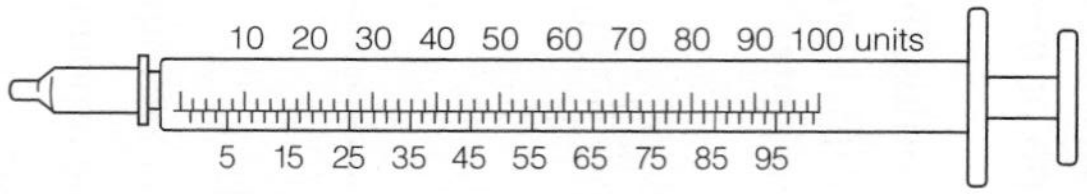 10 20 30 40 50 60 70 80 90 100 units 5 15 25 35 45 55 65 75 85 95 **A**	Nonremovable ⅜ inch 29 gauge	45° or 90°
Intradermal					
Antigens and skin testing Slow absorption	Inner aspect of forearm or scapular area, upper chest, medial thigh	0.1 mL	1 mL tuberculin syringe 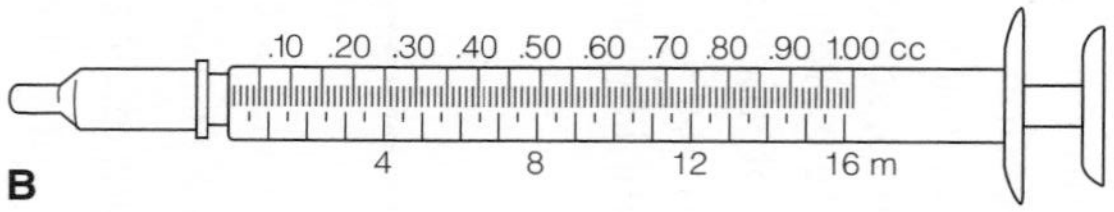 .10 .20 .30 .40 .50 .60 .70 .80 .90 100 cc 4 8 12 16 m **B**	⅜ inch 25–27 gauge	10–15° just under epidermis; bevel of needle up
Subcutaneous					
Absorbed slowly for sustained effect	Abdomen, lateral and posterior aspects of upper arm or thigh, scapular area of back, upper ventrodorsal gluteal areas	1.0 mL	1–3 mL syringe 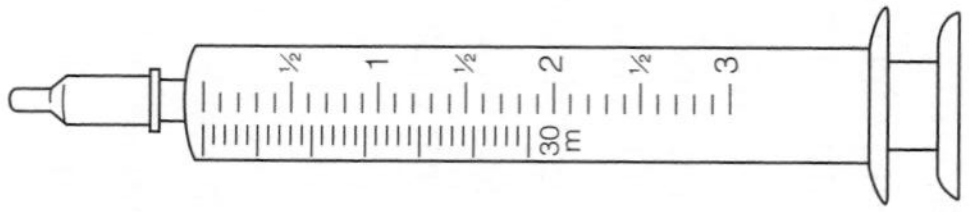 3 2½ 2 1½ 1 ½ 30 U **C**	⅜–⅝ inch 25 gauge	⅝–45° with 1 inch of tissue grasped ⅜ in–90° with 2 inches of tissue grasped
Intramuscular					
Promotes rapid Absorption	Ventrogluteal, vastus lateralis, deltoid *Ventrogluteal*—preferred site for adults *Vastus lateralis*—preferred site for children <7 months of age	*Adult deltoid* 0.5–1 mL *Adult gluteus medius* 1–4 mL	1–5 mL syringe	Deltoid ⅝–1 inch, 23–25 gauge *Vastus lateralis, ventrogluteal,* 1½ inch	90°

Table 11-8	Summary of Injection Sites

Intramuscular

Ventrogluteal

- Place client in side-lying position
- Use right hand for left anterior hip and left hand for right anterior hip
- Place palm over greater trochanter and point index finger toward client's anterior superior iliac spine; spread out index finger from other three fingers to form a "V" area
- Inject at a 90° angle within "V" area

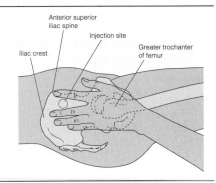

Vastus Lateralis

- Place client in supine position
- Inject at a 90° angle using *anterolateral middle third* of thigh between greater trochanter and lateral femoral condyle

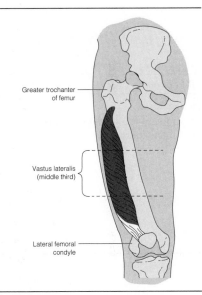

Deltoid

- Palpate lower edge of acromion and midpoint of lateral aspect of arm. Inject at a 90° angle 2 in. below acromion process within triangle between boundaries
- Alternate method—place 4 fingers across deltoid muscle with first finger on acromion process; site is 3 finger breaths below acromion process

Z-Track Injection

- An alternative method of IM injection designed to reduce seepage of medication into subcutaneous tissues
- Prior to injection, displace skin; insert needle at a 90° angle while skin remains displaced; once needle is removed, allow skin to return to a neutral position, thus eliminating an intact needle tract
- This method is used for medications that are irritating to subcutaneous tissues

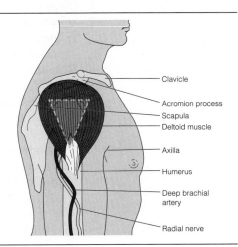

(continued)

Table 11-8	Summary of Injection Sites (Continued)

Subcutaneous

Most common sites

- Lateral posterior aspect of upper arms
- Anterior thighs
- Lower quadrants of abdomen (outside a 2-in. radius of umbilicus): preferred site for heparin

Other site

- Scapular areas

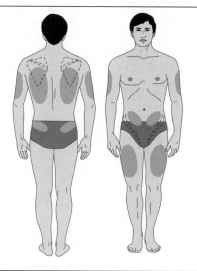

Intradermal

- Forearms
- Upper back beneath scapula
- Upper chest

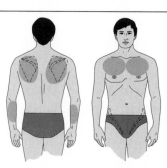

i. Discard syringe and needle into a sharps container
j. Specific information appropriate to injection sites

1) **Intradermal (ID):** gently pull skin taut; do not aspirate (draw back); inject medication slowly and observe for wheal formation and blanching at site

2) **Subcutaneous (subQ):** grasp subQ tissue; hold syringe like a dart (between thumb and forefinger) and insert needle; release subQ tissue; aspirate (except with heparin or insulin) and inject medication slowly if no blood appears (if blood returns withdraw the needle, discard and prepare a new injection); with insulin administration, rotate injection sites in an orderly manner to minimize tissue damage (**lipodystrophy**, atrophy, or hypertrophy of subQ tissue), which affects absorption

3) **Intramuscular (IM):** hold syringe like a dart (between thumb and forefinger); spread skin taught or grasp skin in pediatric and older adult client; use a quick, darting motion to insert needle; aspirate and inject dose slowly unless blood returns; if blood returns, withdraw needle, discard, and prepare a new injection); Z-track technique prevents "tracking" and is used to administer medications that are especially irritating to subcutaneous tissue (e.g., hydroxyzine [Vistaril])—pull skin approximately 1 in. laterally away from injection site, inject medication, withdraw needle, then release tissue

IV. INTRAVENOUS THERAPY

A. Indications

1. The intravenous (IV) route can be used to give medications that are too irritating to give by another route, to avoid discomfort of frequent IM injections, or to maintain a constant therapeutic blood level of a medication
2. In life-threatening situations, it provides access for administration of medications and fluids directly into bloodstream, ensuring prompt onset of action and most complete absorption
3. When client is unable to take fluids by mouth, it provides fluid and electrolyte replacement therapy for clients unable to take oral nourishment (such as with NPO status for diagnostic or surgical procedures, or problems related to swallowing or GI tract)
4. When medications would be destroyed by GI tract
5. When client is unable to digest or absorb a diet or when GI tract is nonfunctional because of an interruption in its continuity or impaired absorptive capacity, nutrition can be provided through venous system, where absorption and digestion of nutrients do not depend on GI tract

B. Types of fluids provided by IV route

1. Hydrating solutions (see Table 11-9)
2. Blood transfusion: administration of whole blood or blood components into venous circulation (see Box 11-4); types of blood products include:
   a. Whole blood: replaces intravascular blood volume and all blood products; contains red blood cells, plasma, plasma proteins, fresh platelets, and other clotting factors
   b. Red blood cells: increase oxygen-carrying capacity of blood; 1 unit of red blood cells increases hematocrit approximately 2–4%
   c. Platelets: play an important role in blood coagulation, homeostasis, and blood thrombus formation
   d. Plasma: liquid part of blood that expands blood volume and provides clotting factors
   e. Albumin: expands blood volume by providing plasma proteins; contains substances that cannot diffuse through capillary walls, resulting in increased plasma volume and increased osmotic pressure causing fluids to move into vascular compartment; used to treat hypovolemic shock
   f. Clotting factors and cryoprecipitate provide different factors involved in blood clotting; cryoprecipitate is prepared from fresh frozen plasma and contains factor VIII, factor XIII, fibronectin, and fibrinogen; it is used to treat hypofibrinogenemia; concentrates of factor VIII and IX are also available
3. Total parenteral nutrition (TPN): solutions that provide all needed calories and contain high dextrose concentrations, water, fat, proteins, electrolytes, vitamins, and trace elements
   a. Hypertonic solutions containing more than 10% dextrose require a high-flow central vein for infusion
   b. Infection control is a high priority because glucose-rich solution promotes bacterial growth
   c. High glucose content requires careful administration and blood glucose monitoring to prevent hypoglycemia or hyperglycemia
   d. TPN is never stopped abruptly because sudden absence of infusion would cause hypoglycemia

C. Equipment needed for IV therapy

1. Catheters/needles
   a. Over-the-needle catheters: plastic catheter fits over needle that is used to pierce skin and vein; once in vein, needle is withdrawn and discarded, leaving catheter in place; available in a variety of lengths and gauges; use smallest length and gauge of catheter appropriate to therapy

Practice to Pass

The nurse is assessing a client receiving a blood transfusion. At what intervals should the nurse monitor the vital signs?

Table 11-9	Hydrating Solutions	
Solution	**Uses**	**Nursing Implications**
Isotonic		
0.9% sodium chloride or NaCl (normal saline or NS) Lactated Ringer's (LR) (Hartmann's solution) 5% dextrose in water (D$_5$W)	Has same concentration of solutes as plasma, so remains in vascular compartment, expanding vascular volume. NS and LR are crystalloid solutions, increase fluid volume in both intravascular and interstitial spaces with minimal fluid volume expansion. NS is the only solution that may be administered with blood products. D$_5$W is isotonic on initial administration but provides free water when glucose is metabolized, expanding intracellular and extracellular fluid volumes.	Assess for signs of hypervolemia: • Bounding pulse • Shortness of breath • Distended neck veins Assess for signs of hypovolemia: • Urine output less than 30 mL/hr • Weak, thready pulse • Subnormal temperature
Hypotonic		
0.45% sodium chloride (½ normal saline, ½ NS) 0.225% sodium chloride or NaCl (¼ normal saline or ¼ NS)	Has lesser concentration of solutes than plasma, therefore treats cellular dehydration through fluid shifting out of vascular compartment into cells; promotes elimination by kidneys.	Do not administer to clients at risk for third-space fluid shift or accumulation (sequestration of extracellular fluid in a body space, resulting in circulatory volume loss and risk for organ failure, or increased intracranial pressure).
Hypertonic		
5% dextrose in normal saline (D$_5$NS) 5% dextrose in 0.45% sodium chloride (D$_5$½NS) 5% dextrose in lactated Ringer's (D$_5$LR) 10% dextrose in water (D$_{10}$W) 20% dextrose in water (D$_{20}$W) 50% dextrose in water (D$_{50}$W)	Has higher concentration of solutes than plasma, therefore causing fluid to shift from the cells into the vascular compartment, expanding vascular volume. 10% dextrose—stand-by solution for clients receiving total parenteral nutrition (TPN) 50% dextrose—used for hypoglycemia	Do not administer to clients with kidney or heart disease or clients who are dehydrated. Monitor for signs of hypervolemia.
Volume Expanders (colloid solutions)		
Albumin 5% (Albumin-5, Buminate 5%) Albumin 25% (Albumin-25, Buminate 25%) Dextran 40 (Gentran 40) Hetastarch (Hespan [HESI]) Plasma protein fraction (Plasmanate, PlasmaPlex, Plasmatein, Protenate)	Colloid solutions—contain substances that cannot diffuse through capillary walls, resulting in increased plasma volume and increased osmotic pressure causing fluids to move into vascular compartment; used to treat hypovolemic shock.	Establish baseline vital signs, lung and heart sounds, and central venous pressure. Repeat per agency protocols. Administer with a large-gauge (18–19 gauge) needle. Monitor intake and output. Monitor for signs of hypervolemia.
Nutrient		
5% dextrose (D$_5$W) 5% dextrose in 0.45% sodium chloride (D$_5$½NS)	Contain some form of carbohydrate (e.g., dextrose or glucose) and water. D$_5$W provides 170 calories per liter.	Useful in preventing dehydration but does not provide sufficient calories to promote wound healing, weight gain, or normal growth in children.
Electrolyte		
0.9% sodium chloride Ringer's solution (contains sodium, chloride, potassium, and calcium) Lactated Ringer's (contains sodium, chloride, potassium, calcium, and lactate) 5% dextrose in 0.45% sodium chloride (D$_5$½NS)	Saline and electrolytes restore vascular volume and replace electrolytes. Lactated Ringer's (LR) is also an alkalinizing solution that treats metabolic acidosis. 5% dextrose in 0.45% sodium chloride is an acidifying solution to treat metabolic alkalosis.	Monitor fluid and electrolytes. Monitor arterial blood gases. Monitor intake and output.

Box 11-4 **Procedure for Blood Administration**	• Verify client consent and obtain baseline vital signs prior to initiating transfusion (some agencies require a provider's order to administer blood with a temperature elevation greater than 100°F). • Ensure a suitable vein and appropriate gauge needle (18 or 20 gauge preferred). • Set up blood infusion equipment. • Obtain a Y-set with a blood filter, using aseptic technique, insert spike into a container of 0.9% normal saline and prime the tubing. Ensure that solution covers filter and ⅓ of drip chamber above filter. Back prime the other Y leg with saline. Never use a solution containing dextrose as that will cause blood to clump. • Start saline solution. • Obtain correct blood component from blood bank comparing requisition form to blood bag label with lab technician. Verify client's name, identification number, blood type (A, B, AB, or O) and Rh group, blood donor number, and expiration date. Note any abnormal color, RBC clumping, gas bubbles, and extraneous material. Return if date is expired or any abnormalities are noted. • Follow general guidelines for medication preparation procedures in Box 11-1. • With another nurse, compare laboratory blood record: client's name and identification number (located on client's blood identiband), number on blood bag label, ABO group and Rh type on blood bag label. If information does not match exactly, notify blood bank and do not administer blood. Sign appropriate form with another nurse according to agency protocol. • Immediately hang blood—blood must be hung within 30 minutes of receipt from blood bank. • Wash hands and don gloves. • Invert blood bag gently several times to mix cells with plasma. • Insert remaining Y-set spike into blood bag. • Open upper clamp on the Y-set arm to blood. • Close upper clamp below IV saline solution and open upper clamp below blood bag to allow blood to run into saline-filled drip chamber. • Begin transfusion at a slow rate of about 2 mL per minute, stay with client and check vital signs every 5–15 minutes for first 50–100 mL of blood transfused, monitoring for reactions: bacterial, allergic, or hemolytic. • After first 15 minutes, increase rate of infusion. A whole unit of blood should be administered within 3–4 hours. • Continue to monitor vital signs throughout blood infusion according to agency protocol. • Document procedure and client's reaction in client's medical record.

    b. Winged needle/butterfly: steel needles with plastic flaps (wings) attached to shaft to facilitate venipuncture; winged needles are commonly used for obtaining some blood samples or for short-term therapy

    c. These devices come in protected needle styles designed to reduce risk of accidental puncture wounds and blood exposure

2. Infusion pumps/electronic delivery devices (EDDs)

    a. Deliver fluids by exerting positive pressure on tubing or on fluid in order to maintain fluid flow despite increased venous resistance

    b. Regulate rate at preset limits and have alarms that are triggered when fluid level is low or there is air in line

    c. Should be utilized when volume needs to be carefully controlled

3. Regulators, controllers, and mechanical infusion devices

    a. Devices designed to aid in monitoring of IV flow rates; they are convenience devices and are not to be used when flow rate must be carefully administered

    b. Because of poorer precision, they are less frequently used today

   4. Tubing: may be vented or nonvented
      a. Vented tubing is used with glass bottles while plastic bags utilize the nonvented tubing
      b. When infusions flow by gravity, tubing's drip chamber determines size of the drop
      c. Drip chambers commonly are rated at 10, 12, or 15 drops per mL; pediatric sets usually are rated at 60 drops per mL
   5. Filters: devices that may be part of infusion set or may be added to infusion line; remove contaminants such as air, bacteria, or particulate matter; not all medications or solutions can or need to be filtered

      a. TPN requires a filter that is changed every 24 hours with the tubing change
      b. Some medications such as phenytoin (Dilantin) and pantoprazole (Protonix) require a filter change with each medication administration
      c. To prime filters, point filter downward so proximal half fills with fluid first, then invert to complete priming the filter
   6. Types of infusions
      a. Peripheral infusion: an IV device whose internal tip terminates in a peripheral vein; in adults, internal tip lies between fingers and shoulder; some fluids and medications cannot be administered by peripheral line because of characteristics of fluids; peripheral devices are often rotated every 3 days but this is determined by agency policy
      b. Central infusion: IV device whose internal tip lies in central venous system, most commonly in superior vena cava; these devices can remain in place for long periods of time; any fluid or medication that can be administered into venous circulation can be administered by central lines; most central lines require sterile dressings to reduce risk of contamination; agency policy and type of dressing determine frequency of dressing changes
      c. Continuous infusion: an infusion which is uninterrupted and runs 24 hours a day
      d. Intermittent infusion: an infusion designed for clients who do not require IV fluid replacement therapy but require an IV access; a saline lock or prn adapter is fitted to end of venous access device providing a connection for intermittent solution or medication administration; these devices require flushing with saline at least once every 8 hours and before and after medication administration; some central lines require a saline flush to be followed by a heparin flush (10 units/mL or 100 units/mL solutions) to maintain the device; follow agency policy
 D. Procedures and skills necessary to start and maintain IV therapy
   1. Peripheral infusion
      a. Start equipment includes:
         1) IV catheter
         2) IV start kit that contains a tourniquet, alcohol and antimicrobial cleansing wipes, sterile tape, and gauze/semipermeable transparent membrane dressing materials
         3) IV fluids and appropriate tubing; filter if indicated
         4) Pump/regulator device if desired or necessary
         5) Gloves
      b. Procedure
         1) Wash hands
         2) Verify type and amount of solution with prescription; note expiration date
         3) Prepare equipment
            a) Obtain needleless adapter to connect to venous access device if device does not include one
            b) Remove outer wrappers from tubing, connect tubing and filter device, and close tubing roller clamp

    c) Remove outer wrapper around IV bag, inspect bag for leaks (small amount of condensation is normal), tears, discoloration, cloudiness, or particulate matter; do not use bag if present

    d) Hang IV bag on pole

    e) Using aseptic technique, remove port cap on IV bag and plastic protector from IV tubing spike (end with drip chamber) and insert spike into IV bag

    f) Squeeze drip chamber until it is partially full

    g) Remove protective cap on tubing if it is not an air-vented cap, open roller clamp on tubing to prime tubing and filter; invert and tap Y injection sites to remove air during priming, replace protective tubing cap

4) Start IV

    a) Follow agency policy when starting and maintaining an IV device; wear gloves for protection from bloodborne pathogens

    b) Prepare client for infusion, explain procedure, and obtain client's permission for procedure

    c) Identify appropriate vein for cannulation: in adults, peripheral IVs are inserted between fingers and shoulders; depending on age, peripheral IVs in children can include the above sites as well as scalp and leg veins; avoid sites where veins are sclerotic, inflamed, or subject to decreased blood flow (as is common in adults following a stroke or mastectomy on that side)

    d) Use tourniquet to distend blood vessel; verify absence of latex allergy before applying tourniquet; in absence of a tourniquet, a blood pressure cuff may be used; some older adults may be accessed without a tourniquet; place tourniquet 4–6 inches above proposed site tightly enough to obstruct venous circulation but not arterial circulation (use gravity and/or topical heat application to aid vein distention)

    e) Prepare skin; typical procedure is to clean site with alcohol followed by an antimicrobial cleanser per agency policy; site is cleaned in a circular manner that removes bacteria from insertion site; the cleansing agent must be allowed to dry on skin

    f) Introduce needle at a 10- to 30-degree angle with bevel up; once blood return occurs, advance catheter until hub is in contact with insertion site

    g) Release tourniquet and remove needle from catheter and dispose of it in a sharps container

    h) Connect catheter to IV tubing and apply a sterile dressing to insertion site; a label on the side of insertion site identifies length and gauge of catheter, date and time of insertion, and nurse's initials

    i) Apply date sticker with time and nurse's initials to tubing

    j) Initiate prescribed flow rate: gravity flow tubing is regulated by drops per minute, and drops delivered per mL of solution vary with different brands and types of infusion sets (drop factor) from 10 to 20 drops/mL; microdrip sets are always 60 drops/mL; to administer 1,000 mL in 8 hours with a drop factor of 15 drops/mL

$$\frac{\text{Total infusion volume} \times \text{drop factor}}{\text{Total time of infusion in minutes}} = \text{drops/minute}$$

$$\frac{1{,}000\,\text{mL} \times 15}{8 \times 60\ \text{min}\ (480\ \text{min})} = 31.25\,\text{drops/min}\ (31)$$

5) Document date, time, solution, amount, infusion device, rate, site location, and condition of site and dressing

6) Maintain IV infusion
  a) Ensure that correct solution is infusing
  b) Check rate of flow every hour or more as per agency policy
  c) Inspect patency of IV tubing and needle
  d) Maintain solution container 3 feet above IV site
  e) Inspect tubing for kinks or obstructions; ensure that it is not dangling below IV site
  f) Lower solution container below IV site and observe for a blood return or gently pinch IV tubing adjacent to needle site causing blood to flow into tubing (flash back), or use a sterile syringe to withdraw fluid from port nearest venipuncture site, causing blood to flow into tubing
  g) Splint a joint if IV site is positional (movement of extremity impedes flow of solution)
  h) Ensure tight connections to prevent leakage
  i) Discontinue solution and remove IV access device if there is no blood return and cannot establish an acceptable drip rate

  j) Inspect insertion site for fluid infiltration (IV access device becomes dislodged from vessel, causing fluid to flow into interstitial tissues); see Table 11-10 for complications of IV therapy
  k) Instruct client to notify nurse if the flow rate changes or solution stops dripping, solution container is nearly empty, if blood is in IV tubing or at insertion site, or there is discomfort or swelling at insertion site

  l) At least every 8 hours document: solution, amount, infusion device, rate, site location, and condition of site and dressing
2. Central venous access devices (CVADs): access a central vein that empties into superior vena cava
  a. Central infusion devices
    1) Percutaneous (nontunneled) catheter: a single or multiple lumen catheter inserted by health care provider at client's bedside
    2) Tunneled catheter: like all central lines, it terminates in central venous system; remainder of catheter passes through a subcutaneous tract and exits on chest wall or abdomen; a dacron cuff on catheter elicits scar formation that prevents ascending tract infection; this catheter does not require a sterile dressing once subcutaneous tract has healed
    3) Peripherally inserted central catheter (PICC): inserted in basilic or cephalic vein just above or below antecubital space of right arm by a provider or specially trained IV therapy nurse and is used for longer term inpatient or outpatient therapy; although insertion site is in periphery, catheter terminates in superior vena cava
    4) Implantable venous access devices or ports: surgically implanted into a small subcutaneous pocket, usually on upper chest using local anesthesia; port is attached to a catheter that terminates in central venous system; most ports are accessed with a Huber needle to preserve life of the port septum
    5) Peripheral access system (PAS) ports are similar to a subcutaneous port except port itself is implanted in antecubital area
  b. The internal tips of all central lines lie within central venous system; placement can occur in numerous settings but all placements must be verified by x-ray
  c. Internal tips: internal tip of catheter comes in 2 versions
    1) Open-tipped: end of catheter opens directly into bloodstream; if flushing techniques are not performed correctly, blood can back up into catheter causing catheter occlusion; there are 2 open-tipped catheters; they must be flushed with saline followed by heparin flush solution to maintain patency when not in use
      a) Hickman: adult form of open-tipped catheter
      b) Broviac: pediatric version, which usually means smaller lumen size

Table 11-10	Complications of IV Therapy
Complication	**Nursing Implications**
Infection (catheter-related) (sepsis)—common occurrence with TPN solutions that have high glucose concentration that invites bacteria; characterized by fever, chills, erythema or drainage at insertion site, elevated white blood count, and possibly septic shock	• Use strict aseptic technique when working with IVs • Change IV solutions at least every 24 hours • Change IV tubing and dressings per agency protocols (TPN tubing every day) • When discontinuing central lines, remove tip of catheter and apply an occlusive dressing; monitor site for 48 hours, the catheter tip may be sent to lab for culture if sepsis is suspected

Air embolism—air is introduced into IV line during catheter insertion, tubing change, or administration of solutions and medications; characterized by respiratory distress, chest pain, dyspnea, hypotension, and weak and rapid pulse	• When changing tubing or reflux valves on CVADs without Groshong valves or catheters, instruct client to perform Valsalva maneuver (forcefully exhale and bear down with mouth closed)
	• Ensure all catheter connections are tight
	• All connections on central lines should be luer lock not slip lock
	• During insertion of a percutaneous central venous catheter, position client in head down position with head turned toward opposite direction of insertion site
	• If an air embolism is suspected:
	  • Clamp catheter
	  • Position client in left Trendelenburg position
	  • Administer oxygen and contact provider

Hypersensitivity reaction—sensitivity to medication; characterized by flushing, itching, and urticaria	• Check client allergies prior to administering medications • Stop infusion • Notify provider • Monitor vital signs
Circulatory overload—fluids administered faster than circulation can accommodate; characterized by cough, dyspnea, crackles, distended neck veins, tachycardia, hypertension, S_3 heart sounds, and cardiac rhythm	• Use IV pumps or controllers to regulate infusion rate • Do not "catch up" with IV solutions • Carefully monitor fluid volumes with administration of multiple concurrent IV solutions or medications • Check client's IV infusion rates at least hourly per agency protocols • Avoid selecting an IV container whose volume is greater than volume ordered • Monitor client's vital signs, intake and output, breath and heart sounds • For signs and symptoms of fluid volume overload: • Slow or stop infusion rate per order • Place client in high-Fowler's position • Administer oxygen and diuretics per order • Notify provider
Infiltration—localized swelling, coolness, pallor, and discomfort at the IV site	• Stop IV and remove venous access device • Apply a warm compress to site of infiltration and elevate extremity on a pillow • Restart infusion at another site
Phlebitis—inflammation of a vein; characterized by warmth, swelling, red streak at vein site, pain along course of vein, and warm to touch	• Inspect and palpate IV site at least every 8 hours for redness; if phlebitis is detected, discontinue infusion and remove venous access device • A prescription is not required to remove and replace a peripheral catheter that shows symptoms of phlebitis • Apply warm compresses to venipuncture site • Select a large vein when administering irritating solutions or medications • Dilute irritating medications (e.g., promethazine [Phenergan]) and administer over prescribed amount of time on an infusion pump; if client reports pain at insertion site, further dilute medication and slow flow rate

(continued)

Table 11-10	Complications of IV Therapy (Continued)
Complication	**Nursing Implications**
Hypoglycemia—decreased blood glucose (BG) level related to TPN being abruptly discontinued or excessive insulin administration; characterized by BG less than 70 mg/dL, hunger, diaphoresis, weakness and anxiety	• Monitor BG level per agency protocols (at least every day) • Gradually decrease infusion when discontinuing TPN • Have 10% dextrose available as stand-by (medical prescription required for prn use)
Hyperglycemia—increased BG related to infusion of TPN or excessive dextrose solutions to diabetic clients; characterized by BG greater than 200 mg/dL, excessive thirst, fatigue, restlessness, confusion, weakness, and diuresis	• Monitor BG per agency protocols (at least every day) • Check medications affecting BG levels (e.g., steroids) • Begin infusion at a slow rate (40 mL/hr) and gradually increase • Do not "catch up" if infusion rate falls behind

    2) Closed-tip catheter or Groshong: this catheter has a valve on its internal tip that prevents backflow of blood; Groshong catheters are routinely flushed with double volumes of saline but do not require instillation of heparin flush solution; advantages of Groshong catheters are:

        a) Decreased risk of air emboli or bleeding

        b) Elimination of heparin flush

        c) Elimination of catheter clamping

        d) Reduced flushing protocols between use

  d. Lumens: central catheters may have a single, double, or triple lumen; each lumen corresponds to a separate catheter and has a separate exit point

    1) Multi-lumens allow for administration of incompatible drugs

    2) Blood drawn from one lumen will not be contaminated by drugs administered through another lumen of catheter

    3) Each lumen is treated as a separate catheter and is flushed according to agency policy

  e. Indications

    1) Long-term IV therapy

    2) Obtaining frequent blood specimens

    3) Central venous pressure (CVP) monitoring

    4) Administration of TPN and medications that are irritating to veins, thus requiring a high-flow vein for rapid dilution

    5) Sclerosed peripheral veins

    6) Limited peripheral venous access

  f. Nursing care involved (dressing, inspection, flushing, etc.): special precautions need to be taken with all central venous devices to ensure asepsis and catheter patency; refer again to Table 11-10 for complications of IV therapy

    1) Site care: subclavian, jugular, and PICC sites

        a) Require air occlusive dressings: dressings should be changed when soiled or loose

        b) Follow agency protocol for frequency of dressing changes—usually every 2 to 7 days; gauze dressings must be changed every 48 hours; semipermeable transparent membrane dressings may remain in place for up to 1 week

        c) Follow agency protocols for cleaning solutions and types of dressings; Chloraprep® (2% chlorhexidine gluconate and 70% isopropyl alcohol) is commonly used to clean insertion site

        d) Using surgical asepsis and a mask, clean an area 2 inches in diameter around site using a swab with Chloraprep, use an up-and-down motion starting at center and working outward; allow Chloraprep to dry before applying air occlusive dressing over entire insertion site

        e) Assess site for redness, swelling, tenderness or drainage, and compare length of external portion of catheter with its documented length to assess for displacement

        f) Document date, condition of site, and dressing

    2) Site care: implantable devices

        a) Follow agency protocols for cleaning solutions and types of dressings; Chloraprep is commonly used to clean insertion site

        b) Before accessing port, using aseptic technique, clean an area 2 inches in diameter around port using a swab with Chloraprep, using an up-and-down motion starting at center and working outward; allow Chloraprep to dry before accessing

        c) Assess site for redness, swelling, tenderness, or drainage

        d) Access site with an appropriate primed needle, usually a Huber needle; assess for patency by aspirating blood and then flushing according to policy

        e) Apply a sterile dressing

    3) Catheter care and flushing

        a) Each lumen of catheter should be flushed according to agency policy; frequency of flush varies among catheters and may be as frequent as once a shift; subcutaneous ports that are not in use may not require flushing more often than once a month

        b) The flushing volume should be at least twice the internal volume of catheter; closed-tip catheters (Groshong) should have flushing volume doubled

        c) The flushing material is usually saline; some medications are incompatible with saline and D_5W may be substituted for saline

        d) For closed-tip catheters, saline flush is followed by a heparin flush instillation; the volume should approximate the internal volume of catheter

        e) Syringes smaller than 10 mL should not be used for flushing as they may contribute to catheter rupture

        f) Blood draws: use distal lumen if possible; discard appropriate amount of blood prior to obtaining sample; following blood aspiration, flush line with a double volume of saline before instilling heplock solution (if appropriate); change injection cap following a blood draw

    4) Client teaching: provide clients with the following instructions:

        a) Do not allow anyone to take a blood pressure on arm with a PICC line or PAS port

        b) Wear a medical identification bracelet if the device will be implanted for a long time

        c) PICC and nonimplanted CVADs: no activity restriction is necessary; do not immerse site in water

        d) Implanted CVADs: no restriction of activities is necessary; there are no restrictions regarding bathing or swimming when device is not accessed

E. IV medication administration

    1. Methods of administering IV medications

        a. Mixtures of medications within large volumes of IV fluids: provide and maintain a constant, well-diluted level of a medication in blood

        1) To add medication to an IV solution, prepare dose from a vial or ampule and draw into a syringe

        2) To add medication to a new IV container

            a) Clean injection port with an alcohol swab and allow to dry for 30 seconds

            b) Remove cap from syringe, insert needle or needleless device through center of injection port, and inject medication into solution

            c) Mix medication and solution by gently rotating bag

d) Complete and attach a medication label to IV solution, with the name and dose of medication, date and time, and nurse's initials

e) Proceed with setting up IV for administration

3) To add medication to an existing infusion

    a) Ensure that there is enough IV solution in container to properly dilute medication

    b) Proceed as with adding a medication to a new IV container

b. Injection by **bolus**, a direct injection of a medication intravenously (push), is used to obtain rapid therapeutic serum concentrations, when medications cannot be diluted, or for administration of emergency drugs

    1) With prn adaptor: when no solutions are running

    2) Prepare medication, draw up into a syringe, and label syringe so that it will not be confused with syringe containing normal saline irrigating solution

    3) Wash hands and put on gloves

    4) Flush IV access device per agency policy

    5) Cleanse infusion port with an alcohol swab and let it dry for 30 seconds

    6) Remove needle from syringe and attach syringe with medication to needleless port access device

    7) Administer medication using recommended IV push rate

    8) Flush IV access device per agency policy

c. Tandem infusion: an intermittent method of administering medications to an existing IV (not frequently used)

    1) Ensure that existing IV solution and intermittent infusion are compatible and that client's condition, vein, and gauge of access device can tolerate volume of fluid

    2) Medication will be administered in a second bag of fluid, usually 50–100 mL, by secondary line into Y port of a continuously running infusion; attach a needleless adapter to tubing of secondary set

    3) Cleanse infusion port of continuous infusion line Y port with an alcohol swab and let it dry 30 seconds

    4) Hang secondary infusion and existing infusion at same level

    5) Maintain existing IV rate and regulate piggyback rate using roller clamp on secondary tubing; the existing and the secondary solutions will run concurrently at their respective rates

d. Piggyback infusion

    1) To administer an intermittent infusion without disconnecting existing IV

        a) Set up secondary set following procedure for setting up an IV

        b) Hang existing infusion set lower than piggyback secondary set

        c) Cleanse uppermost infusion port with an alcohol swab and let it dry for 30 seconds

        d) Connect secondary set to primary set using a needleless access device, above existing IV roller clamp

        e) Maintain existing IV roller clamp position, and regulate piggyback rate using roller clamp on secondary tubing; the piggyback solution will infuse first and when complete, the existing IV will resume at original rate

    2) To administer an intermittent infusion using an infusing pump that is regulating the existing IV:

        a) When intermittent solution is in an IV bag, set up secondary administration set following procedure for setting up an IV; connect infusion tubing to secondary access port on pump; follow protocols for specific pump for administering intermittent medication as either a continuous infusion or an infusion interrupting existing IV

Practice to Pass

The nurse is administering an IV isotonic solution of 0.9% sodium chloride (normal saline). Considering the action of isotonic solutions, what are the nursing assessments specific to this type of fluid?

b) When intermittent solution is in a syringe, connect syringe to secondary access port on pump; follow protocols for specific pump for administering intermittent medication as either a continuous infusion or an infusion interrupting existing IV

e. Syringe pump or mini-infuser: administration of IV medications in a premixed syringe, which is connected to primary IV line via pump or mini-infuser

f. Volume control infusion: administration of small amounts of fluid through a set such as a Buretrol, Soluset, Volutrol, or Pediatrol
1) The 100–150 mL chamber is attached to primary infusion container
2) Allows for delivery of smaller fluid amounts and medications

Case Study

A client was diagnosed with Crohn's disease. A long-term tunneled Groshong CVAD was implanted for long-term total parenteral nutrition (TPN). The nurse is preparing the client and family for discharge. A home care nurse will visit the client each day for the first week to monitor the client's progress in self-administration of her TPN. The client will receive TPN while sleeping at night and will receive no fluids through the CVAD during the daytime. In anticipating the client's discharge learning needs, prepare answers to the following questions.

1. What is total parenteral nutrition (TPN)?
2. What is a tunneled Groshong CVAD?
3. What are the care instructions for a Groshong CVAD?

4. Why is blood glucose monitoring necessary?
5. What are the specific interventions related to TPN?

For suggested responses, see page 309.

POSTTEST

POSTTEST

1 The nurse is to administer 25 mg of promethazine (Phenergan) intramuscularly (IM) to a 150-pound client. The nurse knows that this medication should be given deep into a large muscle mass. Which site should the nurse select as the preferred site to inject the medication?

1. Deltoid
2. Dorsogluteal
3. Vastus lateralis
4. Ventrogluteal

2 The nurse is caring for several clients with central venous access devices (CVADs). While changing the tubing on the central lines, the nurse would need to do which of the following? Select all that apply.

1. Use strict aseptic technique.
2. Use clean technique for the tubing and dressing change.
3. Assess the insertion site for signs of redness and drainage.
4. Document the length of the external portion of the catheter.
5. Remove any sutures at the insertion site if the line has been in place more than 5 days.

POSTTEST

3 The client is receiving 5% dextrose in 0.45% sodium chloride. The provider has prescribed that the client receives 1 unit of packed red blood cells. Prior to hanging the blood, the nurse will prime the blood tubing with which of the following solutions?

1. 5% dextrose in water
2. Lactated Ringer's
3. 0.9% sodium chloride
4. 5% dextrose in 0.45% sodium chloride

4 While assessing a client's intravenous (IV) line, the nurse notes that the area is swollen, cool, pale, and causing the client discomfort. The nurse suspects which of the following problems?

1. Infiltration
2. Phlebitis
3. Infection
4. Air embolism

5 The client is receiving 5% dextrose in 0.45% sodium chloride intravenously (IV) and reports pain at the IV site. The nurse assesses the site and notes erythema and edema. What would be the appropriate action for the nurse to take?

1. Slow the infusion rate.
2. Discontinue the IV and apply a warm compress to the IV site.
3. Apply antibiotic ointment to the IV site.
4. Gently pull back the IV access device to reposition it within the vein.

6 While administering an intramuscular (IM) injection of an analgesic medication, the nurse aspirates and finds blood in the syringe prior to injecting the medication. Which action by the nurse would be appropriate?

1. Continue to administer the medication as it would not have a harmful effect.
2. Continue to administer the medication as the needle has hit a capillary and would not be an intravenous administration.
3. Withdraw the needle, cleanse the needle and the new injection site with alcohol, and administer the medication.
4. Withdraw the needle, discard the medication, and begin again with the medication administration.

7 The nurse is starting a new peripheral intravenous (IV) line in a client. The client reports a latex allergy. The nurse has a typical IV start kit for this procedure. Because of the latex allergy, what action should the nurse take?

1. Obtain a new tourniquet for this client and use standard IV tubing.
2. Utilize a blood pressure cuff to distend the vein.
3. Avoid putting povidone iodine on the skin.
4. Suggest an alternative therapy to a peripheral IV line.

8 The nurse has instructed the client in using a metered-dose inhaler. The nurse determines that the client understands the instructions after observing the client doing which of the following?

1. Administering the 2 puffs rapidly between breaths
2. Holding the inhaler 2 inches away from the mouth
3. Not shaking the canister before puffs
4. Exhaling immediately after administering the puff

9 A client is receiving a continuous enteral feeding via a percutaneous endoscopic gastrostomy (PEG) tube. The provider has prescribed phenytoin (Dilantin) to be administered through the PEG tube. The nurse notes that the medication cannot be administered with tube feedings. What actions should the nurse take at this time? Select all that apply.

1. Contact provider for a prescription to administer Dilantin by another route.
2. Contact provider to change the type of tube feeding to one that is compatible.
3. Stop tube feeding for at least 30 minutes before and after administration of Dilantin.
4. Stop tube feeding, flush the feeding tube with water, administer Dilantin, flush the tube feeding again with water, and continue the tube feeding.
5. Flush tube before and after administering the medication.

10 An alert, competent client refuses to take her daily antihypertensive medication. The nurse has explained to the client why the medication is important and the client states she understands but insists she does not want to take the medication. Which of the following is the best nursing action?

1. Administer the medication anyway because it is important for the client.
2. Inform the client that the medication must be taken until the nurse gets an order to discontinue it.
3. Withhold medication and report it to the provider.
4. Withhold medication and complete an incident report.

➤ *See pages 296–298 for Answers and Rationales.*

ANSWERS & RATIONALES

Pretest

1 **Answer: 3 Rationale:** Under the law, if a medication prescription is written incorrectly, the nurse who administers the incorrect prescription is responsible for the error. This includes both the right medication and the right dose (2 of the 10 rights of medication administration). The other responses are inaccurate conclusions about the case situation in the question. **Cognitive Level:** Analyzing **Client Need:** Management of Care **Integrated Process:** Nursing Process: Evaluation **Content Area:** Fundamentals **Strategy:** The critical words in the question are *NPH insulin* and *IV*. Recall the legal role of the nurse in medication administration and use the process of elimination to make a selection about the nurse's liability. **Reference:** Berman, A., & Snyder, S. J. (2012). *Kozier & Erb's fundamentals of nursing: Concepts, process, and practice* (9th ed.). Upper Saddle River, NJ: Pearson Education, p. 842.

2 **Answer: 1 Rationale:** Because of the thin layer of epithelium and the large network of capillaries under the tongue, sublingual medications such as nitroglycerine absorb rapidly. Medication absorption is slower in the stomach. Absorption is affected by the proximity of the medication to the venous system. Absorption can be delayed or not occur based on stomach contents and acidity. Sublingual medications are never administered in a sustained or timed release form. **Cognitive Level:** Applying **Client Need:** Pharmacological and Parenteral Therapies **Integrated Process:** Teaching and Learning **Content Area:** Fundamentals **Strategy:** The critical words are *sublingual* and *best response*. Recall advantages of various routes of drug administration and use the process of elimination to make a selection. **Reference:** Berman, A., & Snyder, S. J. (2012). *Kozier & Erb's fundamentals of nursing: Concepts, process, and practice* (9th ed.). Upper Saddle River, NJ: Pearson Education, p. 849.

3 **Answer: 2 Rationale:** For a well-developed adult, a 5/8- to 1-inch needle is the appropriate size for an IM deltoid injection. Because this is an obese client, the longer needle (1 inch) is appropriate to ensure it

reaches the muscle. **Cognitive Level:** Applying **Client Need:** Pharmacological and Parenteral Therapies **Integrated Process:** Nursing Process: Planning **Content Area:** Fundamentals **Strategy:** The critical terms are *obese client* and *deltoid*. Use basic nursing knowledge of needle sizes and their associated uses to make a selection. **Reference:** Berman, A., & Snyder, S. J. (2012). *Kozier & Erb's fundamentals of nursing: Concepts, process, and practice* (9th ed.). Upper Saddle River, NJ: Pearson Education, p. 888.

4 **Answer: 4 Rationale:** Z-track technique prevents "tracking" and is used for administering medications that are especially irritating to subcutaneous tissue. With Z-track technique, the skin is pulled approximately 1 inch laterally away from the injection site, the medication is injected, the needle is withdrawn, and the tissue is released. Using a small-gauge needle, injecting at a 45-degree angle, and applying ice to the site would not help prevent irritation to subcutaneous tissue by an irritating medication. **Cognitive Level:** Applying **Client Need:** Pharmacological and Parenteral Therapies **Integrated Process:** Nursing Process: Implementation **Content Area:** Fundamentals **Strategy:** The critical words are *prevent tracking*. Recall the various injection techniques and their indications and use the process of elimination to make a selection. **Reference:** Berman, A., & Snyder, S. J. (2012). *Kozier & Erb's fundamentals of nursing: Concepts, process, and practice* (9th ed.). Upper Saddle River, NJ: Pearson Education, p. 892.

5 **Answer: 4 Rationale:** Eyedrops are placed in the lower conjunctival sac to prevent damage to the cornea and to facilitate coating the eye with the medication. The drops are not applied directly onto the cornea or to the sclera near either the inner or the outer canthus. **Cognitive Level:** Applying **Client Need:** Pharmacological and Parenteral Therapies **Integrated Process:** Nursing Process: Implementation **Content Area:** Fundamentals **Strategy:** The core issue of the question is knowledge of the appropriate area for application of eye drops. Recall critical but basic information about proper technique to make a selection.

Note that all incorrect answers involve applying the medication directly to some area of the eyeball. **Reference:** Berman, A., & Snyder, S. J. (2012). *Kozier & Erb's fundamentals of nursing: Concepts, process, and practice* (9th ed.). Upper Saddle River, NJ: Pearson Education, p. 906.

6 **Answer: 4** **Rationale:** Protein is responsible for a significant portion of the osmotic pressure found in the blood vessels and maintains fluid within the vessels. In burn injuries, protein is lost, allowing fluid to escape into the tissues. Albumin is used to replace the lost proteins and pull fluids from the interstitial space back into the vascular system. It does not contain clotting factors or red blood cells and does not have enough fluid volume to consider it as part of primary fluid resuscitation. **Cognitive Level:** Applying **Client Need:** Pharmacological and Parenteral Therapies **Integrated Process:** Teaching and Learning **Content Area:** Fundamentals **Strategy:** The critical phrase is *rationale for the administration of albumin.* Recall first that albumin is a colloid that can be given intravenously to eliminate the options containing clotting factors and red blood cells. Choose correctly from 2 options, knowing that large volumes of crystalloids are used for fluid resuscitation and that albumin is a colloid. **Reference:** Berman, A., & Snyder, S. J. (2012). *Kozier & Erb's fundamentals of nursing: Concepts, process, and practice* (9th ed.). Upper Saddle River, NJ: Pearson Education, p. 1502.

7 **Answer: 100** **Rationale:** One way to solve the problem is to set it up as follows:

$$\frac{50 \text{ mL}}{30 \text{ min}} = \frac{x \text{ mL}}{60 \text{ min}}$$
$$30x = 3,000$$
$$x = 100 \text{ mL/hour}$$

Cognitive Level: Applying **Client Need:** Pharmacological and Parenteral Therapies **Integrated Process:** Nursing Process: Implementation **Content Area:** Fundamentals **Strategy:** The core issue of the question is knowledge of how to set up and solve an IV problem. Use basic knowledge of pharmacologic math procedures to answer the question. Use the common-sense test to check your answer by reasoning that if 50 mL should infuse in 30 minutes, then that is the equivalent speed of 100 mL infusing in an hour. **Reference:** Berman, A., & Snyder, S. J. (2012). *Kozier & Erb's fundamentals of nursing: Concepts, process, and practice* (9th ed.). Upper Saddle River, NJ: Pearson Education, p. 1493.

8 **Answer: 4** **Rationale:** 0.45% sodium chloride is a hypotonic solution that draws fluid from the vascular compartment into the cells; this type of solution would be used for clients with cellular dehydration. Normal saline and lactated Ringer's solution are isotonic, while 5% dextrose in normal saline is hypertonic until the body metabolizes the dextrose. **Cognitive Level:** Analyzing **Client Need:** Pharmacological and Parenteral Therapies **Integrated Process:** Nursing Process: Planning **Content Area:** Fundamentals

Strategy: The critical term is *hypotonic.* Recall commonly used hydrating solutions and their indications, and use the process of elimination to make a selection. **Reference:** Kozier, B., Erb, G., Berman, A., & Snyder, S. J. (2004). *Fundamentals of nursing: Concepts, process, and practice* (7th ed.). Upper Saddle River, NJ: Pearson Education, p. 1480.

9 **Answer: 2** **Rationale:** The client's body has adjusted to higher blood glucose levels as a result of receiving total parenteral nutrition (TPN) with high dextrose concentrations. Abruptly stopping TPN can result in hypoglycemia. The client is not greatly at risk for hypocalcemia, sepsis, or hyperkalemia because of the dislodgement. **Cognitive Level:** Applying **Client Need:** Pharmacological and Parenteral Therapies **Integrated Process:** Nursing Process: Assessment **Content Area:** Fundamentals **Strategy:** The core issue of the question is knowledge that abrupt cessation of a high-dextrose solution such as total parenteral nutrition (TPN) places the client at risk for rebound hypoglycemia. Use nursing knowledge and the process of elimination to choose correctly. **Reference:** Berman, A., & Snyder, S. J. (2012). *Kozier & Erb's fundamentals of nursing: Concepts, process, and practice* (9th ed.). Upper Saddle River, NJ: Pearson Education, p. 1297.

10 **Answer: 2** **Rationale:** Recall that in the apothecary system, 1 grain = 65 mg. Thus, the 10 grains can be converted to 650 mg. One way to set up the problem is as follows:

$$\frac{650 \text{ mg}}{325 \text{ mg}} = \frac{x}{1}$$
$$325x = 650$$
$$x = 2 \text{ tablets}$$

Cognitive Level: Analyzing **Client Need:** Pharmacological and Parenteral Therapies **Integrated Process:** Nursing Process: Implementation Fundamentals **Strategy:** The core issue of the question is the ability to perform basic pharmacologic math calculations. If this question was difficult, take time to review standard formulas for calculating drug dosages. **Reference:** Berman, A., & Snyder, S. J. (2012). *Kozier & Erb's fundamentals of nursing: Concepts, process, and practice* (9th ed.). Upper Saddle River, NJ: Pearson Education, p. 855.

Posttest

1 **Answer: 4** **Rationale:** For an adult with well-developed muscle mass, the preferred medication administration injection site for medications requiring a large muscle mass is the ventrogluteal area. The vastus lateralis is the preferred IM injection site for children under 7 months of age. The deltoid is not a large muscle and should not be utilized for the administration of promethazine (Phenergan). Medications should not be administered in the dorsogluteal area due to the risk of injury of the sciatic nerve. **Cognitive Level:** Applying

Client Need: Pharmacological and Parenteral Therapies **Integrated Process:** Nursing Process: Implementation **Content Area:** Fundamentals **Strategy:** The critical terms are *150-pound client* and *preferred site of injection.* Use knowledge of the advantages and disadvantages of each injection site to answer the question. **Reference:** Berman, A., & Snyder, S. J. (2012). *Kozier & Erb's fundamentals of nursing: Concepts, process, and practice* (9th ed.). Upper Saddle River, NJ: Pearson Education, pp. 868–869.

2 Answers: 1, 3, 4 Rationale: Strict aseptic technique is always required for the changing of central line tubing and/or dressings to prevent bloodborne infection. The catheter length should be documented to assess possible displacement. Removing sutures that secure the line would be inappropriate. All venous access sites should be assessed on a regular basis for signs of inflammation or infection. Clean technique would be appropriate for changing peripheral IV tubing in most cases, but not central lines. **Cognitive Level:** Applying **Client Need:** Pharmacological and Parenteral Therapies **Integrated Process:** Nursing Process: Implementation **Content Area:** Fundamentals **Strategy:** The core issue of the question is knowledge of principles of safe care when working with a central venous access device (CVAD). Recall that the catheter is placed into a central vein to reason that strict aseptic technique is necessary and that other general assessments of intravenous lines would also be important. **Reference:** Berman, A., & Snyder, S. J. (2012). *Kozier & Erb's fundamentals of nursing: Concepts, process, and practice* (9th ed.). Upper Saddle River, NJ: Pearson Education, p. 1485.

3 Answer: 3 Rationale: 0.9% sodium chloride (normal saline) is the only solution that can be administered with blood or blood products. Other solutions may cause the blood cells to clump or cause clotting, making the other options incorrect. **Cognitive Level:** Applying **Client Need:** Pharmacological and Parenteral Therapies **Integrated Process:** Nursing Process: Implementation **Content Area:** Fundamentals **Strategy:** The critical phrase is *prime the blood tubing.* Recall information about correct techniques for blood administration to answer the question. If this question was difficult, memorize that normal saline is the only solution compatible with blood products. **Reference:** Berman, A., & Snyder, S. J. (2012). *Kozier & Erb's fundamentals of nursing: Concepts, process, and practice* (9th ed.). Upper Saddle River, NJ: Pearson Education, pp. 1505–1507.

4 Answer: 1 Rationale: Infiltration is leakage of fluids into the surrounding tissues, resulting in edema around the insertion site, blanching, and coolness of skin around the site. Phlebitis and infection would result in redness, heat, and discomfort to the client at the site. Air embolism would result in sudden respiratory distress. **Cognitive Level:** Analyzing **Client Need:** Pharmacological and Parenteral Therapies **Integrated Process:** Nursing Process: Diagnosis **Content Area:** Fundamentals **Strategy:** The core issue of the question is the

ability to recognize common complications of IV therapy, such as infiltration. Use this knowledge and the process of elimination to make a selection. **Reference:** Berman, A., & Snyder, S. J. (2012). *Kozier & Erb's fundamentals of nursing: Concepts, process, and practice* (9th ed.). Upper Saddle River, NJ: Pearson Education, pp. 1495–1496.

5 Answer: 2 Rationale: Erythema and edema are consistent with phlebitis, an inflammation of the vein wall. Continuing the infusion at that site would only worsen the phlebitis. The IV should be discontinued and restarted at a new site. Applying a warm compress to an area of phlebitis dilates the vessel, improves circulation, and reduces the resistance to blood flow from within the vein reducing the pain. The other options are inaccurate statements about the method of treatment for phlebitis. **Cognitive Level:** Analyzing **Client Need:** Pharmacological and Parenteral Therapies **Integrated Process:** Nursing Process: Implementation **Content Area:** Fundamentals **Strategy:** The core issue of the question is recognition that the client has developed phlebitis at the IV site and the ability to determine the appropriate actions. Review this basic information if this question was difficult. **Reference:** Berman, A., & Snyder, S. J. (2012). *Kozier & Erb's fundamentals of nursing: Concepts, process, and practice* (9th ed.). Upper Saddle River, NJ: Pearson Education, pp. 1495–1496.

6 Answer: 4 Rationale: If blood returns while aspirating during an IM injection, the nurse should discard and prepare a new injection. Blood indicates that the needle has entered a blood vessel, and medication injected directly into the bloodstream may be dangerous. **Cognitive Level:** Applying **Client Need:** Pharmacological and Parenteral Therapies **Integrated Process:** Nursing Process: Implementation **Content Area:** Fundamentals **Strategy:** The critical phrase is *blood in the syringe.* Eliminate 2 options because they are similar and a third because it violates principles of aseptic technique for medication administration using needles. **Reference:** Berman, A., & Snyder, S. J. (2012). *Kozier & Erb's fundamentals of nursing: Concepts, process, and practice* (9th ed.). Upper Saddle River, NJ: Pearson Education, pp. 888–893.

7 Answer: 2 Rationale: Tourniquets and the ports of standard IV tubing are made of latex. A blood pressure cuff can be used as an alternative method of vein distention. Povidone iodine is an unrelated item, and it is not the nurse's role to suggest alternatives to IV therapy when appropriate equipment can be obtained. **Cognitive Level:** Analyzing **Client Need:** Safety and Infection Control **Integrated Process:** Nursing Process: Implementation **Content Area:** Fundamentals **Strategy:** The critical words are *latex allergy* and *typical IV start kit.* Recall what equipment contains latex and choose the option that eliminates it from contact with the client. All equipment made of rubber will cause signs and symptoms of allergy. **Reference:** Berman, A., & Snyder, S. J. (2012). *Kozier & Erb's fundamentals of nursing: Concepts, process, and practice* (9th ed.). Upper Saddle River, NJ: Pearson Education, pp. 1487–1491.

ANSWERS & RATIONALES

8 **Answer: 2** **Rationale:** Clients should be instructed to hold inhaler 2 inches away from mouth, hold the breath for 10 seconds after inhalation, slowly exhale through pursed lips, and wait 2 minutes between puffs. The other options describe incorrect actions. **Cognitive Level:** Applying **Client Need:** Pharmacological and Parenteral Therapies **Integrated Process:** Teaching and Learning **Content Area:** Fundamentals **Strategy:** The core issue of the question is correct administration of a dose of medication using an inhaler. Recall basic administration principles for this medication route and use the process of elimination to make a selection. **Reference:** Berman, A., & Snyder, S. J. (2012). *Kozier & Erb's fundamentals of nursing: Concepts, process, and practice* (9th ed.). Upper Saddle River, NJ: Pearson Education, pp. 912–913.

9 **Answers: 3, 5** **Rationale:** When medications are administered enterally and cannot be administered with tube feedings, it is best to stop the tube feedings for at least 30 minutes prior to and after the administration of the medication. A time period of 30 minutes allows for the tube feeding to clear the GI tract and therefore not mix with the medication. The tube should be flushed before and after the dose to prevent the medication from coming in contact with the feeding. The actions listed in the other options do not provide for safe medication administration based on the incompatibility. **Cognitive Level:** Applying **Client Need:** Pharmacological and

Parenteral Therapies **Integrated Process:** Nursing Process: Implementation **Content Area:** Fundamentals **Strategy:** The core issue of the question is knowledge of safe medication administration technique via a feeding tube when medication and feeding are incompatible. Choose the options that physically separate the feeding from the medication to avoid their interaction. **Reference:** Berman, A., & Snyder, S. J. (2012). *Kozier & Erb's fundamentals of nursing: Concepts, process, and practice* (9th ed.). Upper Saddle River, NJ: Pearson Education, p. 871.

10 **Answer: 3** **Rational:** A client has the right to refuse a medication regardless of how important it may be to his or her health. Withholding the medication because of client refusal is not an incident and does not require an incident report, but it should be documented and reported to the provider. **Cognitive Level:** Applying **Client Need:** Management of Care **Integrated Process:** Communication and Documentation **Content Area:** Fundamentals **Strategy:** The core issue of the question is the ability to apply client rights to the procedure of medication administration. Recall the principle of client autonomy to make a selection and also realize that the prescriber should be informed of the event. **Reference:** Berman, A., & Snyder, S. J. (2012). *Kozier & Erb's fundamentals of nursing: Concepts, process, and practice* (9th ed.). Upper Saddle River, NJ: Pearson Education, p. 82.

References

Adam, M. P. & Koch, R. (2010). *Pharmacology connections to nursing practice.* Upper Saddle River, NJ: Pearson Education.

Berman, A., & Snyder, S. J. (2012). *Kozier & Erb's fundamentals of nursing: Concepts, process, and practice* (9th ed.). Upper Saddle River, NJ: Pearson Education, pp. 840–917, 1449–1511.

LeMone, P. Burke, K., & Bauldoff, G. (2012). *Medical-surgical nursing: Critical thinking in patient care* (5th ed.). Upper Saddle River, NJ: Pearson Education.

Smith, R. S., Duell, D. J., & Martin, B. C. (2012). *Clinical nursing skills: Basic to advanced skills* (8th ed.). Upper Saddle River, NJ: Pearson Education.

Zimmerman, P. G. (2010). Revisiting IM injections. *American Journal of Nursing.* 11(2), 60–61/ doi: 10.1097/01. NAJ 0000368058.72729. c6.

ANSWERS & RATIONALES

Appendix

➤ *Practice to Pass Suggested Answers*

Chapter 1

Page 9: *Suggested Answer*—

Open: "Can you describe your pain for me?"

Closed: "On a scale of 0 to 10, with 10 being the worst pain you have ever felt, how would you rank your pain?"

Page 13: *Suggested Answer*—

- Knowledge Deficit related to medication regimen; Ineffective Health Maintenance related to ineffective individual coping; Noncompliance related to knowledge and skill related to the regimen behavior
- Impaired Skin Integrity related to immobility

Page 15: *Suggested Answer*—

- PO intake will be 700 mL per 8 hours
- Urine specific gravity, weight, and laboratory studies will remain within age-appropriate parameters
- Respiratory rate will be 12 to 18 breaths per minute
- Client will remain afebrile

Page 16: *Suggested Answer*—

- Call you to assess his coccyx.
- Turn and position him so there is no weight on his coccyx.
- Cleanse reddened area gently, dry well, and do not massage it.

Page 20: *Suggested Answer*—

- When did you go to sleep?
- When did you wake up?
- Do you feel rested?

Chapter 2

Page 31: *Suggested Answer*—The interview is an important process in which the nurse attempts to extrapolate information from the client to determine health care needs. The nurse should first establish a rapport and attempt to make the client comfortable with the process. The nurse can use multiple skills to elicit data. The use of good communication skills and proceeding in a systematic, nonthreatening manner will facilitate the process.

Page 32: *Suggested Answer*—Clues provided by the client's complaint include:

- Client's overall health
- Client's health prior to initiating health care
- Client's perspective of health concerns
- Client's attempt to treat the disorder
- Client's perception of health needs
- Client's perception of how the health care team can assist the client's return to health

Page 32: *Suggested Answer*—The family history is crucial in relaying significant medical information to the health care team. The overall health and illnesses of a close relation will lead the health care team to investigate multiple areas of potential concern. All factors are significant as the health care team begins to build a picture of the client's current and future health status.

Page 35: *Suggested Answer*—The nurse can help alleviate the client's psychological discomfort by providing privacy, providing a gown to change into, and by ensuring that only the body part being examined is exposed at any given time. A matter-of-fact but understanding manner will also be reassuring to the client.

Page 43: *Suggested Answer*—Once the nurse detects the client has adventitious breath sounds, identification of the sounds will assist the health care team to choose the course of therapy. The nurse should continue to perform respiratory assessments by noting the rate, character, and depth of the respirations. Inspecting the client's mucous membranes, nail beds, and lips will indicate if the periphery of the body is being oxygenated. In addition, the nurse can percuss for diaphragmatic excursion and areas of dullness, resonance, or hyperresonance. As the assessment proceeds, the nurse questions the client about the overall state of health, duration of the symptoms, any related symptoms, cough, mucus production, chest pain, palpitation, urine output, respiratory distress, and additional illnesses. The nurse can also ask the client for family history, smoking history, and exposure to asbestos.

Page 50: *Suggested Answer*—

- Brain: controls thoughts, emotions, speech
- Limbic system: emotional and behavioral responses to environmental stimuli
- Reticular formation: wake–sleep cycle
- Spinal cord: sensory and motor functions

- Peripheral nervous system: receives and transmits impulses from environment
- Autonomic nervous system: regulates internal environment
- Sympathetic nervous system: affects target organs (pupils, secretions, sweat, heart rate and rhythm, coronary arteries, bronchioles, digestion, liver, urine output, abdominal and skin blood vessels, blood clotting, metabolic rate, mental alertness)
- Parasympathetic nervous system: regulates digestion, elimination, and other activities (pupils, glandular secretions, heart rate, coronary arteries, bronchioles, peristalsis, and gastric secretions)

Chapter 3

Page 62: *Suggested Answer*—An unconscious client may hear what is being said because hearing is believed to be the last sense lost. The nurse should act as if the client can hear and should talk in a normal tone of voice. Communication should be simple and concrete.

The client should be spoken to before the nurse provides touch. Touching is a form of communication and should be done gently and smoothly. The nurse should ask closed questions that call for a simple response; for example, "If you can hear me, squeeze my hand" or "Move your head." Unavoidable environmental noises should be explained. Environmental noises should be decreased when possible to help the client focus on communication. Information regarding orientation and client care needs to be repeated frequently. Clients should be given sufficient time to respond to questions.

Page 64: *Suggested Answer*—Reduce environmental noise when possible. Decreasing environmental stimuli is likely to have a calming effect on the client. Allow the client to express his or her feelings as long as the client is not a danger to self or others. Approach the client by using his or her name. Appear accepting and not challenging. To appear nonthreatening, keep posture relaxed and have minimum eye contact. Do not react to the client's loud voice or aggressive behavior; however, listen carefully to what is said. Using simple and direct communication, explain all care measures before implementing them.

Page 65: *Suggested Answer*—Reduce environmental noise. Orient the client before initiating verbal communication. Face the client and talk in a low-pitched voice using simple sentences. Use gestures or environmental cues to augment verbal messages. Use a word board or written messages to help convey information. Explain all procedures using pantomime as appropriate. Ensure that hearing aids are in working order.

Page 68: *Suggested Answer*—Draw a single line through the mistaken entry; write "void" or "error" above the line and initial this entry. Sign the record as per policy.

Page 68: *Suggested Answer*—Information should be complete, accurate, and relevant. Record assessment data objectively and avoid including the nurse's interpretation. Note problems as they occur, as well as nursing interventions and client

options. It is not enough to document a problem without addressing it. Avoid unclear terms like "good" and "appears to be." Interventions should be documented immediately after they occur and signed by the person performing them.

Page 70: *Suggested Answer*—Important information to report would include:

- Information to identify client and medical diagnosis or major medical procedures
- Physician name, including consulting services
- Significant assessment findings, including vital signs
- Diagnostic and laboratory tests scheduled, as well as results of tests done
- Information related to maintaining client safety, use of restraints, and/or sensory impairments
- Specific treatments ordered such as dressing changes, tube feedings, and intravenous therapy

Page 72: *Suggested Answer*—The nurse should consider:

- The client's developmental level
- The client's emotional state
- The client's motivation
- The client's reading ability
- What the client needs to know
- What the client already knows

Chapter 4

Page 82: *Suggested Answer*—Effective leaders adapt their style of leadership to the situation. Therefore, situational leadership is regarded as the style most compatible with a professional staff. The nurse in charge should not have to use an autocratic style to offer direction; a professional staff would be involved in making decisions and facilitating the organization in meeting its goals. A professional staff would be internally motivated, capable of making decisions, and value independence. Moreover, a style that offers no direction at all (*laissez-faire*) is incompatible with attempts to meet personal and organizational goals. Therefore, the situational leadership style would allow input from the staff and cooperation in many situations but could revert to autocratic in emergency situations.

Page 83: *Suggested Answer*—The management process provides a framework for managers and leaders to use in order to be successful in attaining organizational goals. Management functions include planning, organizing, directing, and controlling. These activities promote successful attainment of organizational goals.

Page 84: *Suggested Answer*—A new graduate does not have expert or positional power but can have referent power. As the graduate matures, the expert power can emerge. Power that is vested in the registered nurse's position generates the ability to delegate tasks and responsibilities.

Page 86: *Suggested Answer*—Delegation is the transfer of responsibility for the completion of a task. The RN should consider the nature of the task to be delegated. It should not be too complex, and it should be part of the unlicensed assistive personnel's area of responsibility. The nurse must communicate the task and responsibility to be delegated and offer guidance. The nurse retains accountability for the task and must monitor the performance of the task and its outcome.

Page 86: *Suggested Answer*—The ANA Code for Nurses is a group statement of the values held by the group. This code serves as a standard for practice and provides guidance for the professional nurse. It offers parameters for the protection of both the client and the family.

Page 88: *Suggested Answer*—Unless there is malpractice a nurse cannot be held liable for stopping to render assistance as any other reasonably prudent person would.

Page 89: *Suggested Answer*—The nurse can avoid malpractice by abiding by the ANA Code for Nurses and the state Nurse Practice Act. The nurse must be familiar with the Nurse Practice Act of the state, because it defines the practice of all nurses. In addition, the nurse will follow the policies and procedures of the agency as long as the policies are in compliance with state law. When the nurse accepts employment, the nurse must consider personal abilities versus job requirements and determine personal ability to function in a role. The nurse must communicate with supervisors when aspects of the job fall beyond the nurse's ability. The nurse should maintain a good rapport with the client—every client should be treated with kindness and respect. Also, it is crucial that the nurse participates in continuing education programs and serves as an advocate for the client and the family.

Chapter 5

Page 103: *Suggested Answer*—The client will demonstrate adaptation to current life situation, express acceptance of self, acknowledge changes in self-concept, and develop a realistic plan for adapting to life after mastectomy.

Page 105: *Suggested Answer*—Testicular cancer is the most common cancer in men aged 15 to 35. Testicular self-examination (TSE) should be done monthly on a specific day. The best place for TSE is the shower. Index and middle fingers should be under the testicle while the thumb is on top. Roll the testicle, feeling for lumps, thickenings, or hardened areas. Repeat on the other testicle. Also palpate the epididymis and the vas deferens. After the shower, use a mirror to check for swelling or changes in skin texture. The physician should be notified of any unusual findings.

Page 111: *Suggested Answer*—Interpreters should be objective and seek to provide accurate translation of information. It is best to avoid using family members as translators because of lack of objectivity. Gender and age should be similar to that of the client in order to avoid embarrassment in sensitive issues. The interpreter should be socially and politically compatible with the client. The nurse should speak directly to the

client and not the interpreter. The nurse should speak slowly and with clarity. Observe nonverbal communication from the client to validate the verbal response.

Page 113: *Suggested Answer*—Parents or guardians should be asked what religious beliefs have been taught to the preschooler. Ask the preschooler "Who is God?", "What is heaven?", "Do you pray?", "If so, can you tell me how you pray?" Ask the child about what he or she believes about religious holidays, such as Christmas, Hanukkah, or others.

Page 114: *Suggested Answer*—The nurse's response should be customized for the parent following an assessment of her grief level. Answers should be direct without detail, but sufficient to allow the parent to recognize approaching death. Symptoms of approaching death include loss of muscle tone, bowel and bladder incontinence (although urine output greatly decreases), difficulty swallowing, lack of appetite, dry mucous membranes, and low-grade fever; extremities are cyanotic, mottled, cool and clammy, or may be perspiring; respirations become slow and labored often with loud lung sounds, disorientation, blurred vision, and diminished blink reflex. Ensure that the parents know that hearing is the last sense to go and encourage them to talk to their child throughout the experience.

Chapter 6

Page 126: *Suggested Answer*—General assessment data that indicate a client may be more susceptible to pathogens include:

- Poor hygiene practices
- Inadequate nutrition
- Being underweight or overweight
- Having negative lifestyle habits such as cigarette smoking and lack of physical activity

Physical assessment data that may indicate a client is susceptible to pathogens may include:

- Generalized pallor
- Poor peripheral circulation
- Abnormal respiratory rate with decreased lung expansion
- Nail clubbing
- Presence of abnormal heart sounds
- Skin and mucous membranes not intact
- History of chronic illness

Page 131: *Suggested Answer*—

- The parents should be given information about proper hand hygiene techniques and basic infection control information.
- Information should be provided about the importance of immunizations and about accident prevention specific to the child's age.
- Parents should be instructed to seek medical treatment early in the event the child becomes ill.

- Food preparation should be discussed, including washing all fresh vegetables and fruits and ensuring meat is cooked at proper temperatures.
- Environmental controls should be discussed to prevent the spread of microorganisms. For example, toys should be washed periodically and soiled diapers handled appropriately.

Page 135: *Suggested Answer*—

- Client conditions that may cause the body temperature to be lower than normal include shock, accidental exposure to cold temperature, and postsurgical procedures. In addition, age is a factor as older adult clients experience integumentary changes and infants have immature temperature regulatory mechanisms.
- Interventions to prevent heat loss include increasing environmental temperature, providing extra blankets, keeping the client's head covered, providing warm liquids, and avoiding exposure of the skin during care.

Page 139: *Suggested Answer*—The nurse needs to consider the client's age, body type, and build. The assessment should include the client's emotional heath and evaluation of the client's stressors. Physical assessment criteria would include a body system assessment to ensure proper functioning. For instance, if the client's general color is normal, lungs are clear to auscultation, heart sounds are normal, nail beds blanch well, and urinary and bowel elimination are within normal limits, the client probably has compensated for the abnormal blood pressure measurement.

Page 140: *Suggested Answer*—The nurse could anticipate that the body temperature would be below normal. The pulse will be weak and rapid if blood loss is not too extensive. As the client loses more blood, the pulse may become very slow and difficult to palpate. The blood pressure will be slightly elevated at first as the body tries to compensate. The systolic pressure will decrease more in comparison to the diastolic, with the pulse pressure narrowing. The blood pressure will fall rapidly as the client changes position. As blood loss continues, the blood pressure continues to decline.

Chapter 7

Page 160: *Suggested Answer*—

- Provide a clutter-free environment. Depending on the degree and extensiveness of the burn, the child may try to investigate the environment. Young children are very curious and will handle anything within reach.
- Follow clean and aseptic precautions strictly (isolation, if ordered; use of sterile gloves, mask, and gown when in contact with client).
- Provide crib or bed with side rails. Sides may be padded. A toddler may need a crib that prevents him or her from crawling over the top of the rails.
- Assess child's risk for injury. The child may pull at dressings, damage blisters that form over burn area, or contaminate wounds. The child will need assistance with positioning. If needed, may use mitt or elbow restraints.

Page 165: *Suggested Answer*—

- Maintain the water seal and patency of the drainage system: tape connector sites; provide a straight line of tubing from bed to the collection system; ensure there are no kinks in tubing; do not use pins or restrain tubing.
- Assess client's vital signs and respiratory and cardiovascular status regularly.
- Maintain integrity of the drainage system: disposable system or suction bottles below level of bed; maintain suction control to create gentle bubbling.
- Strip chest tubes only with physician's orders; excessive negative pressure can damage lung tissue. If ordered, strip by pinching tube close to client chest with one hand, lubricate thumb and forefinger to compress and slide down toward the receptacle.
- Keep rubber-tipped clamps (if indicated by policy) and a sterile occlusive dressing near the client. In case connections are broken or air leaks occur, the chest tube may need to be clamped immediately or an underwater seal may need to be reestablished. If the chest tube is pulled out inadvertently, apply an occlusive dressing to the wound immediately.
- Mark drainage on the receptacle every shift and read at eye level. Report if drainage exceeds 100 mL/hr.

Page 167: *Suggested Answer*—The nurse should question the client about these common factors that interfere with sleep: heavy meals just prior to bedtime, caffeine, nicotine, or other stimulants, and environmental factors such as light, noise, and television.

Page 169: *Suggested Answer*—

- Ensure appropriate lighting, ventilation, and temperature. Keep noise level to a minimum.
- Promote rituals or routines that people are accustomed to in order to promote relaxation and encourage sleep.
- Avoid heavy meals 3 hours before bedtime, decrease fluid intake 2 hours before sleep, and avoid alcohol, caffeine, or heavily spiced foods.
- Get adequate exercise during the day to reduce stress. Pursue a nonstrenuous activity prior to sleep.
- Medications are to be used as a last resort and be taken on prn (as necessary) basis. Clients need to be aware of the actions and desired and adverse effects of medications used to aid sleep. Sedatives and hypnotics have different onset and duration of actions. Regular use may lead to tolerance of the drug, which can lead to rebound insomnia.

Page 173: *Suggested Answer*—

- Appears tired and fatigued; listless; may be overweight or underweight; slowing of reflexes; motor restlessness; confusion, disorientation
- Lack of appetite (anorexia); nausea, vomiting, overeating; indigestion; constipation

- Dry, dull, sparse, brittle hair; loss of hair color; dry, flaky, or scaly skin; pale or pigmented skin; presence of petechiae or bruising; lack of subcutaneous fat; poor skin turgor; brittle, pale, ridged, or spoon-shaped nails
- Facial edema; any swelling in the neck (enlarged lymph nodes)
- Swollen lips, red cracks at side of mouth (angular stomatitis), vertical fissures (cheilosis); dry mucous membranes in the oral cavity
- Tongue: swollen, beefy, red or magenta-colored; coated; smooth appearance; increase or decrease in size
- Teeth: dental caries; gums inflamed (gingivitis), spongy, bleed easily
- Eyes: pale or red conjunctiva; dryness (xerophthalmia); soft cornea (keratomalacia); dull cornea
- Numbness, tingling, edema of legs and feet; underdeveloped, flaccid, soft, wasting muscles

Page 177: *Suggested Answer—*

- Drink eight 8-ounce glasses of water daily.
- Empty bladder at least every 2 to 4 hours while awake, avoiding voluntary retention.
- For women: wear cotton briefs; cleanse perineal area from front to back after voiding and defecating; void before and after sexual intercourse; avoid bubble baths, feminine hygiene sprays, and douches.
- Unless contraindicated, teach client to maintain acidity in urine by taking vitamin C or drinking at least 2 glasses of cranberry juice per day; avoiding excess milk products and sodium bicarbonate.
- Teach symptoms of urinary tract infection and measures to prevent it or to report promptly.

Page 180: *Suggested Answer—*

- Dietary teaching should include information on foods that cause stool odor (asparagus, beans, eggs, fish, onions, garlic); foods that increase gas; foods that thicken stool (applesauce, bananas, rice, tapioca, cheese, yogurt) and foods that loosen stool (chocolate, dried beans, fried foods, highly spiced foods, leafy green vegetables, raw fruits and vegetables).
- Skin care will need to be taught. The client will need information on protecting the exposed skin as well as changing colostomy bags. The client should be taught to assess skin and report changes.

Chapter 8

Page 191: *Suggested Answer—* In addition to trauma or surgical interventions, any of the following serve as potential sources of pain stimuli:

- Microorganisms
- Inflammation
- Impaired blood flow
- Invasive tumor
- Radiation

- Heat
- Electricity
- Compression
- Decreased movement
- Stretching/straining
- Swelling
- Chemicals

Page 193: *Suggested Answer—* Ask the client about tolerance to pain, and assess pain location, intensity, quality, pattern, aggravating and alleviating factors, medication history, and expectations for pain relief.

Page 193: *Suggested Answer—* Acute pain usually is accompanied by fear and anxiety, while chronic pain can result in depression, despair, hopelessness, and fatigue.

Page 196: *Suggested Answer—* Common barriers include the following:

- Inadequate knowledge of pain management
- Poor assessment of pain
- Concern about regulation of controlled substances
- Fear of client addiction
- Concern about adverse effects of analgesics
- Concern about clients becoming tolerant to analgesics

Page 197: *Suggested Answer—* The client most likely is experiencing a nociceptive type of pain known as somatic.

Page 203: *Suggested Answer—* NSAIDs, tricyclic antidepressants, antiepileptics, local anesthetics, corticosteroids, Baclofen (muscle relaxant), and capsaicin (Zostrix) can be used.

Page 206: *Suggested Answer—* The nurse should discuss with the client TENS, cutaneous stimulation, heat and cold therapy, distraction, relaxation, acupuncture, and biofeedback.

Chapter 9

Page 220: *Suggested Answer—*

- Diagnostic surgery is done to diagnose or confirm a diagnosis. In some cases, the procedure may rule out a disease process. An example of a diagnostic surgical procedure would be a breast biopsy or a craniotomy to diagnose the location of a brain tumor.
- Palliative surgery is performed to reduce or relieve symptoms of a disease. It is not performed to cure a disease. A client with a brain tumor may have surgery to insert a ventriculoperitoneal shunt to reinstate ventricular flow and relieve (temporarily) the increased intracranial pressure.
- Ablative surgery is a surgical procedure to remove a diseased body part. An example of this would be an appendectomy or hysterectomy.
- Reconstructive surgery is performed to restore body appearance or function or to create a more normal appearance or function. An example of reconstructive surgery would be cleft lip surgery or relief of adhesions in a client with burn injuries.

- Transplant surgery replaces malfunctioning tissues (e.g., heart, kidney).

Page 221: *Suggested Answer*—

- Medication history, including current medications taken and previous medications, especially those with side effects or allergic reactions.
- Tobacco use, as it can affect the respiratory system and the client's response to anesthesia.
- Allergies, including food and medications. Contact allergies should be discussed. The nurse needs to particularly question the client about latex allergies because the client will be exposed during the surgical procedure from gloves and other equipment in use. Clients with a history of many surgeries and those with a history of spina bifida are at higher risk for latex allergies.
- Alcohol use, including type and frequency of use. The nurse should be aware of the risk of withdrawal.
- Previous surgical experiences including anesthesia. The nurse can discuss the previous experiences, which may influence how the client perceives this surgery. In addition, types of anesthesia used previously with any complications that occurred would be important to note.
- Psychosocial factors such as culture, support systems, and anxieties. Culture can influence a client's beliefs and values. For instance, if the culture values large families, a woman having a hysterectomy can have emotional distress. The adequacy of support systems will affect the client's needs for emotional support during periods of stress. Anxieties and fears (such as those related to body image) can make the stress of surgery greater for the client.

Page 222: *Suggested Answer*—

- Integumentary: rashes may indicate an infection. Poor skin turgor may indicate dehydration.
- Lungs: crackles and rhonchi heard on auscultation could indicate a respiratory infection.
- Cardiovascular: murmurs could indicate a heart defect that may interfere with the effectiveness of circulation. Clients with heart defects may be at greater risk for the development of subacute bacterial endocarditis. Prophylactic antibiotics are used to prevent this infection.
- Gastrointestinal: obesity can interfere with the body's ability to heal. The cardiovascular system can be affected by obesity and makes the client more prone to postoperative complications.
- Genitourinary/reproductive system: urinary frequency can indicate a urinary tract infection.
- Neurologic: difficulty with memory may interfere with the client's ability to understand the procedure and postoperative teaching.

Page 223: *Suggested Answer*—

- The client's consent is voluntary. The client is not being forced or coerced to sign the consent form.
- The client's mental status allows him or her to understand the procedure to be done and make a rational decision.

- The client has the authority to consent. This means the client is by law allowed to make decisions for his or her own care. The client would be of legal age in the state where the procedure is being performed.
- The client has received the information necessary to make an informed decision.

Page 227: *Suggested Answer*—To prevent hypothermia in the surgical client, the OR nurse should cover the client's head, use warm blankets and warm IV fluids, and minimize body surface area exposures.

Page 230: *Suggested Answer*—Client goal: the lungs remain clear to auscultation.

Nursing interventions:

- Turn and reposition the client every 2 hours while awake.
- Encourage the client to use an incentive spirometer every 2 hours while awake.
- Auscultate the lungs every 4 hours.

Chapter 10

Page 243: *Suggested Answer*—The nurse should assess the wound for healing. The wound edges should be well approximated; sutures may or may not be present at this stage. Dehiscence and evisceration are less likely to occur at this stage; the time for these complications is usually 4 to 5 days postoperative. At this stage, the wound should be in the proliferative phase, which extends from day 3 to 21 after injury. The fibroblasts that surround the wound have begun to synthesize collagen. A raised "healing ridge" may be noted. The presence of granulation tissue (translucent red tissue) will be noted.

The nurse will also observe for drainage from the wound. Purulent exudate, thick pus with varying colors including yellow and green, would be present if the wound was infected. The nurse would note the color of the drainage as that may provide information on the causative organism. Clear discharge (serous) may be noted during the early stages of healing.

Page 245: *Suggested Answer*—In this stage of a pressure ulcer, there is no broken skin. The wound care would be to keep the area clean and dry. To keep pressure off the area, turn and position the client frequently. Encourage the client to remain in side-lying positions whenever possible. When moving the client up in bed, try to prevent dragging the client as this creates shearing pressure that can promote skin breakdown. Skin prep is a spray that could be used to toughen the skin. Specialty mattresses can be added to the bed that reduce pressure by means of distributing body weight more evenly or by alternating pressure on different portions of the skin. The client should avoid using doughnuts and rings that interfere with circulation to the area. Good nutrition is important; include high amounts of protein and vitamin C in food choices.

Page 247: *Suggested Answer*—Factors that add to sensory overload are pain, anxiety, and lack of sleep. The nurse would want to avoid excessive light and noise. Provide clocks and calendars in the client's line of vision. Allow for uninterrupted rest periods. Eliminate noxious odors.

Page 250: *Suggested Answer*—The nurse should face the client and speak directly facing him. The nurse should not have anything in the mouth while speaking. The voice should be kept at a moderate volume, the nurse should not shout, as that distorts the words. The nurse should avoid making excessive mouth and face movements. Use nonverbal cues whenever possible. Eliminate background noise if possible.

Page 254: *Suggested Answer*—Have the client squeeze a rubber ball several times a day. Have the client flex and extend the arms. Move from a supine to a sitting position by flexing elbows and pushing hands against the bed. Lift the body off the bed by pushing down with the palms of the hands and extending the elbow.

Chapter 11

Page 264: *Suggested Answer*—In the United States and Canada, the federal government regulates the production, prescription, distribution, and administration of drugs. Each state legislates a Nurse Practice Act for RNs and LVN/LPNs. Nurse Practice Act defines the nurses' boundaries and responsibilities regarding medications. Law also governs nursing practice involving use and management of controlled substances. It is the responsibility of local health care facilities to establish and implement policies and procedures that conform to their state's regulations. When the laws or regulations of a community, state, or institution differ from the federal laws, the stricter law generally prevails.

Page 265: *Suggested Answer*—The client is most probably experiencing an idiosyncratic effect: unexpected and unpredictable individual response to a drug manifested as an under-response, over-response, or completely different response. The nurse should withhold further doses of the medication and notify the physician.

Page 266: *Suggested Answer*—1 kilogram = 2.2 pounds. 160 pounds = 72.73 kilograms. 0.5 micrograms × 72.73 = 36.365 micrograms/kg/min.

Page 268: *Suggested Answer*—The nurse should discuss the medication with the client to ensure that the client is basing her decision on accurate information about the medication and how it relates to her condition, and that she is mentally competent to make an informed decision. Despite the client's medical condition warranting the need for the medication, the client has the right to refuse to take a medication and the nurse should honor the client's wishes and report this to the physician.

Page 272: *Suggested Answer*—The client should be instructed about the action and use of the drug as it pertains to his condition; adverse effects and what to do should he experience any of these effects; route; dose; frequency; and how long he should take the medication. If he received a dose of the medication in the health care agency, the nurse should advise him when the next dose is due.

Page 279: *Suggested Answer*—You will need a syringe appropriate for the volume of medication (generally a tuberculin syringe), #25 gauge, ⅜- to ⅝-inch needle, clean gloves, and an alcohol swab. Administer the medication in the lower abdomen fat pad at least 2 fingerbreadths from the umbilicus and above the iliac crest. Gently pinch an inch of subcutaneous tissue, inject at a 90-degree angle, and administer the medication slowly without aspirating.

Page 283: *Suggested Answer*—The nurse should take initial vital signs before starting the transfusion. The nurse should stay with the client, taking vital signs every 5 to 15 minutes for the first 50 mL of the transfusion.

➤ Case Study Suggested Answers

Chapter 1

1. Critical assessment data includes:
   - Thorough pain assessment (using a pain scale, location of pain, characteristics of pain, onset of pain, associated signs and symptoms, aggravating factors, relieving factors, treatments tried and their effects)
   - Physical examination of abdomen and gastrointestinal system
   - Vital signs to obtain objective data related to signs and symptoms of pain
2. Nursing diagnoses could include: Pain incisional (location) related to . . . and Nausea related to . . .
3. Client outcomes could include:
   - Client will state pain at or below 3 on a 0-to-10 scale within 30 minutes after administration of pain medication and repositioning.
   - Client will deny nausea 30 minutes after administration of antiemetic medication.
   - Client will not vomit throughout shift.
4. Independent and interdependent interventions include:
   - Independent: reposition for comfort; teach coughing and deep-breathing techniques, relaxation techniques, and splinting of abdomen when changing positions
   - Interdependent: Obtain physician's order for pain and antiemetic medication; administer as ordered
5. Criteria used for evaluation:
   - Objective data: vital signs, numerical pain scale (or Wong-Baker Faces pain scale if client has language or developmental barriers), presence or absence of nausea and/or vomiting
   - Subjective data related to pain, nausea

Chapter 2

1. The nurse must first establish a rapport with the client; the appearance of warmth and understanding provides her with some comfort. Additionally, the nurse must demonstrate a professional attitude and demeanor.

2. The health history is crucial in helping to determine the origin and critical nature of the client's symptoms. The nurse must be prepared before beginning the health history. A complete knowledge of the mechanics of the health history as well as methods to promote communication are essential as the client and nurse work together to investigate the health problem. The history as well as the physical must be done in a methodical, systematic manner.

3. As the nurse commences with the history and physical, some of the symptoms and physical manifestations can be linked with the chief complaint. An in-depth knowledge of anatomy and physiology will assist the nurse to link the symptoms to possible etiologies of the client's difficulties.

4. When a client has external pressures and stress, symptoms can exacerbate because of the stimulation of the sympathetic nervous system.

5. The nurse must return the client to bed and raise the head of the bed. Vital signs must be taken and compared to normal values and the client's normal values. The nurse begins to assess her while asking pointed questions about her "spell." The nurse utilizes inspection, palpation, auscultation and percussion to determine normal and abnormal findings.

Chapter 3

1. Learning objectives that focus on client behavior need to be identified. The nurse needs to establish the content for each objective and identify the method of instruction based on the clients' learning ability. The teaching plan should include skills taught, strategies to be used, time framework, and content.

 The following is a list of items to include in the plan for this client:

Learning Objectives
- Client will verbalize basic anatomy of urinary system before discharge.
- Client will verbalize reason for catheterization in own terms before discharge.
- Client will describe measures to prevent urinary tract infection before discharge.
- Client will identify signs and symptoms that require medical care before discharge.
- Client will demonstrate self-catheterization technique before discharge.

Content
- Explanation of anatomy as relates to client's medical condition
- Signs and symptoms of infection and urinary retention
- Client behaviors to decrease incidence of urinary tract infection
- Equipment required
- Preparation for procedure guidelines

Methods
- Audiovisuals: diagrams of system, video on procedure
- Discussion
- Demonstration
- Return demonstration

The parts of the teaching process that should be documented in the client's chart include diagnosed learning needs, learning objectives, topics taught and client outcomes, need for additional teaching, and resources provided.

2. The nurse needs to evaluate the client's willingness to learn as well as what the client views as important. The nurse needs to evaluate the client's knowledge about the problem and how the problem affects his life. The nurse needs to evaluate the client's sensory abilities and physical state, which may affect the learning process. Finally, the nurse should assess the client's preferred learning style.

3. The nurse should begin with open-ended questions that are associated with the impact his health problem has on his life, for example, "How has your bladder problem affected the things you enjoy doing?" The nurse should validate the client's option. The nurse could also begin by restating what the daughter has told the nurse, for example, "Your daughter has told me that recently you have not attended church or gone to the high school to help the students, and that you also have talked more about death." Then allow the client sufficient time to respond.

4. Possible nursing diagnoses include:
- Deficient Knowledge related to how to perform self-catheterization
- Death Anxiety related to increased discussion with daughter
- Potential for Enhanced Spiritual Well-Being related to past history of church attendance daily
- Hopelessness (alteration in health has altered client's church attendance and mentoring of high school students)

5. Criteria to evaluate the nursing diagnosis of Deficient Knowledge would be client's verbalization of the health problem and cause, client's ability to perform the procedure correctly, client's verbalization of signs and symptoms to report to doctor, and client's verbalization of the need to maintain adequate fluid intake.

 Criteria to evaluate Death Anxiety could be verbalization of feelings, preparation for end of life, identification of unresolved issues, and planning funeral.

 Criteria to evaluate Potential for Enhanced Spiritual Well-Being could be verbalizing importance of church in his own life, identifying an alternative to church attendance to enhance spirituality, or identifying plans to attend church again.

 Criteria to evaluate Hopelessness could be the client's verbalization how learning this new procedure will improve his quality of life so that he can resume normal activities.

Chapter 4

1. The registered nurse does not have a legal obligation to stop at the scene of the accident unless the state has a duty-to-rescue statute.

2. Good Samaritan laws differ from state to state. It is important the RN understands the state law.

3. The situation must be considered an emergency if there will be loss of life or limb without immediate assistance. The Good Samaritan law does not cover providing care in a nonemergent situation.

4. If someone willfully injures the victim, the Good Samaritan law will not protect him or her from liability.

5. The nurse can leave the scene when someone with appropriate skills such as a paramedic or EMT arrives at the scene. Until then, the nurse is bound to stay and continue assistance.

Chapter 5

1. Determine if she is serious about suicide. If so, suicide precautions are in order. If not, a spiritual assessment is the priority. Determine what religious practices are important to the client. Ask what her faith means to her. Does her faith bring her strength? Look around the home for religious artifacts. Observe for support people in the client's life and whether they visit, call, or write her notes.

2. Spiritual Distress related to concerns about disease state

3. The client will renew relationships to strengthen her; find meaning in her spiritual being; and express positive feelings regarding the future.

4. Help the client gather strength from her faith by supporting her religious practices.
   - Encourage the client to have increased contact with the support people in her life.
   - Allocate more time per visit to listen closely to the client.
   - Ask the client if you may call her priest for a home visit. If she agrees, make the call and encourage him to make a visit with the client a priority.

5. Observe and inquire whether relationships have helped to strengthen the client; discuss with the client the utilization and effectiveness of her spiritual practices; inquire whether the client's perception of the future has been modified.

Chapter 6

1. The tests likely to be ordered for this client include culture and sensitivity of the wound exudate, erythrocyte sedimentation rate, white blood count with differential, and fasting blood glucose. The fasting blood glucose will be ordered to determine if the client's blood glucose level is within normal limits because a high level promotes pathogen growth.

2. The body defense mechanism activated was the inflammatory response. In response to injury, dilatation of the blood vessels caused increased permeability of fluids and an influx of leukocytes to the site. This allowed phagocytosis to occur, resulting in destruction of the pathogen. The inflammatory response accounts for some of the symptoms the client is experiencing.

3. Possible diagnoses include:
   - Risk for Injury: criteria to support this diagnosis are presence of a wound on the bottom of foot interfering with normal gait, and client statement of pain.
   - Impaired Tissue Integrity: the criterion to support this diagnosis is a wound at bottom of foot.
   - Impaired Mobility: criteria to support this diagnosis are wound on bottom of foot, swollen foot, and statement of pain.

4. Expected outcomes include:
   - Pain: the criterion to support this diagnosis is the client's statement of pain.
   - Expected outcome for Risk for Injury: client will be free of injury.
   - Expected outcome for Impaired Tissue Integrity: client's foot will show signs of healing by discharge as indicated by decreased redness and decreasing size of wound.
   - Expected outcome for Pain: client will verbalize decreased pain each hospitalized day.
   - Expected outcome for Impaired Mobility: client will demonstrate walking with assistance of cane until foot is healed.

5. Implementation of standard precautions and medical asepsis including hand hygiene, use of gloves when in contact with body fluids, proper disposal of soiled dressings and linens, and following procedures for disinfecting room. In addition, ensure that the client does not use a communal shower or bathtub. Sterile (surgical aseptic) technique should be used with any dressing changes ordered for client.

Chapter 7

1. Assessments about client's ability to meet basic needs:
   - Self-care abilities for hygiene and toileting
   - Risk factors related to safety: poor eyesight; use of equipment such as a cane; use of medications that cause postural hypotension and changes in mental status; environmental factors such as presence of clutter, ability to use call bell, use of side rails
   - Factors affecting sleep: illnesses, emotional stress, drugs and other substances, exercise, usual sleep patterns
   - Factors affecting air exchange: lifestyle factors (exercise, smoking, anxiety)
   - Self-care abilities for nutrition, urinary and bowel elimination
   - Factors affecting nutrition: ability to chew, special or therapeutic diets, drugs
   - Factors affecting urinary and bowel elimination: fluid intake, activity, psychological factors, personal habits, and problems

2. Measures to ensure safety:
   - Give clear instructions to client regarding use of call bell, necessity of side rails
   - Provide a nightlight

- Make frequent checks on client
- Have a clutter-free environment
- Follow protocol for safe medication administration
- Use preventive measures for fire safety
- Do proper maintenance of equipment
- Keep needed objects within client's reach

3. Interventions to promote sleep:
   - Alleviate pain: relaxation techniques, back massage, medication
   - Assist in performing bedtime rituals
   - Encourage toileting prior to bedtime
   - Avoid strenuous exercise or anxiety-producing conversations immediately prior to bedtime
   - Make environment conducive for sleep
   - Avoid heavy meal 3 hours before bedtime
   - Decrease fluid intake 2 hours before sleep
   - Avoid alcohol, caffeine, or heavily spiced foods

4. Measures to assist with adequate air exchange:
   - Assess client's respiratory and cardiovascular status
   - Assist client to a Fowler's position to promote adequate chest expansion
   - If client has dyspnea, instruct client to do slow, rhythmic breathing and assist with relaxation
   - If pain interferes with breathing, use pain distraction methods

5. Promote healthy urinary elimination:
   - Instruct about sufficient (2 liters) fluid intake
   - Teach Kegel exercises; contract perineal muscles and hold for a count of 3 to 5 seconds and relax; do 10 contractions 5 times daily
   - Empty bladder at least every 2 to 4 hours while awake, avoiding voluntary retention; for bladder training if client is incontinent, instruct to void according to a timetable rather than urge to void
   - Unless contraindicated, teach client to maintain acidity in urine by drinking at least 2 glasses of cranberry juice per day or taking vitamin C; avoiding excess milk products and sodium bicarbonate

Chapter 8

1. Common physiologic responses for acute pain includes nausea and vomiting, tachycardia, rapid, shallow respirations, hypertension, sweating, pallor, and dilated pupils.

2. Due to the type of trauma (a fractured hip), this client may benefit from medications having anti-inflammatory effects such as NSAIDs and corticosteroids. In addition, a muscle relaxant such as Baclofen may be helpful.

3. The initial priority is client teaching about the purpose and correct use of the device, and to provide information regarding any questions the client or family members have. The control button must always be in reach for client use. The nurse should provide regular pain assessments, including vital signs, and check the pump settings to assure accuracy of the physician's orders. Side effects such as pruritis, sedation, and respiratory compromise need to be monitored and documented according to agency policies.

4. Application of cold, repositioning, massage, and a variety of distraction techniques may be helpful.

5. Based on the information provided, the following nursing diagnoses could be anticipated:
   - Ineffective Coping related to persistent pain that may add stress affecting the client's ability to cope
   - Deficient Knowledge related to lack of information or misinformation regarding pain treatment strategies
   - Impaired Physical Mobility related to movement limited by pain
   - Disturbed Sleep Pattern related to persistent pain
   - Anxiety related to loss of control
   - Fear related to pain
   - Activity Intolerance related to pain and/or depression
   - Self-Care Deficit (total or partial) related to pain

Chapter 9

1. This client is not allowed by law to make decisions about her own care. However, because of her age and mental capacity, the nurse would want to ensure that the client is included with the parents when information is shared related to her condition and proposed treatments. The nurse would encourage communication between the girl and her parents that allow both sides to express their feelings and concerns.

2. The nurse would want to ask the usual questions about her medical/surgical history including medications, previous illnesses, chronic illnesses, and alcohol and drug use including tobacco. The nurse would want to ask the client about her concerns and fears related to the surgery. This discussion should be done in private to allow the client to express thoughts she may be unwilling to share with her parents. In addition to the usual lab tests, a pregnancy test might be indicated if there is evidence the client is sexually active. The client will be allowed to select the support person that stays with her as allowed by hospital policies.

3. Two preoperative diagnoses would include:
   - Deficient Knowledge related to the postoperative experience
   - Anxiety related to the uncertainty of the diagnosis and surgical outcome

4. Postoperative care to be taught would include the need for coughing and deep breathing in the postoperative period. The use of an incentive spirometer would be taught, as well as abdominal splinting. The client will also receive initial instructions about the expected wound appearance. Pain control methods will be discussed, and she will be assured that her needs will be met.

5. The nurse will discuss what occurs as the anesthesia is being administered, as well as what she will see and hear during the induction and as she is coming out of anesthesia.

Chapter 10

1. The compression bandage should be applied from the bottom aspect of the foot going upward toward the calf in even spiral turns. In order to properly apply a compression bandage to an extremity, you must go from distal to proximal (in the flow of venous return).
2. Teach the 3-point gait. The client must be able to bear the entire weight on the unaffected (uninjured) leg. The 2 crutches and the unaffected leg are used to walk and bear weight alternately.
3. To obtain a proper fit, the client should lay in a supine position. The nurse should measure from the anterior fold of the axilla to the heel and add 2.5 cm. Alternately, have the client stand erect holding the crutch in position. The arm rest should fall 3 finger widths below the axilla.
4. The client had a closed wound. There was no break in the skin. Inflammation can take up to 10 days to resolve.
5. Teach the client to wear nonskid shoes and to make sure crutches have rubber tips to help prevent falls. Using good lighting and keeping the environment free of clutter are other general measures to prevent falls.

Chapter 11

1. Total parenteral nutrition (TPN) are solutions that provide all needed calories and contain high-dextrose concentrations, water, fat, proteins, electrolytes, vitamins, and trace elements. Hypertonic solutions containing greater than 10% dextrose require a high-flow central vein for infusion. Infection control is a high priority because the glucose-rich solution invites bacteria. The high-glucose content requires careful administration and blood glucose monitoring to prevent hypoglycemia or hyperglycemia.
2. A tunneled Groshong CVAD is a catheter that provides long-term access to a central vein for the purpose of medication administration, blood draws, or hyperalimentation administration. The tip is inserted into a central vein and advanced to the superior vena cava. The remainder of the catheter passes through a subcutaneous track and exits on the chest wall or abdomen. It contains a 3-way pressure-sensitive valve that remains closed at normal vena caval pressure. When closed, it restricts air from entering the venous system or a backflow of blood from the catheter. Advantages of the Groshong valve and catheter include:
   - Decreased risk of air emboli or bleeding
   - Elimination of heparin flush
   - Elimination of catheter clamping
   - Reduced flushing protocols between use
3. Caring for the Groshong catheter involves:
   - Maintenance flush—according to agency policy, usually 10 to 20 mL saline vigorously weekly
   - Medication flush—5 to 10 mL saline before and vigorously after medication administration
   - Blood draws—double the normal flushing volume of saline with 10 mL saline after blood sampling
     - Waste—5 mL blood for routine sampling
     - Waste—10 mL blood for PT or PTT
     - TPN—flush with 20 mL saline before blood sampling
   - TPN flush—20 mL saline vigorously upon discontinuing TPN
   - Always use a 10 mL or larger size syringe
   - All lumens must have a luer-locked cap or needleless adaptor with reflux valves
   - Lumens *do not* require clamping when not in use
   - Does not require heparin
4. TPN has a high dextrose concentration, thus increasing blood glucose levels. It is therefore important to test blood glucose per agency protocols (at least once each day) to ensure that the values remain within normal limits (70–110). Should the client's blood glucose levels consistently be elevated, frequently insulin will be added to the TPN solution to maintain a normal serum glucose level.
5. Interventions include:
   - If the dextrose solution is greater than 10 percent, a high flow central vessel is required for administration
   - Blood glucose monitoring per agency protocols (at least once each day)
   - Requires a filter
   - Tubing and filter changes every 24 hours
   - Air occlusive dressings
   - Sterile technique for dressing changes at a frequency per agency protocol (usually every 3–7 days)
   - Change solution every 24 hours
   - Gradually increase and decrease the rate when instantiating and discontinuing the treatment

Index

Page numbers followed by b indicate box; those followed by f indicate figure; those followed by t indicate table.